VOLUME SEVENTY NINE

ADVANCES IN PHARMACOLOGY

VOLUME SEVENTY NINE

Advances in PHARMACOLOGY

Ion Channels DownUnder

Edited by

DOMINIC P. GERAGHTY

School of Health Sciences, Faculty of Health, University of Tasmania, Launceston, Australia

LACHLAN D. RASH

School of Biomedical Science, Faculty of Medicine, University of Queensland, Brisbane, Australia

Serial Editor

S.J. ENNA

University of Kansas Medical Center, Kansas City, Kansas, United States

Managing Editor

LYNN LECOUNT

University of Kansas Medical Center School of Medicine, Kansas City, Kansas, United States

ELSEVIER

ACADEMIC PRESS

An imprint of Elsevier

Academic Press is an imprint of Elsevier
50 Hampshire Street, 5th Floor, Cambridge, MA 02139, United States
525 B Street, Suite 1800, San Diego, CA 92101-4495, United States
The Boulevard, Langford Lane, Kidlington, Oxford OX5 1GB, United Kingdom
125 London Wall, London, EC2Y 5AS, United Kingdom

First edition 2017

ISBN: 978-0-12-810413-2
ISSN: 1054-3589

For information on all Academic Press publications
visit our website at https://www.elsevier.com/books-and-journals

Publisher: Zoe Kruze
Acquisition Editor: Zoe Kruze
Editorial Project Manager: Shellie Bryant
Production Project Manager: Vignesh Tamil
Cover Designer: Christian J. Bilbow

Typeset by SPi Global, India

CONTENTS

CONTRIBUTORS

Murray J. Adams
School of Health Sciences, University of Tasmania, Launceston, TAS, Australia

John J. Bassett
School of Pharmacy, The University of Queensland, Brisbane, QLD, Australia

Nicole A. Beard
John Curtin School of Medical Research, Australian National University, Canberra; Health Research Institute, Faculty of Education Science Technology and Mathematics, University of Canberra, Bruce, ACT, Australia

Philip G. Board
John Curtin School of Medical Research, Australian National University, Canberra, ACT, Australia

Amanda Buyan
Research School of Biology, Australian National University, Canberra, ACT, Australia

Marco G. Casarotto
John Curtin School of Medical Research, Australian National University, Canberra, ACT, Australia

Mary Chebib
Faculty of Pharmacy, The University of Sydney, Sydney, NSW, Australia

Rong Chen
Research School of Biology, Australian National University, Canberra, ACT, Australia

Han Chow Chua
Faculty of Pharmacy, The University of Sydney, Sydney, NSW, Australia

Ben Corry
Research School of Biology, Australian National University, Canberra, ACT, Australia

Jennifer R. Deuis
Centre for Pain Research, Institute for Molecular Bioscience, The University of Queensland, Brisbane, QLD, Australia

Angela F. Dulhunty
John Curtin School of Medical Research, Australian National University, Canberra, ACT, Australia

Argel Estrada-Mondragon
Queensland Brain Institute, University of Queensland, Brisbane, QLD, Australia

Dominic P. Geraghty
School of Health Sciences, University of Tasmania, Launceston, TAS, Australia

Mathilde R. Israel
Centre for Pain Research, Institute for Molecular Bioscience, The University of Queensland, Brisbane, QLD, Australia

Joseph W. Lynch
Queensland Brain Institute; School of Biomedical Sciences, University of Queensland, Brisbane, QLD, Australia

Mehdi Mobli
Centre for Advanced Imaging, St Lucia, QLD, Australia

Gregory R. Monteith
School of Pharmacy; Mater Research, The University of Queensland, Brisbane, QLD, Australia

Sofia A. Omari
School of Health Sciences, University of Tasmania, Launceston, TAS, Australia

Daniel P. Poole
Monash Institute of Pharmaceutical Sciences, Monash University, Melbourne; Australian Research Council Centre of Excellence in Convergent Bio-Nano Science and Technology; The University of Melbourne, Parkville, VIC, Australia

Pradeep Rajasekhar
Monash Institute of Pharmaceutical Sciences, Monash University, Melbourne; Australian Research Council Centre of Excellence in Convergent Bio-Nano Science and Technology, Parkville, VIC, Australia

Lachlan D. Rash
School of Biomedical Sciences, The University of Queensland, St Lucia, QLD, Australia

Sahil Talwar
Queensland Brain Institute, University of Queensland, Brisbane, QLD, Australia

Bryan Tay
Centre for Pain Research, Institute for Molecular Bioscience, The University of Queensland, Brisbane, QLD, Australia

Eivind A.B. Undheim
Centre for Advanced Imaging, St Lucia, QLD, Australia

Nicholas A. Veldhuis
Monash Institute of Pharmaceutical Sciences, Monash University, Melbourne; Australian Research Council Centre of Excellence in Convergent Bio-Nano Science and Technology; The University of Melbourne, Parkville, VIC, Australia

Irina Vetter
Centre for Pain Research, Institute for Molecular Bioscience; School of Pharmacy, The University of Queensland, Brisbane, QLD, Australia

Yan Zhang
Queensland Brain Institute, University of Queensland, Brisbane, QLD, Australia

PREFACE

Ion channels are the fastest cellular signaling system, underlying rapid processes such as axon conduction and synaptic transmission. However, ion channels are also found in nonexcitable cells and are indispensable for processes such as secretion, gene expression, and cell division. With over 140 members, ion channels are the second largest family of signaling molecules in the body and are activated by a diverse range of stimuli such as ligands, membrane voltage changes, temperature, stretch, and changes in pH. As "first responders," a detailed understanding of ion channels is crucial to understanding how cells initially respond to changes in their environment.

There have been spectacular advances in this area in the past two decades, highlighted by the award of the 2003 Nobel Prize in Chemistry to Roderick MacKinnon for his determination of the 3D structure of a voltage-gated potassium channel. Despite the recent leaps and bounds of progress made in the area of ion channel structural biology (e.g., cryo-EM), it is our ability to selectively modulate ion channel function in vitro and in vivo that holds the key to unlocking the physiological and pathological roles of ion channels. To this end, high-quality ion channel pharmacology will provide the tools and therapeutic leads to address many unmet medical needs. The chapters in this volume demonstrate that the momentum has not changed and, indeed, has increased. Whether dissecting the activation of ryanodine receptors, describing the development of subunit-selective ligands for glycine and GABA receptors, or the contribution of calcium imaging in high-throughput identification of drug leads, the contributors have used state-of-the-art techniques and provided narratives and insights that will generate new ideas for years to come.

We wish to thank the many contributors to this volume. They have covered the pharmacology and role of a large number of channels in health and disease, and included some uniquely Australian research, such as employing peptides from our (many) venomous animals. You will no doubt agree that *Ion Channels DownUnder* demonstrates the depth and breadth of excellent research being undertaken on the pharmacology ion channels around Australia.

Dominic P. Geraghty, PhD
School of Health Sciences, Faculty of Health,
University of Tasmania, Launceston, Australia
Lachlan D. Rash, PhD
School of Biomedical Science, Faculty of Medicine,
University of Queensland, Brisbane, Australia

CHAPTER ONE

$GABA_A$ Receptors and the Diversity in their Structure and Pharmacology

Han Chow Chua, Mary Chebib[1]
Faculty of Pharmacy, The University of Sydney, Sydney, NSW, Australia
[1]Corresponding author: e-mail address: mary.collins@sydney.edu.au

Contents

Abstract

$GABA_A$ receptors ($GABA_AR$s) are a class of ligand-gated ion channels with high physiological and therapeutic significance. In the brain, these pentameric receptors occur with diverse subunit composition, which confers highly complex pharmacology to this receptor class. An impressive range of clinically used therapeutics are known to bind to distinct sites found on $GABA_AR$s to modulate receptor function. Numerous experimental approaches have been used over the years to elucidate the binding sites of these drugs, but unequivocal identification is challenging due to subtype- and ligand-dependent pharmacology. Here, we review the current structural and pharmacological understanding of $GABA_AR$s, besides highlighting recent evidence which has revealed greater complexity than previously anticipated.

Advances in Pharmacology, Volume 79
ISSN 1054-3589
http://dx.doi.org/10.1016/bs.apha.2017.03.003

ABBREVIATIONS

CS read counter-clockwise when viewed from the extracellular side

1. INTRODUCTION

γ-Aminobutyric acid (GABA), the major inhibitory neurotransmitter in the mammalian central nervous system (CNS), is the conductor of an intricate inhibitory orchestra fundamental to the harmonious coordination of brain function. The inhibitory effects of GABA rely on two types of receptors—the fast-acting, Cl^--conducting ionotropic $GABA_A$ receptors ($GABA_ARs$) and the slower-acting, G protein-coupled metabotropic $GABA_B$ receptors ($GABA_BRs$) (Note: GABA- and GABAR-mediated actions may be excitatory under certain circumstances, but these actions are not discussed in this chapter). $GABA_ARs$ are ubiquitously expressed throughout the mammalian CNS and have indispensable physiological roles emphasized by a few lines of evidence. First, the mutation or deletion of various genes encoding for $GABA_AR$ subunits in mice is highly disruptive to the normal phenotype, causing developmental defects, sensorimotor dysfunction, hypersensitive behavior, anxiety, epilepsy, and/or reduced lifespan (DeLorey et al., 1998; Gunther et al., 1995; Homanics et al., 1997; Vien et al., 2015). Second, aberrant $GABA_AR$ trafficking, expression and/or gating effects have been implicated in autism (Fatemi, Reutiman, Folsom, & Thuras, 2009), schizophrenia (Mueller, Haroutunian, & Meador-Woodruff, 2014), and a range of idiopathic epileptic syndromes (Hirose, 2014) in humans. Furthermore, genetic association studies have also linked $GABA_AR$ subunit genes with alcohol dependence (Li et al., 2014), eating disorder outcomes (Bloss et al., 2011), autism (Collins et al., 2006; Ma et al., 2005), and bipolar disorders (Ament et al., 2015; Craddock et al., 2010).

$GABA_ARs$ are also important drug targets, as evidenced by the successful clinical utilization of $GABA_AR$ modulators in the treatment of CNS-related disorders such as insomnia, anxiety, and epilepsy, as well as in the induction of anesthesia in surgical patients (Sieghart, 2015). While clinically useful, the misuse of these drugs poses risks of dependence, addiction, abuse, and life-threatening conditions associated with overdose or withdrawal. Hence, understanding the functions of $GABA_ARs$ and the underlying mechanisms of the clinical and undesirable effects of $GABA_AR$-targeting drugs to improve the selectivity and safety of these therapeutics are topics of intensive research (Atack, 2010; Rudolph & Knoflach, 2011). However, the striking structural and functional heterogeneity of these channels pose major challenges in the study of $GABA_ARs$. In this chapter, we provide an overview of the structure and pharmacology of $GABA_ARs$. We also discuss recent evidence which highlights the potential for greater diversity in $GABA_AR$ pharmacology due to subunit stoichiometric and arrangement differences.

2. ARCHITECTURE OF $GABA_ARs$

$GABA_ARs$ are members of the pentameric ligand-gated ion channel (pLGIC) superfamily, which includes the nicotinic acetylcholine receptors (nAChRs), 5-hydroxytryptamine type 3 receptors ($5\text{-}HT_3Rs$), and glycine receptors. These receptors are made up of five homologous subunits that surround a central ion-conducting pore, a structure which is often likened to a barrel with five staves. Each receptor subunit has an extracellular domain (ECD), a transmembrane domain (TMD), and an intracellular domain (ICD). The ECDs are mostly made up of β-sheets and contribute to agonist binding sites, whereas the TMDs consist of the pore-forming α-helices and the structurally variable ICDs are involved in receptor assembly, trafficking and clustering.

The recent determination of a three-dimensional crystal structure of the β3 homomeric $GABA_AR$ captures structural details at 3 Å resolution (Miller & Aricescu, 2014). This receptor subtype is unlikely to be physiologically relevant, but its functional expression in heterologous systems is well known, and has been used as a model to study heteromeric $GABA_ARs$ (Taylor et al., 1999; Yip et al., 2013). The receptor stands approximately 110 Å in height when viewed parallel to the membrane (Fig. 1A). The five subunits assemble in a doughnut-like shape with a diameter around 80 Å, when viewed from the extracellular space, down the channel pore (Fig. 1B). The large ECD (~65 Å in height) of each subunit is made up of an N-terminal α-helix followed by a β-sandwich core with 10 antiparallel β-sheets (Fig. 1C). The TMD consists of four membrane-spanning α-helices (M1–M4), with the M2 helices of all five subunits arranging themselves to form a tapered ion-conducting pore (Fig. 1B and C). The outermost M4 helix harbors the C-terminus on the extracellular end. The ICD contains a small M1–M2 loop and a much larger M3–M4 loop (G333–N446; residue numbering follows sequence of P28472 in UniProt) which was replaced with a 7-amino acid linker for the crystallization of this structure (Fig. 1C).

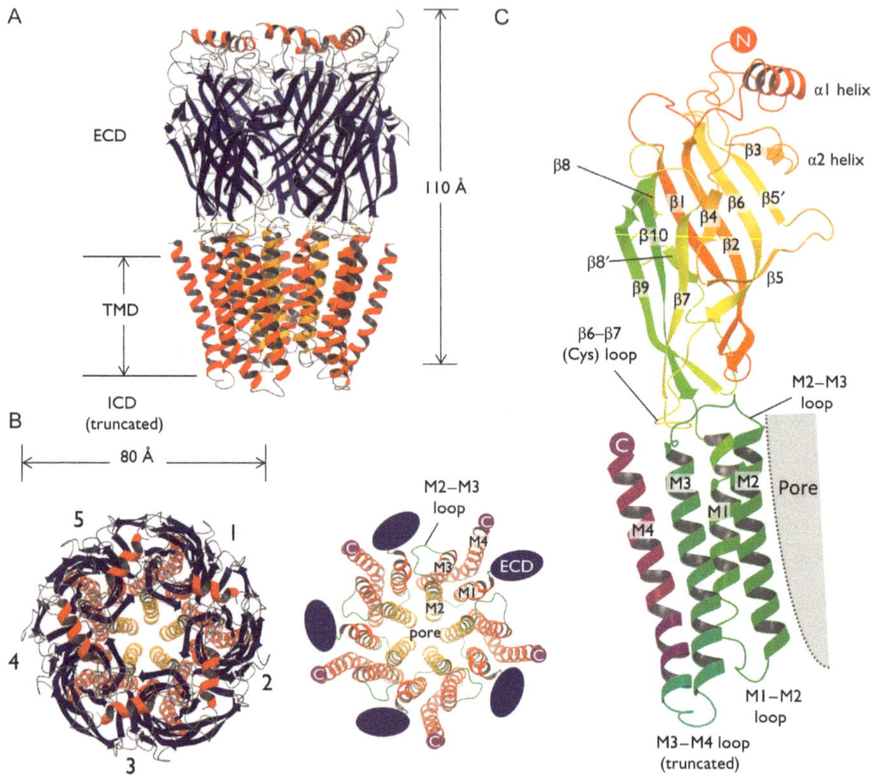

Fig. 1 The crystal structure of a human β3 homomeric $GABA_AR$ (PDB: 4COF). (A) Cartoon representation of $GABA_AR$ viewed parallel to the membrane, colored according to secondary structures (α-helices are in *red* except for the pore-forming helices (*orange*), β-sheets are in *blue*). (B) *Left*, $GABA_AR$ viewed from the extracellular space, with the five subunits labeled 1–5. *Right*, Transmembrane region of $GABA_AR$, with the ECDs simplified as *blue ovals* for clarity. The arrangement of the four TMDs (M1–M4), the C-terminus (*purple circles*), and the M2–M3 loop (*green*) are illustrated. (C) Topology of a single subunit of $GABA_AR$, *rainbow* colored from the N-terminus (*red*) to the C-terminus (*purple*). The β-sheets of the ECD, the α-helices of the TMDs, the characteristic Cys-loop, and other relevant loops are indicated. *Note*: the intracellular M3–M4 loop (G333–N446) was replaced with a 7-amino acid linker for crystallization. Figures were prepared using Maestro, v. 9.5.014, Schrödinger, LLC.

3. $GABA_AR$ ASSEMBLY: SELECTIVE SUBUNIT OLIGOMERIZATION

Human genome sequencing has identified at least 19 $GABA_AR$ subunit genes (α1–6, β1–3, γ1–3, δ, ε, θ, π, and ρ1–3). Given the heteromeric nature of $GABA_ARs$ in vivo, this long list of subunits, together with the splice variants of some of the subunits allow for an enormous range of theoretically possible subunit combinations. Yet, experimental evidence suggests that only a few dozen combinations exist in vivo (see Section 4), indicating that GABA$_A$R assembly is a selective, and not a random process. A hierarchical assembly mechanism has been proposed, in which certain subunits are preferred over others to form dimeric intermediates that ultimately assemble into pentameric complexes (Sarto-Jackson & Sieghart, 2008).

Different methods have been used to define the rules underlying receptor assembly. In concert, data obtained using functional, immunoimaging, and sucrose gradient centrifugation techniques suggest that both α and β subunits are obligatory for the surface expression of fully functional pentameric receptors in heterologous cell systems (Angelotti, Uhler, & Macdonald, 1993; Connor, Boileau, & Czajkowski, 1998; Gorrie et al., 1997). The additional third γ subunit has been shown to enhance the efficiency of receptor assembly (Tretter, Ehya, Fuchs, & Sieghart, 1997). In contrast, the recombinant expression of individual α, β, and γ subunits, and the αγ and βγ combinations mainly yielded di-, tri-, and tetrameric oligomers which were retained in the endoplasmic reticulum (Connolly, Krishek, McDonald, Smart, & Moss, 1996; Gorrie et al., 1997). There are a few notable exceptions, however, with the homomeric β1 and β3 and the heteromeric β3γ2 receptors expressing readily in heterologous systems (Chua, Absalom, Hanrahan, Viswas, & Chebib, 2015; Sanna et al., 1999; Taylor et al., 1999; Wooltorton, Moss, & Smart, 1997).

Amino acid residues important for assembly have been identified in several studies using the chimeric receptor and site-directed mutagenesis approaches (Sarto-Jackson & Sieghart, 2008). These residues are found mainly in the ECD, and to a lesser extent in the intracellular M3–M4 loop. In accordance with these data, the β3 GABA$_A$R crystal structure revealed extensive energetically favorable interactions such as hydrogen bonds, salt bridges, and van der Waals forces along the interfaces between subunit ECDs (Miller & Aricescu, 2014). Disruption to these interactions could affect receptor assembly, and may be the reason for impaired GABA$_A$R surface expression with epilepsy-associated mutations found in the N-terminal regions such as β3G32R and γ2R43Q (Frugier et al., 2007; Gurba, Hernandez, Hu, & Macdonald, 2012; Sancar & Czajkowski, 2004).

While considerable insights have been provided by these studies, the molecular determinants could not be firmly established for several reasons. First, these determinants differ depending on the partner subunits.

For example, four residues in the ECD of the β3 subunit (G171, K173, E179, and R180) have been identified to be critical for the assembly of β3 and β3γ2 receptors, but they are not compulsory for the assembly of αβ receptors (Taylor et al., 1999). In another study that investigated the role of the N-terminal regions in the expression of α1β2γ2 $GABA_AR$s, subunit-specific contributions to receptor assembly were found (Wong, Tae, & Cromer, 2015). When deleted, the N-terminus of the α1 subunit had the most prominent effect on the expression of α1β2γ2 receptors, whereas deletion in similar regions of the β2 and γ2 subunits had minimal effect on surface expression. Second, multiple residues may be involved in oligomerization with the same neighboring subunit (Sarto et al., 2002). As such, when a putative binding residue is mutated and has no effect on receptor expression, it does not necessarily indicate no participation in intersubunit linking. Conversely, an expression-impairing mutation does not validate its significance in subunit oligomerization, as the residue may indirectly contribute to this process (e.g., by stabilizing interacting regions). All in all, $GABA_AR$ assembly is a highly complex, multistep process which involves subunit-specific determinants that govern the subunit composition of $GABA_AR$s found natively.

4. MULTIPLE SUBTYPES, LOCATIONS, AND ACTIONS OF $GABA_AR$s

In recent years, it has become evident that the multiplicity in $GABA_AR$ subunit composition (or subtypes) is one of the main reasons for the heterogeneity observed in their cellular and subcellular distributions, biophysical characteristics, pharmacological properties, in addition to physiological functions (Farrant & Nusser, 2005; Jacob, Moss, & Jurd, 2008; Rudolph, Crestani, & Möhler, 2001). Furthermore, the subunit composition of $GABA_AR$s is plastic. Alterations in brain $GABA_AR$ subtypes have been reported under various developmental and pathological conditions (Brooks-Kayal, Shumate, Jin, Rikhter, & Coulter, 1998; Fritschy, Paysan, Enna, & Mohler, 1994; Steiger & Russek, 2004). As such, answering the question "which $GABA_AR$ subtypes actually occur in vivo?" is essential to understanding the diverse roles played by GABAergic inhibition.

Currently, existing experimental techniques are unable to unequivocally identify $GABA_AR$ subunit composition in neurons. To help determine the likelihood of a receptor subtype being expressed physiologically, the IUPHAR committee has introduced five classification criteria (Olsen &

Sieghart, 2008). Briefly, (1) the expression and coassembly of the subunit proteins of a receptor candidate must be demonstrated in heterologous systems, along with (2) the characterization of its biophysical and pharmacological properties. In the brain, (3) the subunit mRNAs or proteins should colocalize on the cellular and subcellular levels, and (4) the coprecipitation of these subunits would provide stronger evidence. More importantly, (5) a receptor candidate has to show unique functional characteristics that match those of the recombinant receptor subtype, and disruption to the expression of this receptor subtype in genetically engineered mice should lead to altered receptor responses and behavioral profile.

A working list of native $GABA_AR$ subtypes was proposed following stringent consideration of the criteria discussed (Table 1). These receptors are categorized as "identified," "existence with high probability," or "tentative." Evidence from immunochemical, pharmacological, and genetic studies collectively indicate that the majority of $GABA_ARs$ are composed of α, β, and γ2 subunits in the CNS. The α1β2γ2 subtype is the most prevalent isoform (approximately 50%–60% of all $GABA_ARs$), and are expressed in almost all brain regions. The γ2 subunit also coassembles with other α and β variants in the brain, but these receptors are found in considerably less abundance and are restricted in their regional (e.g., α5-containing receptors are expressed in high density in hippocampus) and cellular (e.g., the α2β3γ2 and α3β3γ2 subtypes are highly enriched in hippocampal pyramidal neurons and cholinergic neurons of the basal forebrain, respectively) distributions.

Table 1 The Working List of Native $GABA_AR$ Subtypes Categorized Based on the Strength of Evidence Proposed by Olsen and Sieghart (2008)

Identified	High Probability	Tentative
α1β2γ2	α1β3γ2	αβγ1
α2βγ2	α1βδ	αβγ3
α3βγ2	α5β3γ2	αβθ
α4βγ2	αβ1γ/αβ1δ	αβε
α5βγ2	αβ	αβπ
α6βγ2	α1α6βγ/α1α6βδ	αxαyβγ2[a]
α4β2/3δ		
α6β2/3δ		

[a]αxαy represents two different α subunit isoforms (α1–6).

In addition to the region- and cell-specific expression patterns, these receptors also show distinct subcellular localization. The α1βγ2, α2βγ2, and α3βγ2 isoforms are typically found postsynaptically, whereas the α4βγ2, α5βγ2, and α6βγ2 isoforms are found extrasynaptically. In contrast, the δ subunit which preferentially assembles with the α6 and β2/3 subunits in the cerebellar granule cells (Nusser, Sieghart, & Somogyi, 1998), and with the α4 and β2/3 subunits in the forebrain (Peng et al., 2002), are exclusively expressed at extrasynaptic sites. Due to their proximity to the site of vesicle release, synaptic $GABA_ARs$ are exposed to saturating GABA concentrations (~1–3 mM) that diffuse away from the synaptic cleft rapidly (clearance time < 1 ms) (Mozrzymas, Barberis, Michalak, & Cherubini, 1999; Mozrzymas, Żarmowska, Pytel, & Mercik, 2003). This transient activation of synaptic $GABA_ARs$ is responsible for phasic inhibition, a form of fast, point-to-point synaptic communication used to control the flow of specific signals. Extrasynaptic $GABA_ARs$, on the other hand, are randomly activated by low levels of ambient GABA (low micromolar range) which has escaped from the synaptic cleft on the same or nearby neurons. These receptors are persistently activated, thus provide a basal inhibitory conductance, termed tonic inhibition, which is believed to be important in the regulation of the overall excitability in the brain (Farrant & Nusser, 2005). Synaptic and extrasynaptic $GABA_ARs$ are equipped with distinct properties that facilitate their unique roles in their local environments. For example, δ subunit-containing receptors display characteristics such as higher GABA affinity, minimal desensitization, and longer channel open time, which are ideal for continual activation with sustained exposure to low levels of GABA (Bianchi & Macdonald, 2002). On the other hand, synaptic αβγ isoforms have lower GABA sensitivity, and rapid activation and desensitization kinetics, making them well suited to mediate responses of the phasic vesicular release of GABA (Mortensen, Patel, & Smart, 2012). It is also worth noting that a recent study has shown that synaptic receptors are activated by low ambient concentrations of GABA and are modulated by clinical concentrations of anesthetics, raising the possibility that the distinction between synaptic and extrasynaptic $GABA_ARs$ may not be as clear as previously thought (Li & Akk, 2015).

Contrary to the belief that binary αβ combination has no physiological relevance, there is ample evidence suggesting that these receptors are highly probable to be found in vivo. The defining characteristics of these receptors such as low conductance states and high sensitivity to Zn^{2+} inhibition have been detected in single-channel recordings conducted in rat neurons

(Brickley, Cull-Candy, & Farrant, 1999; Mortensen & Smart, 2006; Yeung et al., 2003). Besides that, receptors consisting only of α and β subunits have also been immunoprecipitated from brain membranes derived from normal or mutant rodents (Bencsits, Ebert, Tretter, & Sieghart, 1999; Gunther et al., 1995; Ogris et al., 2006; Tretter et al., 2001). The exact α and β isoforms that make up these receptors remains unclear, but they are thought to constitute a small portion of GABA$_A$Rs, likely to be expressed at extrasynaptic sites in the brain (Mortensen & Smart, 2006). To add to the diversity, GABA$_A$Rs comprised of different types of α subunits (αxαyβγ2) have also been detected in the CNS, with high prevalence suggested in the spinal cord (Ralvenius, Benke, Acuna, Rudolph, & Zeilhofer, 2015). Other combinations that incorporate the minor subunits (γ1, γ3, θ, ε, or π) are likely to occur in vivo, but more evidence is required to confirm their presence. It is expected that the list of native GABA$_A$R subtypes will expand as the identification techniques continue to improve over time.

5. SUBUNIT STOICHIOMETRY AND ARRANGEMENT OF GABA$_A$Rs

Theoretically, a pentameric GABA$_A$R composed of three types of subunits (e.g., αβγ) will have six configurations with different subunit stoichiometry (i.e., the number of each subunit in each receptor)—1α:1β:3γ, 2α:1β:2γ, 3α:1β:1γ, 1α:2β:2γ, 1α:3β:1γ, and 2α:2β:1γ. A greater number of unique configurations arise when the subunit arrangement (i.e., the spatial orientation of subunits around the channel pore) is taken into consideration. For instance, a receptor with a 2α:2β:1γ subunit stoichiometry can have up to six different arrangements of γ-α-α-β-β, γ-α-β-α-β, γ-α-β-β-α, γ-β-β-α-α, γ-β-α-β-α, and γ-β-α-α-β in a counter-clockwise direction around the pore when viewed from the extracellular side. These configurations vary in the number and type of subunit interfaces, and as almost all known ligand binding sites are located interfacially, establishing the physiologically relevant configuration(s) is a prerequisite to understanding the mechanisms of receptor activation and modulation.

Over the last two decades, considerable effort has been devoted to the elucidation of GABA$_A$R subunit stoichiometry and arrangement. Numerous approaches such as mutagenesis in combination with electrophysiological recording (Backus et al., 1993; Chang, Wang, Barot, & Weiss, 1996), subunit counting in combination with immunoprecipitation (Tretter et al., 1997), fluorescence energy transfer microscopy (Farrar, Whiting,

Bonnert, & McKernan, 1999), and flow cytometry (Botzolakis et al., 2016) have aided in the determination of $GABA_AR$ subunit stoichiometry. However, as these methods do not provide any information on the spatial arrangement of subunits in a receptor complex, researchers have resorted to subunit concatenation to define subunit orientation. By combining subunit genes with a linker of optimized length joining the C-terminus of a preceding subunit to the N-terminus of a following subunit, subunit concatenation allows multiple subunits to be engineered as a single polypeptide with predetermined orientation, thus constraining the stoichiometry and arrangement of receptors expressed. This approach, while powerful in tackling the complicated structural issues of multimeric proteins, has several caveats that may confound data interpretation. Hence, the results described below for various $GABA_AR$ subtypes should be interpreted with two things in mind—(1) the drawbacks with existing methods in elucidating the subunit stoichiometry and arrangement and (2) the vast potential of structural diversity in this receptor class.

For the most abundant αβγ subtype, data obtained using various approaches collectively indicate a 2α:2β:1γ stoichiometry. Earlier studies expressing various di-, tri-, and pentameric concatemers in heterologous systems suggested that only the γ-β-α-β-α arrangement (read counterclockwise when viewed from the extracellular side; abbreviated hereafter as CS) yielded receptors with similar pharmacological and kinetic properties established in receptors assembled from free subunits (Baumann, Baur, & Sigel, 2001, 2002, 2003; Boileau, Pearce, & Czajkowski, 2005). Following these reports, there is an overwhelming consensus that the αβγ subtype has a 2α:2β:1γ stoichiometry, arranged γ-β-α-β-α CS. However, more recently, using the same set of concatemers characterized in a series of studies performed by Erwin Sigel's laboratory previously, another group has identified two additional functional configurations—3α:1β:1γ (γ-α-α-β-α CS) and 2α:1β:2γ (γ-α-γ-β-α CS) (Fig. 2), raising the possibility that alternate stoichiometries and arrangements may exist for the αβγ subtype (Botzolakis et al., 2016).

For δ-containing receptors, the accurate determination of the exact number and arrangement of the subunits is hindered by the promiscuous assembly properties of the δ subunit. Several studies suggest that αβδ receptors share similar stoichiometry and arrangement as αβγ receptors, with the δ subunit replacing the γ subunit (2α:2β:1δ; δ-β-α-β-α CS; Fig. 2) (Barrera et al., 2008; Patel, Mortensen, & Smart, 2014). However, 1α:1β:3δ, 1α:2β:2δ, 1α:3β:1δ, and 2α:1β:2δ stoichiometries have also been detected

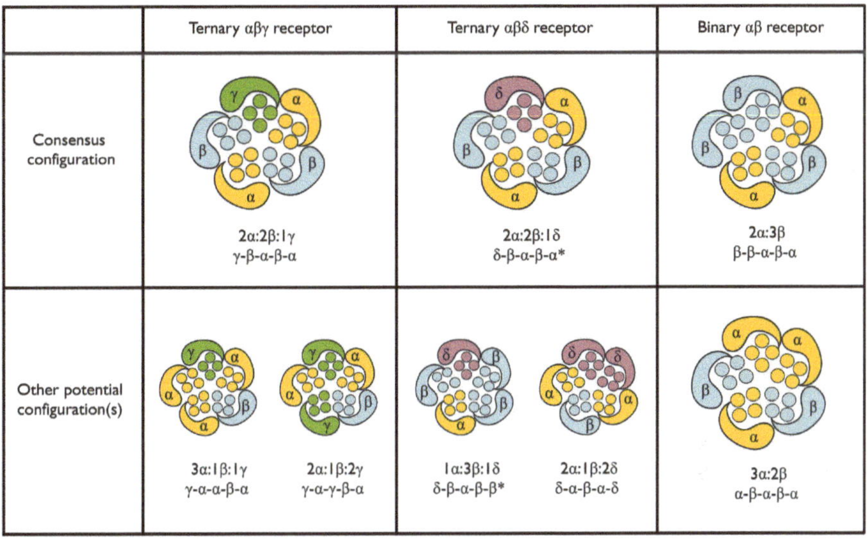

Fig. 2 Model structures of the ternary αβγ, αβδ, and binary αβ GABA$_A$Rs demonstrating their consensus and other potential configurations. The most prevalent native GABA$_A$R subtype αβγ has a stoichiometry of 2α:2β:1γ, arranged γ-β-α-β-α counter-clockwise around the pore when viewed from the extracellular side. The 3α:1β:1γ (γ-α-α-β-α) and 2α:1β:2γ (γ-α-γ-β-α) configurations have also been shown to be functional in vitro (Botzolakis et al., 2016). The δ subunit-containing GABA$_A$Rs are thought to have a 2α:2β:1δ stoichiometry, arranged δ-β-α-β-α. The 1α:3β:1δ (δ-β-α-β-β) and 2α:1β:2δ (δ-α-β-α-δ) configurations have also been reported as well. * Denotes more than one arrangement have been proposed. The binary αβ receptors have been shown to assemble in two different stoichiometries of 2α:3β or 3α:2β, with a β-β-α-β-α or α-β-α-β-α arrangement, respectively.

with the subunit-counting and concatemer strategies (Baur, Kaur, & Sigel, 2009; Kaur, Baur, & Sigel, 2009; Shu et al., 2012; Wagoner & Czajkowski, 2010). To make things more complicated, the δ subunit is flexible in its positioning in the pentameric complex, producing receptors with diverse pharmacological properties (Eaton et al., 2014; Wongsamitkul, Baur, & Sigel, 2016).

In the case of the binary αβ receptors, functional concatemers with 2α:3β (β-β-α-β-α CS) and 3α:2β (α-β-α-β-α CS) stoichiometries have both been reported (Fig. 2) (Baumann et al., 2001; Boileau et al., 2005; Im, Pregenzer, Binder, Dillon, & Alberts, 1995). Interestingly, most studies have only reported one of the two configurations, despite both configurations being functional. Of growing interest is the 3α:2β (α-β-α-β-α CS) stoichiometry as a recent study found that clinically relevant concentrations of zolpidem can differentiate between the two subunit stoichiometries (Che Has et al.,

2016), and this configuration may in part contribute to the physiological effects of zolpidem observed under distinct physiological and clinical conditions. Despite these observations, it remains unclear whether one stoichiometry predominantly forms or both stoichiometries coexist when these subunits are allowed to assemble freely.

6. PHARMACOLOGY OF GABA$_A$Rs

GABA$_A$Rs are well known for their diverse pharmacology. The orthosteric GABA binding sites aside, it has been estimated that there are more than 10 potential ligand binding sites which are distributed at various locations throughout the receptor (Fig. 3). A range of ligands, such as benzodiazepines, barbiturates, anesthetics, neurosteroids, and convulsants, can bind to distinct allosteric (nonorthosteric) sites to exert their physiological or clinical effects by influencing GABA$_A$R function, either by causing or by stabilizing conformational changes in the receptor. Some of these sites are found at specific receptor subtypes, which define the unique pharmacological signatures of these receptors. The properties of the GABA binding sites and several well-studied allosteric binding sites, as well as surfacing

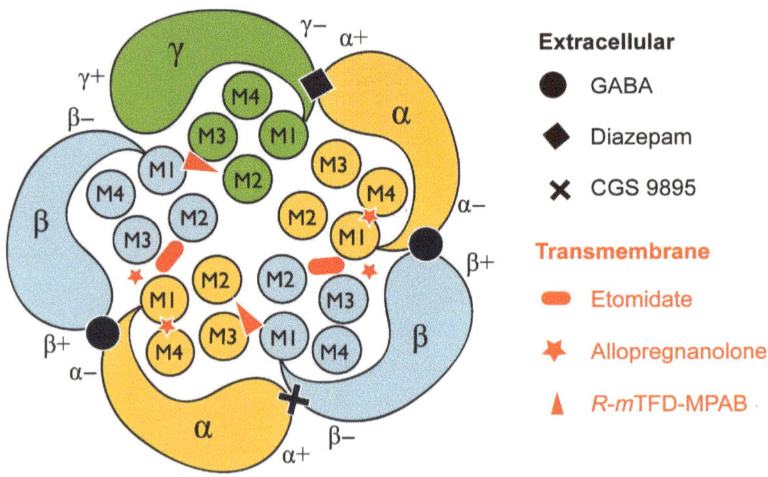

Fig. 3 Schematic illustration of an αβγ GABA$_A$R with a canonical 2α:2β:1γ stoichiometry, γ-β-α-β-α arrangement (read counter-clockwise when viewed from the extracellular side) highlighting the orthosteric and allosteric binding sites. For the purpose of discussion, the approximate binding site locations are indicated by the prototype ligands. The principal (+) and complementary (−) faces of each subunit are also labeled.

evidence indicating the possibility of noncanonical pharmacology are discussed later.

6.1 Orthosteric GABA Binding Sites

6.1.1 Extracellular $\beta + \alpha -$ Interfaces

A common feature of Cys-loop receptors is that the neurotransmitter binding pocket is located at the extracellular interface between two adjacent subunits. Each subunit contributes three (in some cases four) noncontiguous regions that form the binding site. By convention, the principal (+) face of the neurotransmitter binding site is made up of three loops (named loops A, B, and C) and the complementary (−) face has three β-strands and/or one loop (loops D, E, F, and/or G; Fig. 4A) (Lynagh & Pless, 2014). For GABA$_A$Rs, the β and α subunits bear the principal and complementary components of the GABA binding site, respectively. In the most prevalent αβγ subtype (2α:2β:1γ; γ-β-α-β-α), there are two GABA binding sites per receptor at the $\beta + \alpha -$ interfaces (Fig. 3). Channel opening occurs with GABA occupying just one site, but the probability increases greatly when both sites are engaged (Baumann et al., 2003; Macdonald, Rogers, & Twyman, 1989; Twyman, Rogers, & Macdonald, 1990). These identical

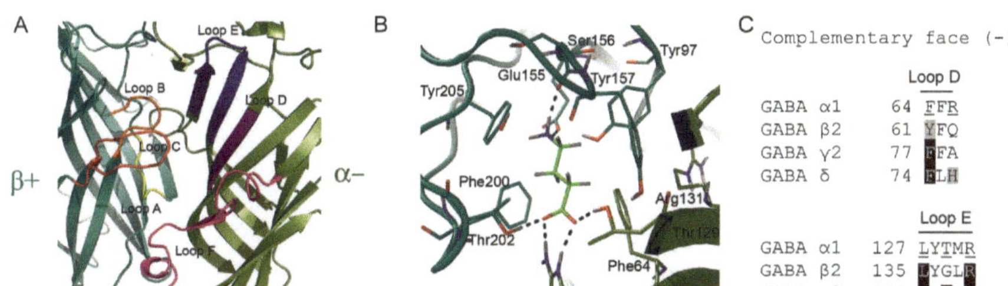

Fig. 4 Homology model of the GABA binding site at α1β2γ2 receptors. (A) The GABA binding site is located at the $\beta + \alpha -$ extracellular interface. The principal (loops A, B, and C) and the complementary (loops D, E, and F) components which form the binding pocket are highlighted in *different colors.* (B) GABA (*green*; ionized form) binding mode predicted by induced fit docking. Residues on both the β and α subunits that are implicated in GABA binding are indicated. (C) Alignment of amino acid residues in loops D and E of α1, β2, γ2, and δ subunits. Critical binding residues on the α1-face are *underlined.* Identical corresponding residues in β2, γ2, and δ subunits are highlighted in *black*, whereas functionally conserved residues are highlighted in *gray*. *Panel (B) Figures were adapted from Bergmann, R., Kongsbak, K., Sorensen, P. L., Sander, T., & Balle, T. (2013). A unified model of the GABAA receptor comprising agonist and benzodiazepine binding sites. PLoS One, 8(1), e52323. doi:10.1371/journal.pone.0052323.*

sites contribute asymmetrically to receptor activation, a phenomenon which has been tentatively correlated with the binding sites assuming different conformations depending on their flanking subunits (one site sits between γ and β, the other sits between α and γ; Fig. 3) (Baumann et al., 2003).

Mutational, radioligand binding, and photoaffinity labeling studies have identified residues with aromatic, hydroxylated, and charged side chains on both the α and β subunits that are critical determinants in GABA sensitivity (Lummis, 2009; Smith & Olsen, 1995). It is currently inconclusive how these residues are located spatially to interact with GABA, but homology modeling has shed some light on the GABA binding mode. In 2013, a model of the α1β2γ2 $GABA_AR$ was created based on the *C. elegans* GluClα and ELIC crystal structures (Bergmann, Kongsbak, Sorensen, Sander, & Balle, 2013). When docked into the orthosteric binding site, GABA forms (1) salt bridges with α1Arg66 and β2Glu155, (2) hydrogen bonds with α1Thr129 and β2Thr202, and (3) cation–π interaction with β2Tyr205 (Fig. 4B). These predictions are in good agreement with experimental evidence, but crystal structures of GABA-bound $GABA_ARs$ will be necessary for validation.

Besides GABA, other structurally similar chemicals can access the orthosteric binding sites to elicit distinct functional responses. Some prototypical ligands include agonists muscimol, partial agonists THIP/gaboxadol, and competitive antagonists bicuculline (Fig. 5). The classification of ligands as agonists or partial agonists is not absolute and is relative to the function of GABA, which is dependent on receptor subtype. For instance, GABA is known to act as a partial agonist at αβδ receptors, exhibiting higher affinity and lower intrinsic efficacy, unlike its full agonist activity at αβγ receptors (Bianchi & Macdonald, 2003; Brown, Kerby, Bonnert, Whiting, & Wafford, 2002). Such functional difference has resulted in the agonist muscimol and partial agonist THIP (at αβγ receptors) to exhibit superagonism (higher maximal efficacy than GABA) at αβδ receptors (Mortensen, Ebert, Wafford, & Smart, 2010; Stórustovu & Ebert, 2006).

6.1.2 Alternative GABA-Binding Interfaces?

A strong consensus that GABA can only bind to the β + α − interfaces has formed since the elucidation of the GABA binding sites. Nonetheless, over the years, numerous individual in vitro studies demonstrating functional receptors lacking the α subunit (e.g., homomeric β, binary βγ and βδ) have accumulated (Amin, Brooks-Kayal, & Weiss, 1997; Bell-Horner, Dibas, Huang, Drewe, & Dillon, 2000; Boileau, Kucken, Evers, & Czajkowski, 1998; Bollan et al., 2003; Chang, Xie, & Weiss, 2001; Chua et al., 2015;

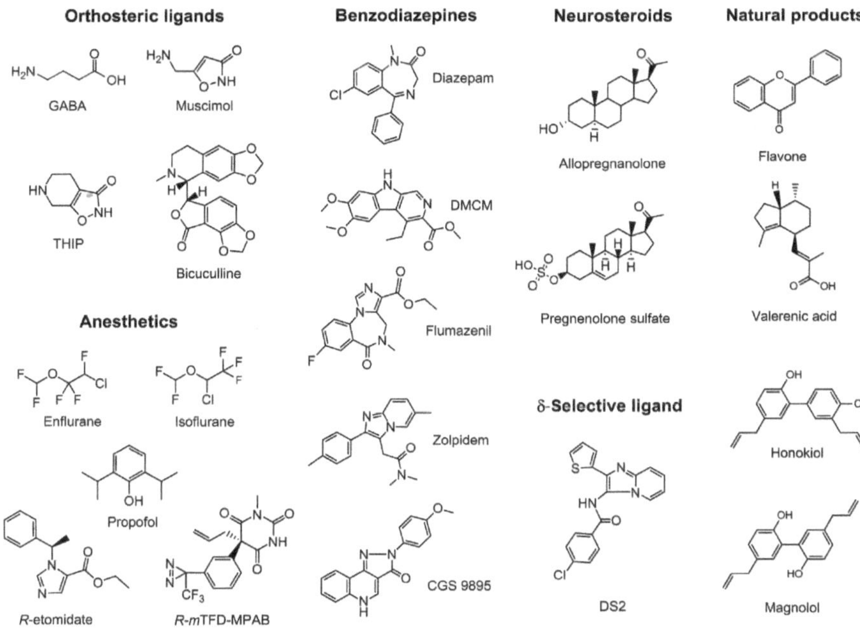

Fig. 5 Chemical structures of various classes of ligands that bind to the orthosteric and allosteric binding sites at GABA$_A$Rs.

Hoerbelt, Lindsley, & Fleck, 2015; Lee et al., 2016; Sanna et al., 1999; Taylor et al., 1999; Whittemore, Yang, Drewe, & Woodward, 1996; Yamaura, Kiyonaka, Numata, Inoue, & Hamachi, 2016). The ability of GABA to activate receptors without the canonical GABA binding sites is unanticipated and raises the question whether additional agonist binding sites exist. While it is possible that hitherto unidentified structurally distinct agonist binding sites are responsible for these unexpected responses, a more logical explanation would be the structural requirement for GABA binding sites is more flexible than they are generally perceived (i.e., homologous interfacial subunit sites exist).

We propose that homologous orthosteric binding sites exist in alternative subunit interfaces for two reasons. (1) The conventional $\beta + \alpha -$ interface has an aromatic box formed by βY97, βY157, βF200, βY205, and αF64 residues, a common feature among the Cys-loop receptors which is essential in agonist recognition (Bergmann et al., 2013; Laha & Tran, 2013; Lynagh & Pless, 2014). The integrity of this aromatic box is maintained at the $\beta + \beta -$, $\beta + \gamma -$, and $\beta + \delta -$ interfaces, as the aromatic side chain of the complementary face is conserved at homologous positions in the β, γ, and δ subunits (α1F64; β2Y61; γ2F77; δF74; Fig. 4C). (2) Other α subunit residues implicated in GABA binding/function such as L127, T129, and R131 are also mostly conserved at the corresponding positions in the β, γ, and δ subunits (Fig. 4C). Therefore, it is possible that the overall architecture of the agonist binding site is maintained across most β + X− subunit interfaces. However, differences in other critical binding residues may alter the GABA binding affinity of these interfaces. For instance, the α1R66 was previously predicted to form salt bridges with GABA within the β + α− cavity (Bergmann et al., 2013), but as the bidentate arginine is replaced with a nonpolar alanine residue in the γ2 subunit (γ2A79), this interaction is unlikely to occur, which may underlie the lower GABA potency reported at βγ receptors (Chua et al., 2016; Whittemore et al., 1996).

The physiological relevance of these alternative GABA binding interfaces is an open question. However, given the ongoing nature of the native $GABA_AR$ subtypes identification process, the whole picture of their structural heterogeneity awaits further substantiation and completion (Olsen & Sieghart, 2008). Moreover, the fact that GABA is still able to bind and activate ELIC, the prokaryotic pLGIC despite high divergence in sequence highlights the potential for homologous GABA binding sites in other subunit interfaces (Spurny et al., 2012). Whether GABA accesses these noncanonical sites and how these sites may contribute to receptor activation are some of the interesting questions to be investigated in future studies.

6.2 Benzodiazepine Binding Sites

6.2.1 High-Affinity Site: Extracellular α + γ − Interface

Homologous to the β + α− GABA binding sites, a structurally related pocket exists at the extracellular α + γ− interface (Fig. 3). This allosteric site is commonly referred to as the benzodiazepine binding site, named after the prototype drugs. Benzodiazepines do not directly activate $GABA_ARs$, but they are able to modulate receptor function. Benzodiazepine site agonists (e.g., diazepam; Fig. 5) potentiate $GABA_ARs$ to produce clinically useful effects such as sedation (for insomnia), anxiolysis (for anxiety), anticonvulsant (for epilepsy), myorelaxant (for muscle spasms), and amnesia (for invasive medical procedures). Conversely, benzodiazepine site inverse agonists (e.g., DMCM) inhibit $GABA_ARs$ to exert anxiogenic, convulsant, and memory-enhancing effects. Benzodiazepine site competitive antagonists (e.g., flumazenil) block the actions of other benzodiazepines and can be used clinically as antidote for benzodiazepine toxicity. Ligands that are structurally unrelated to the benzodiazepines can also access the high-affinity benzodiazepine site (e.g., zolpidem) to elicit similar responses.

Extensive effort has gone into the delineation of benzodiazepine pharmacology using the representative ligand diazepam. It is now clear that diazepam, at low concentrations, indiscriminately modulates α1βγ2, α2βγ2, α3βγ2, and α5βγ2 $GABA_A$Rs, and is insensitive at α4βγ2 and α6βγ2 $GABA_A$Rs. A conserved histidine residue found in the α1, α2, α3, and α5 subunits confers high-affinity diazepam sensitivity, whereas the homologous arginine in the α4 and α6 subunits renders these receptors diazepam insensitive. The histidine-to-arginine mutation has been shown to selectively abolish diazepam activity at α1H101Rβ2γ2, α2H101Rβ2γ2, α3H126Rβ2γ2, and α5H105Rβ2γ2 recombinant receptors, and the reverse mutation produced diazepam-responsive α4R99Hβ2γ2 and α6R100Hβ2γ2 receptors (Benson, Löw, Keist, Mohler, & Rudolph, 1998; Wieland & Luddens, 1994; Wieland, Lüddens, & Seeburg, 1992). Genetic studies have exploited this functional switch to engineer point-mutated mice bearing diazepam-insensitive α1, α2, α3, and/or α5 subunits. Behavioral analysis of single point-mutated (only one type of diazepam-insensitive α subunit) and triple point-mutated (only one type of diazepam-sensitive α subunit) mice in response to diazepam has helped define the functional role(s) of individual α subunits (Ralvenius et al., 2015; Rudolph et al., 2001; Rudolph & Möhler, 2004). Taken together, these studies strongly suggest that sedation is primarily mediated by α1βγ2, anxiolysis by α2βγ2, myorelaxant by both α2- and α3βγ2, and amnesia by α5βγ2 $GABA_A$Rs. In light of these findings, as well as the fact that the α1-preferring zolpidem displays mainly sedative hypnotic effects, there is a surge of interest in the development of subtype-selective benzodiazepine site agonists with improved therapeutic profiles (Rudolph & Knoflach, 2011). In particular, α2-selective modulators with anxioselectivity devoid of sedating property are highly sought after (Skolnick, 2012).

It is also worth mentioning that while the α4- and α6-containing receptors lack high sensitivity to diazepam, it does not mean that the high-affinity benzodiazepine site is absent altogether. Indeed, members of the same ligand class such as bretazenil and Ro 15–4513 are able to bind to both diazepam-sensitive and -insensitive $GABA_A$Rs with high affinities (Pym, Cook, Rosahl, McKernan, & Atack, 2005). Furthermore, the molecular determinants of these benzodiazepines are different from those of diazepam, as their functions are not diminished when the conserved histidine is mutated to arginine (Benson et al., 1998). Interestingly, a high-affinity zolpidem binding site at the α1–α1 has also been proposed following detection of zolpidem modulation at α1β3 binary receptors with a 3α:2β subunit stoichiometry (Che Has et al., 2016). However, the molecular detail of this binding site is still unclear and awaits further investigation.

6.2.2 Low-Affinity Benzodiazepine Binding Site(s)

Many benzodiazepines also display additional low-affinity components at $GABA_ARs$. The binding site(s) responsible for these actions are poorly characterized, but evidence thus far suggests that the receptor responses mediated by these site(s) do not require the γ subunit, and may vary depending on the ligand, the concentration tested, and the type of subunits present (Sieghart, 2015). The classical benzodiazepine diazepam, for instance, modulates α1β2γ2 $GABA_ARs$ via two distinct mechanisms manifested as a biphasic potentiation with nanomolar and micromolar potencies (Walters, Hadley, Morris, & Amin, 2000). The nanomolar component is mediated by the high-affinity benzodiazepine site and can be selectively blocked by the antagonist flumazenil. The micromolar component, however, is flumazenil insensitive and has been shown to be affected by mutations in the TMD where anesthetics usually bind (Section 6.3). The physiological function of the low-affinity component is unclear, but has been postulated to underlie diazepam's anesthetic property. Like diazepam, CGS 9895 (Fig. 5), has high- and low-affinity components at α1β3γ2 $GABA_ARs$ (Ramerstorfer et al., 2011). At nanomolar concentrations, CGS 9895 acts as a neutralizing modulator to block diazepam action. At micromolar concentrations, CGS 9896 potentiates $GABA_ARs$, an effect selectively mediated by a cluster of residues found on the α and β subunits (α1V211, α1S204, and β3Q64). Homology modeling has located this low-affinity benzodiazepine site on the extracellular α + β− interfaces, homologous to the classical benzodiazepine site (Fig. 3). The therapeutical potential for subtype-selective ligands targeting this site is an area of interest (Sieghart, Ramerstorfer, Sarto-Jackson, Varagic, & Ernst, 2012; Varagic, Ramerstorfer et al., 2013; Varagic, Wimmer et al., 2013).

6.3 Anesthetic Binding Sites in the TMD

The transmembrane region of $GABA_ARs$ harbors many solvent-accessible pockets which are the site of action for a range of structurally diverse chemicals including volatile anesthetics (e.g., enflurane, isoflurane), general anesthetics (e.g., etomidate, propofol), anticonvulsants (e.g., barbiturates, loreclezole), and sedative hypnotics (e.g., methaqualone) (Fig. 5). These chemicals exhibit multiphasic activity at GABA$_A$Rs, enhancing GABA-elicited current at clinical concentrations, directly activate receptors at high micromolar concentrations, and in some cases, act as open-channel blockers at even higher concentrations (Feng, Bianchi, & Macdonald, 2004; Feng & Macdonald, 2004; Hill-Venning, Belelli, Peters, & Lambert, 1997). These binding sites are traditionally described in the context of their prototypical ligands. However, as more experimental evidence has become available to indicate that these sites are not unique to the prototype drugs, it is more appropriate to address them according to their locations.

6.3.1 Transmembrane $\beta + \alpha -$ Interfaces

Two key approaches have hitherto contributed to the elucidation of the first class of anesthetic binding sites, commonly referred to as the etomidate binding sites. First, using photoreactive analogues of etomidate ([^{3}H]azietomidate and [^{3}H]TDBzl-etomidate) which covalently label binding residues upon UV irradiation, photoaffinity labeling studies have jointly identified the βM286 (located in the M3 domain) and αM236 (located in the M1 domain) residues (Chiara et al., 2012; Li et al., 2006). Etomidate is able to inhibit the photolabeling of these residues in a concentration-dependent manner, further supporting etomidate's interaction with both residues. Second, conventional and cysteine-substitution mutagenesis studies have also demonstrated that these methionine residues are important determinants of etomidate binding and function (Stewart, Desai, Cheng, Liu, & Forman, 2008; Stewart, Hotta, Desai & Forman, 2013; Stewart, Hotta, Li, et al., 2013). With the help of homology models based on various crystal structures of related receptors, βM286 and αM236 are predicted to be located at the $\beta + \alpha -$ interfaces in the TMD, just below the orthosteric binding sites (Fig. 3). Other residues in the vicinity implicated in etomidate binding include βF289 (M3), βV290 (M3), αL232 (M1), αT237 (M1), and αI239 (M1) (Chiara et al., 2012; Stewart, Hotta, Li, et al., 2013).

6.3.2 Transmembrane $\alpha + \beta -$ and $\gamma + \beta -$ Interfaces

Another class of anesthetic binding sites has recently been identified in α1β3γ2 GABA$_A$Rs using *R*-[^{3}H]*m*TFD-MPAB, a photoreactive barbiturate analogue (Chiara et al., 2013). These binding pockets are located at the $\alpha + \beta -$ and $\gamma + \beta -$ interfaces, in homologous positions to the etomidate binding sites (Fig. 3). Binding residues labeled by *R*-[^{3}H]*m*TFD-MPAB include αA291 (M3; equivalent to βM286), αY294 (M3), and γS301

(M3; equivalent to βM286) found on the principal faces of the respective subunits, whereas the βM227 (M1; equivalent to αL232) is found on the complementary face.

6.3.3 Transmembrane *β* + *β* − Interface

Studies conducted in α1β3 $GABA_A$Rs have also demonstrated that the photoreactive etomidate analogues and *R*-[^{3}H]*m*TFD-MPAB which preferentially label β+ and β− residues, respectively, also contact residues found on the opposite faces (Chiara et al., 2012; Jayakar et al., 2014). [^{3}H]Azietomidate and [^{3}H]TDBzl-etomidate have been shown to photolabel βM227 on the complementary side, whereas *R*-[^{3}H]*m*TFD-MPAB also photolabeled βM286 and βF289 located on the principal face. These findings suggest that a homologous cavity at the β + β− interface, which is absent in the αβγ subtypes is also accessible to these anesthetics. The existence of the transmembrane β + β− anesthetic binding site is also corroborated by evidence obtained from photoaffinity labeling, structural modeling, and functional studies focusing on propofol actions at β3 homomeric $GABA_A$Rs (Eaton et al., 2015; Franks, 2015; Yip et al., 2013).

6.3.4 The Promiscuity of Anesthetics Binding

While [^{3}H]azietomidate and [^{3}H]TDBzl-etomidate are highly selective for the β + α− interfaces, and *R*-[^{3}H]*m*TFD-MPAB prefers the α+/γ + β− interfaces, the different classes of binding pockets are not exclusive to etomidate or barbiturates. Structurally dissimilar anesthetics are able to compete with these photoreactive analogues to prevent residue photolabeling (Chiara et al., 2013; Li, Chiara, Cohen, & Olsen, 2010). Evidence from mutagenesis studies are in concordance with these findings. The substitution of methionine by tryptophan at residue 286 of the β subunit (βM286W) attenuates etomidate, propofol, volatile anesthetics, and methaqualone activity at $GABA_A$Rs (Hammer et al., 2015; Krasowski et al., 1998; Siegwart, Krähenbühl, Lambert, & Rudolph, 2003). Moreover, the substituted cysteine accessibility method (SCAM) has also revealed that propofol protects the modification of α1M236C and β2M286C mutants by sulfhydryl-reactive reagent, indicating that propofol also contacts these residues (Bali & Akabas, 2004; Stewart, Pierce, Hotta, Stern, & Forman, 2014). Also, we and others have demonstrated that general anesthetics such as etomidate and propofol, initially believed to bind only to the β + α− interfaces are able to activate the α-lacking βγ receptors (Chua et al., 2015; Sanna et al., 1999).

Thus, it appears that a structurally diverse set of chemicals including, but most likely not limited to the ligands investigated to date are able to access different number and classes of interfacial anesthetic binding sites to exert their clinical effects. This heterogeneity is best exemplified by the convulsant *S*-*m*TFD-MPAB which selectively binds to the $\gamma + \beta-$ interface to inhibit $GABA_ARs$ (Jayakar et al., 2015), and the general anesthetic propofol that binds nonselectively to the $\beta + \alpha-$, $\alpha + \beta-$, $\gamma + \beta-$, and $\beta + \beta-$ interfaces to potentiate $GABA_ARs$ (Chiara et al., 2013; Jayakar et al., 2014). More complexity is likely as other binding sites in the $\alpha + \gamma-$ transmembrane region, intrasubunit helical bundles, and intracellular loop have also been suggested (Sieghart, 2015). However, due to limitations associated with available experimental techniques, and the lack of crystal structures of anesthetic-bound $GABA_ARs$, their existence remains to be confirmed.

6.4 Neurosteroid Binding Sites in the TMD

Endogenous steroids such as allopregnanolone (Fig. 5) and their synthetic analogues have neuroactive effects such as anxiolysis, analgesia, sedation, anticonvulsant, and anesthesia mediated via $GABA_ARs$ (Belelli & Lambert, 2005). These neurosteroids potently enhance $GABA_AR$ function at low nanomolar concentrations and activate $GABA_ARs$ at submicromolar-to-micromolar concentrations. The mechanism(s) of action of neurosteroids are different from those of benzodiazepines and anesthetics as demonstrated in mutational (Siegwart et al., 2003), kinetic (Akk et al., 2004), photoaffinity labeling (Li, Chiara, Cohen & Olsen, 2009), and transgenic mice behavioral studies (Jurd et al., 2003; Rudolph et al., 1999). The precise locations of the neurosteroid binding sites remain to be confirmed, but several residues in the TMDs have been demonstrated to influence distinct actions of neurosteroids. For instance, residues such as αS240 (M1), αQ241 (M1), αN407 (M4), and αY410 (M4) have been shown to be implicated in neurosteroid potentiation, whereas αT236 (M1) and βY284 (M3) mediate neurosteroid activation (Akk et al., 2008; Hosie, Wilkins, da Silva, & Smart, 2006; Li, Bandyopadhyaya, Covey, Steinbach & Akk, 2009). Homology modeling located the modulatory site at the M1–M4 interface within the α subunit, and the activation site occurs at the $\beta + \alpha-$ interfaces, between the M3 and M1 domains of the β and α subunits, respectively (Fig. 3). These residues are conserved in all α and β subunits, which may explain the lack of subtype selectivity in neurosteroid activity (Hosie, Wilkins, & Smart, 2007).

Naturally occurring neurosteroids that block $GABA_ARs$ (e.g., pregnenolone sulfate) also exist, but their physiological actions are not well defined. Evidence from binding and mutational studies suggest that inhibitory neurosteroids do not share the same sites with neurosteroids that augment $GABA_AR$ function (Akk et al., 2008). A residue found in the M2 domain of the α1 subunit (V256) which is located further down the channel pore has been implicated, but this putative inhibitory neurosteroid binding cavity is controversial and awaits further clarification (Akk, Bracamontes, & Steinbach, 2001; Seljeset, Laverty, & Smart, 2015). All in all, neurosteroids appear to interact in a complex manner with at least three distinct transmembrane sites to potentiate, activate, and inhibit $GABA_ARs$.

6.5 Variable Pharmacology of δ-Containing $GABA_ARs$

The exclusivity of the δ subunit in extrasynaptic $GABA_ARs$, a group of receptors responsible for tonic GABAergic inhibition has generated immense research and therapeutical interests. However, (1) the scarcity of δ-selective ligands and (2) the promiscuous assembly properties of the δ subunit are hampering the progress in establishing the pharmacology of these receptors.

Numerous compounds have been claimed to be selective for the δ subunit. The hypnotic drug THIP/gaboxadol directly activates αβδ with higher potency and efficacy than αβγ $GABA_ARs$ (relative to GABA), but does not discriminate between αβ and αβδ receptors (Brown et al., 2002; Stórustovu & Ebert, 2006). Similar to THIP, anesthetics (Feng & Macdonald, 2004), neurosteroids (Bianchi & Macdonald, 2003), ketamine (Hevers, Hadley, Lüddens, & Amin, 2008), and AA29504 (Hoestgaard-Jensen et al., 2010) also show more pronounced action at δ-containing $GABA_ARs$, but as their activity is independent of subunit composition, these compounds are not considered to be δ-selective. In contrast, 4-chloro-*N*-(2-thiophen-2-ylimidazo[1,2-*a*]pyridin-3-yl)benzamide (DS2; Fig. 5) was found to predominantly act as an efficacious positive modulator at α4/6βδ, has limited relative efficacy at αβγ, and is inactive at αβ $GABA_ARs$ (Jensen et al., 2013). Following these findings, there is a prevailing view that DS2 is a δ-selective ligand. However, this premise has been challenged recently by Ahring et al. (2016), who argued that conventional ligand characterization approach is biased in comparing ligand activity at $GABA_ARs$ with divergent intrinsic properties, leading to inaccurate determination of ligand selectivity (Ahring et al., 2016). As such, the quest for δ-defining ligands continues.

Unlike αβγ, the expression of α, β, and δ subunits has led to inconsistent pharmacological profile in heterologous systems, a phenomenon which has been attributed to the flexible stoichiometry and arrangement of αβδ receptors. Discrepancy in GABA activity ranging from potency, intrinsic efficacy, and current level can be found in the literature, despite comparable experimental conditions (Eaton et al., 2014; Hartiadi, Ahring, Chebib, & Absalom, 2016; Hoestgaard-Jensen et al., 2014; Karim et al., 2012). This variability in receptor properties is not only limited to agonists, and conflicting results with allosteric ligands are not uncommon. For instance, while it is generally agreed that DS2 acts as a positive modulator with no agonist activity at α4β2δ receptors, Hartiadi et al. (2016) have shown that a functionally distinct subtype of α4β2δ receptors expressed in *Xenopus* oocytes can be directly activated by DS2 (Hartiadi et al., 2016). A study by Eaton et al. (2014) also reported similar observation with the neurosteroid alfaxalone at α4β2δ receptors (Eaton et al., 2014). Thus, it appears that a comprehensive pharmacological characterization of δ-containing $GABA_ARs$ is inherently challenging to achieve, and it is expected that with more evidence coming from studies employing concatenated constructs will help clarify their enigmatic pharmacology.

6.6 Natural Products of Plant Origin

$GABA_ARs$ are the molecular target for a remarkable range of natural products of plant origin. Prominent examples of these plant-derived ligands include the $GABA_AR$-defining antagonist bicuculline (from *Dicentra cucullaria*), the potent psychoactive agonist muscimol (from the intoxicating mushroom *Amanita muscaria*), and the pore-blocking convulsant picrotoxin (from the *Menispermaceae* family). Given the long history of herbal medicine use in alleviating symptoms associated with CNS-related disorders implicating $GABA_ARs$ such as anxiety and insomnia, the pharmacologically active constituents of these herbs are of great therapeutical interest. Several families of natural products-inspired $GABA_AR$ ligands such as the flavonoids (Hanrahan, Chebib, & Johnston, 2011; Johnston, Hanrahan, Chebib, Duke, & Mewett, 2006), valerenic acids (Khom et al., 2007; Khom et al., 2010), honokiol, and magnolol (Alexeev, Grosenbaugh, Mott, & Fisher, 2012; Fuchs, Baur, Schoeder, Sigel, & Müller, 2014; Taferner et al., 2011) derivatives have emerged over the years. These compounds exhibit diverse pharmacology mediated by known (reviewed earlier) and unknown binding sites. The potential for the clinical application of several of these compounds is currently being explored (Hintersteiner et al., 2014).

7. CONCLUSION

There is now strong evidence indicating more complex $GABA_AR$ pharmacology than previously anticipated as a consequence of the vast potential heterogeneity in the subunit composition, stoichiometry, and arrangement. Nevertheless, most of this evidence has not received significant attention, perhaps due to the reluctance to accept results that contradict general consensus. In our view, it is of utmost importance for future drug discovery and structure–function analysis efforts targeting $GABA_ARs$ to be designed and interpreted with this complexity in mind.

CONFLICT OF INTEREST

The authors have no conflicts of interest to declare.

ACKNOWLEDGMENTS

H.C.C. acknowledges the International Postgraduate Research Scholarship and John Lamberton Scholarship for financial support. M.C. acknowledges the National Health and Medical Research Council of Australia for financial support (APP 1069201 and APP1081733). M.C. also wishes to acknowledge her $GABA_A$ receptor collaborators past and present and specifically Graham A.R. Johnson, Jane R. Hanrahan, Nathan Absalom, Petra van Nieuwenhuijzen, Thomas Balle, and Philip Ahring.

REFERENCES

Ahring, P. K., Bang, L. H., Jensen, M. L., Strøbæk, D., Hartiadi, L. Y., Chebib, M., et al. (2016). A pharmacological assessment of agonists and modulators at α4β2γ2 and α4β2δ $GABA_A$ receptors: The challenge in comparing apples with oranges. *Pharmacological Research*, *111*, 563–576. http://dx.doi.org/10.1016/j.phrs.2016.05.014.

Akk, G., Bracamontes, J. R., Covey, D. F., Evers, A., Dao, T., & Steinbach, J. H. (2004). Neuroactive steroids have multiple actions to potentiate $GABA_A$ receptors. *The Journal of Physiology*, *558*(1), 59–74. http://dx.doi.org/10.1113/jphysiol.2004.066571.

Akk, G., Bracamontes, J., & Steinbach, J. H. (2001). Pregnenolone sulfate block of $GABA_A$ receptors: Mechanism and involvement of a residue in the M2 region of the α subunit. *The Journal of Physiology*, *532*(3), 673–684. http://dx.doi.org/10.1111/j.1469-7793.2001.0673e.x.

Akk, G., Li, P., Bracamontes, J., Reichert, D. E., Covey, D. F., & Steinbach, J. H. (2008). Mutations of the GABA-A receptor α1 subunit M1 domain reveal unexpected complexity for modulation by neuroactive steroids. *Molecular Pharmacology*, *74*(3), 614–627. http://dx.doi.org/10.1124/mol.108.048520.

Alexeev, M., Grosenbaugh, D. K., Mott, D. D., & Fisher, J. L. (2012). The natural products magnolol and honokiol are positive allosteric modulators of both synaptic and extra-synaptic $GABA_A$ receptors. *Neuropharmacology*, *62*(8), 2507–2514. http://dx.doi.org/10.1016/j.neuropharm.2012.03.002.

Ament, S. A., Szelinger, S., Glusman, G., Ashworth, J., Hou, L., Akula, N., et al. (2015). Rare variants in neuronal excitability genes influence risk for bipolar disorder. *Proceedings of the National Academy of Sciences of the United States of America*, *112*(11), 3576–3581. http://dx.doi.org/10.1073/pnas.1424958112.

Amin, J., Brooks-Kayal, A., & Weiss, D. S. (1997). Two tyrosine residues on the α subunit are crucial for benzodiazepine binding and allosteric modulation of γ-aminobutyric acid$_A$ receptors. *Molecular Pharmacology*, *51*(5), 833–841. http://dx.doi.org/10.1124/mol.51.5.833.

Angelotti, T. P., Uhler, M. D., & Macdonald, R. L. (1993). Assembly of GABA$_A$ receptor subunits: Analysis of transient single-cell expression utilizing a fluorescent substrate/marker gene technique. *The Journal of Neuroscience*, *13*(4), 1418–1428.

Atack, J. R. (2010). Development of subtype-selective GABA$_A$ receptor compounds for the treatment of anxiety, sleep disorders and epilepsy. In J. M. Monti, S. R. Pandi-Perumal, & H. Möhler (Eds.), *GABA and sleep: Molecular, functional and clinical aspects* (pp. 25–72). Basel: Springer Basel.

Backus, K. H., Arigoni, M., Drescher, U., Scheurer, L., Malherbe, P., Mohler, H., et al. (1993). Stoichiometry of a recombinant GABA$_A$ receptor deduced from mutation-induced rectification. *Neuroreport*, *5*(3), 285–288.

Bali, M., & Akabas, M. H. (2004). Defining the propofol binding site location on the GABA$_A$ receptor. *Molecular Pharmacology*, *65*(1), 68–76. http://dx.doi.org/10.1124/mol.65.1.68.

Barrera, N. P., Betts, J., You, H., Henderson, R. M., Martin, I. L., Dunn, S. M. J., et al. (2008). Atomic force microscopy reveals the stoichiometry and subunit arrangement of the α4β3δ GABA$_A$ receptor. *Molecular Pharmacology*, *73*(3), 960–967. http://dx.doi.org/10.1124/mol.107.042481.

Baumann, S. W., Baur, R., & Sigel, E. (2001). Subunit arrangement of γ-aminobutyric acid type a receptors. *Journal of Biological Chemistry*, *276*(39), 36275–36280. http://dx.doi.org/10.1074/jbc.M105240200.

Baumann, S. W., Baur, R., & Sigel, E. (2002). Forced subunit assembly in α1β2γ2 GABA$_A$ receptors: Insight into the absolute arrangement. *Journal of Biological Chemistry*, *277*(48), 46020–46025. http://dx.doi.org/10.1074/jbc.M207663200.

Baumann, S. W., Baur, R., & Sigel, E. (2003). Individual properties of the two functional agonist sites in GABA$_A$ receptors. *The Journal of Neuroscience*, *23*(35), 11158–11166.

Baur, R., Kaur, K. H., & Sigel, E. (2009). Structure of α6β3δ GABA$_A$ receptors and their lack of ethanol sensitivity. *Journal of Neurochemistry*, *111*(5), 1172–1181. http://dx.doi.org/10.1111/j.1471-4159.2009.06387.x.

Belelli, D., & Lambert, J. J. (2005). Neurosteroids: Endogenous regulators of the GABA$_A$ receptor. *Nature Reviews Neuroscience*, *6*(7), 565–575.

Bell-Horner, C. L., Dibas, M., Huang, R.-Q., Drewe, J. A., & Dillon, G. H. (2000). Influence of subunit configuration on the interaction of picrotoxin-site ligands with recombinant GABA$_A$ receptors. *Molecular Brain Research*, *76*(1), 47–55. http://dx.doi.org/10.1016/S0169-328X(99)00330-7.

Bencsits, E., Ebert, V., Tretter, V., & Sieghart, W. (1999). A significant part of native γ-aminobutyric acid$_A$ receptors containing α4 subunits do not contain γ or δ subunits. *Journal of Biological Chemistry*, *274*(28), 19613–19616. http://dx.doi.org/10.1074/jbc.274.28.19613.

Benson, J. A., Löw, K., Keist, R., Mohler, H., & Rudolph, U. (1998). Pharmacology of recombinant γ-aminobutyric acid$_A$ receptors rendered diazepam-insensitive by point-mutated α-subunits. *FEBS Letters*, *431*(3), 400–404. http://dx.doi.org/10.1016/S0014-5793(98)00803-5.

Bergmann, R., Kongsbak, K., Sorensen, P. L., Sander, T., & Balle, T. (2013). A unified model of the GABA$_A$ receptor comprising agonist and benzodiazepine binding sites. *PLoS One*, *8*(1), e52323. http://dx.doi.org/10.1371/journal.pone.0052323.

Bianchi, M. T., & Macdonald, R. L. (2002). Slow phases of $GABA_A$ receptor desensitization: Structural determinants and possible relevance for synaptic function. *The Journal of Physiology, 544*(Pt 1), 3–18. http://dx.doi.org/10.1113/jphysiol.2002.020255.

Bianchi, M. T., & Macdonald, R. L. (2003). Neurosteroids shift partial agonist activation of $GABA_A$ receptor channels from low- to high-efficacy gating patterns. *The Journal of Neuroscience, 23*(34), 10934–10943.

Bloss, C. S., Berrettini, W., Bergen, A. W., Magistretti, P., Duvvuri, V., Strober, M., et al. (2011). Genetic association of recovery from eating disorders: The role of GABA receptor SNPs. *Neuropsychopharmacology, 36*(11), 2222–2232. http://dx.doi.org/10.1038/npp.2011.108.

Boileau, A. J., Kucken, A. M., Evers, A. R., & Czajkowski, C. (1998). Molecular dissection of benzodiazepine binding and allosteric coupling using chimeric γ-aminobutyric $acid_A$ receptor subunits. *Molecular Pharmacology, 53*(2), 295–303.

Boileau, A. J., Pearce, R. A., & Czajkowski, C. (2005). Tandem subunits effectively constrain $GABA_A$ receptor stoichiometry and recapitulate receptor kinetics but are insensitive to $GABA_A$ receptor-associated protein. *The Journal of Neuroscience, 25*(49), 11219–11230. http://dx.doi.org/10.1523/jneurosci.3751-05.2005.

Bollan, K., King, D., Robertson, L. A., Brown, K., Taylor, P. M., Moss, S. J., et al. (2003). $GABA_A$ receptor composition is determined by distinct assembly signals within α and β subunits. *Journal of Biological Chemistry, 278*(7), 4747–4755. http://dx.doi.org/10.1074/jbc.M210229200.

Botzolakis, E. J., Gurba, K. N., Lagrange, A. H., Feng, H.-J., Stanic, A. K., Hu, N., et al. (2016). Comparison of γ-aminobutyric acid, type a ($GABA_A$), receptor αβγ and αβδ expression using flow cytometry and electrophysiology: Evidence for alternative subunit Stoichiometries and arrangements. *Journal of Biological Chemistry, 291*(39), 20440–20461. http://dx.doi.org/10.1074/jbc.M115.698860.

Brickley, S. G., Cull-Candy, S. G., & Farrant, M. (1999). Single-channel properties of synaptic and extrasynaptic $GABA_A$ receptors suggest differential targeting of receptor subtypes. *The Journal of Neuroscience, 19*(8), 2960–2973.

Brooks-Kayal, A. R., Shumate, M. D., Jin, H., Rikhter, T. Y., & Coulter, D. A. (1998). Selective changes in single cell $GABA_A$ receptor subunit expression and function in temporal lobe epilepsy. *Nature Medicine, 4*(10), 1166–1172.

Brown, N., Kerby, J., Bonnert, T. P., Whiting, P. J., & Wafford, K. A. (2002). Pharmacological characterization of a novel cell line expressing human α4β3δ $GABA_A$ receptors. *British Journal of Pharmacology, 136*(7), 965–974. http://dx.doi.org/10.1038/sj.bjp.0704795.

Chang, Y., Wang, R., Barot, S., & Weiss, D. S. (1996). Stoichiometry of a recombinant $GABA_A$ receptor. *The Journal of Neuroscience, 16*(17), 5415–5424.

Chang, Y., Xie, Y., & Weiss, D. S. (2001). Positive allosteric modulation by ultraviolet irradiation on $GABA_A$, but not $GABA_C$, receptors expressed in *Xenopus* oocytes. *The Journal of Physiology, 536*(2), 471–478. http://dx.doi.org/10.1111/j.1469-7793.2001.0471c.xd.

Che Has, A. T., Absalom, N., van Nieuwenhuijzen, P. S., Clarkson, A. N., Ahring, P. K., & Chebib, M. (2016). Zolpidem is a potent stoichiometry-selective modulator of α1β3 $GABA_A$ receptors: Evidence of a novel benzodiazepine site in the α1-α1 interface. *Scientific Reports, 6*, 28674. http://dx.doi.org/10.1038/srep28674.

Chiara, D. C., Dostalova, Z., Jayakar, S. S., Zhou, X., Miller, K. W., & Cohen, J. B. (2012). Mapping general anesthetic binding site(s) in human α1β3 γ-aminobutyric acid type a receptors with [^{3}H]TDBzl-etomidate, a photoreactive etomidate analogue. *Biochemistry, 51*(4), 836–847. http://dx.doi.org/10.1021/bi201772m.

Chiara, D. C., Jayakar, S. S., Zhou, X., Zhang, X., Savechenkov, P. Y., Bruzik, K. S., et al. (2013). Specificity of intersubunit general anesthetic-binding sites in the transmembrane domain of the human α1β3γ2 γ-aminobutyric acid type a (GABA$_A$) receptor. *Journal of Biological Chemistry*, *288*(27), 19343–19357. http://dx.doi.org/10.1074/jbc.M113.479725.

Chua, H. C., Absalom, N. L., Hanrahan, J. R., Viswas, R., & Chebib, M. (2015). The direct actions of GABA, 2′-methoxy-6-methylflavone and general anaesthetics at β3γ2L GABA$_A$ receptors: Evidence for receptors with different subunit stoichiometries. *PLoS One*, *10*(10). e0141359. http://dx.doi.org/10.1371/journal.pone.0141359.

Chua, H. C., Christensen, E. T. H., Hoestgaard-Jensen, K., Hartiadi, L. Y., Ramzan, I., Jensen, A. A., et al. (2016). Kavain, the major constituent of the anxiolytic kava extract, potentiates GABA$_A$ receptors: Functional characteristics and molecular mechanism. *PLoS One*, *11*(6). e0157700. http://dx.doi.org/10.1371/journal.pone.0157700.

Collins, A. L., Ma, D., Whitehead, P. L., Martin, E. R., Wright, H. H., Abramson, R. K., et al. (2006). Investigation of autism and GABA receptor subunit genes in multiple ethnic groups. *Neurogenetics*, 7(3), 167–174. http://dx.doi.org/10.1007/s10048-006-0045-1.

Connolly, C. N., Krishek, B. J., McDonald, B. J., Smart, T. G., & Moss, S. J. (1996). Assembly and cell surface expression of heteromeric and homomeric γ-aminobutyric acid type a receptors. *Journal of Biological Chemistry*, *271*(1), 89–96. http://dx.doi.org/10.1074/jbc.271.1.89.

Connor, J. X., Boileau, A. J., & Czajkowski, C. (1998). A GABA$_A$ receptor α1 subunit tagged with green fluorescent protein requires a β subunit for functional surface expression. *Journal of Biological Chemistry*, *273*(44), 28906–28911. http://dx.doi.org/10.1074/jbc.273.44.28906.

Craddock, N., Jones, L., Jones, I. R., Kirov, G., Green, E. K., Grozeva, D., et al. (2010). Strong genetic evidence for a selective influence of GABA$_A$ receptors on a component of the bipolar disorder phenotype. *Molecular Psychiatry*, *15*(2), 146–153. http://dx.doi.org/10.1038/mp.2008.66.

DeLorey, T. M., Handforth, A., Anagnostaras, S. G., Homanics, G. E., Minassian, B. A., Asatourian, A., et al. (1998). Mice lacking the β3 subunit of the GABA$_A$ receptor have the epilepsy phenotype and many of the behavioral characteristics of Angelman syndrome. *The Journal of Neuroscience*, *18*(20), 8505–8514.

Eaton, M., Bracamontes, J., Shu, H.-J., Li, P., Mennerick, S. J., Steinbach, J. H., et al. (2014). GABA$_A$ α4, β2 and δ subunits assemble to produce more than one functionally distinct receptor type. *Molecular Pharmacology*, *86*(6), 647–656. http://dx.doi.org/10.1124/mol.114.094813.

Eaton, M. M., Cao, L. Q., Chen, Z., Franks, N. P., Evers, A. S., & Akk, G. (2015). Mutational analysis of the putative high-affinity propofol binding site in human β3 homomeric GABA$_A$ receptors. *Molecular Pharmacology*, *88*(4), 736–745. http://dx.doi.org/10.1124/mol.115.100347.

Farrant, M., & Nusser, Z. (2005). Variations on an inhibitory theme: Phasic and tonic activation of GABA$_A$ receptors. *Nature Reviews Neuroscience*, *6*(3), 215–229.

Farrar, S. J., Whiting, P. J., Bonnert, T. P., & McKernan, R. M. (1999). Stoichiometry of a ligand-gated ion channel determined by fluorescence energy transfer. *Journal of Biological Chemistry*, *274*(15), 10100–10104. http://dx.doi.org/10.1074/jbc.274.15.10100.

Fatemi, S. H., Reutiman, T., Folsom, T., & Thuras, P. (2009). GABA$_A$ receptor downregulation in brains of subjects with autism. *Journal of Autism and Developmental Disorders*, *39*(2), 223–230. http://dx.doi.org/10.1007/s10803-008-0646-7.

Feng, H.-J., Bianchi, M. T., & Macdonald, R. L. (2004). Pentobarbital differentially modulates α1β3δ and α1β3γ2L GABA$_A$ receptor currents. *Molecular Pharmacology*, *66*(4), 988–1003. http://dx.doi.org/10.1124/mol.104.002543.

Feng, H.-J., & Macdonald, R. L. (2004). Multiple actions of propofol on αβγ and αβδ GABA$_A$ receptors. *Molecular Pharmacology*, *66*(6), 1517–1524. http://dx.doi.org/10.1124/mol.104.003426.

Franks, N. P. (2015). Structural comparisons of ligand-gated ion channels in open, closed, and desensitized states identify a novel propofol-binding site on mammalian γ-aminobutyric acid type a receptors. *Anesthesiology, 122*, 787–794. http://dx.doi.org/10.1097/ALN.0000000000000588.

Fritschy, J. M., Paysan, J., Enna, A., & Mohler, H. (1994). Switch in the expression of rat $GABA_A$-receptor subtypes during postnatal development: An immunohistochemical study. *The Journal of Neuroscience, 14*(9), 5302–5324.

Frugier, G., Coussen, F., Giraud, M.-F., Odessa, M.-F., Emerit, M. B., Boué-Grabot, E., et al. (2007). A γ2(R43Q) mutation, linked to epilepsy in humans, alters $GABA_A$ receptor assembly and modifies subunit composition on the cell surface. *Journal of Biological Chemistry, 282*(6), 3819–3828. http://dx.doi.org/10.1074/jbc.M608910200.

Fuchs, A., Baur, R., Schoeder, C., Sigel, E., & Müller, C. E. (2014). Structural analogues of the natural products magnolol and honokiol as potent allosteric potentiators of $GABA_A$ receptors. *Bioorganic & Medicinal Chemistry, 22*(24), 6908–6917. http://dx.doi.org/10.1016/j.bmc.2014.10.027.

Gorrie, G. H., Vallis, Y., Stephenson, A., Whitfield, J., Browning, B., Smart, T. G., et al. (1997). Assembly of $GABA_A$ receptors composed of α1 and β2 subunits in both cultured neurons and fibroblasts. *The Journal of Neuroscience, 17*(17), 6587–6596.

Gunther, U., Benson, J., Benke, D., Fritschy, J. M., Reyes, G., Knoflach, F., et al. (1995). Benzodiazepine-insensitive mice generated by targeted disruption of the γ2 subunit gene of γ-aminobutyric acid type a receptors. *Proceedings of the National Academy of Sciences of the United States of America, 92*(17), 7749–7753.

Gurba, K. N., Hernandez, C. C., Hu, N., & Macdonald, R. L. (2012). GABRB3 mutation, G32R, associated with childhood absence epilepsy alters α1β3γ2L $GABA_A$ receptor expression and channel gating. *Journal of Biological Chemistry, 287*(15), 12083–12097. http://dx.doi.org/10.1074/jbc.M111.332528.

Hammer, H., Bader, B. M., Ehnert, C., Bundgaard, C., Bunch, L., Hoestgaard-Jensen, K., et al. (2015). A multifaceted $GABA_A$ receptor modulator: Functional properties and mechanism of action of the sedative-hypnotic and recreational drug methaqualone (Quaalude). *Molecular Pharmacology, 88*(2), 401–420. http://dx.doi.org/10.1124/mol.115.099291.

Hanrahan, J. R., Chebib, M., & Johnston, G. A. R. (2011). Flavonoid modulation of $GABA_A$ eceptors. *British Journal of Pharmacology, 163*(2), 234–245. http://dx.doi.org/10.1111/j.1476-5381.2011.01228.x.

Hartiadi, L. Y., Ahring, P. K., Chebib, M., & Absalom, N. L. (2016). High and low GABA sensitivity α4β2δ $GABA_A$ receptors are expressed in *Xenopus laevis* oocytes with divergent stoichiometries. *Biochemical Pharmacology, 103*, 98–108. http://dx.doi.org/10.1016/j.bcp.2015.12.021.

Hevers, W., Hadley, S. H., Lüddens, H., & Amin, J. (2008). Ketamine, but not phencyclidine, selectively modulates cerebellar $GABA_A$ receptors containing α6 and δ subunits. *The Journal of Neuroscience, 28*(20), 5383–5393. http://dx.doi.org/10.1523/jneurosci.5443-07.2008.

Hill-Venning, C., Belelli, D., Peters, J. A., & Lambert, J. J. (1997). Subunit-dependent interaction of the general anaesthetic etomidate with the γ-aminobutyric acid type a receptor. *British Journal of Pharmacology, 120*(5), 749–756. http://dx.doi.org/10.1038/sj.bjp.0700927.

Hintersteiner, J., Haider, M., Luger, D., Schwarzer, C., Reznicek, G., Jäger, W., et al. (2014). Esters of valerenic acid as potential prodrugs. *European Journal of Pharmacology, 735*, 123–131. http://dx.doi.org/10.1016/j.ejphar.2014.03.019.

Hirose, S. (2014). Chapter 3—Mutant $GABA_A$ receptor subunits in genetic (idiopathic) epilepsy. In K. S. Ortrud (Ed.), *Progress in brain research: Vol. 213* (pp. 55–85). Amsterdam, The Netherlands: Elsevier B.V.

Hoerbelt, P., Lindsley, T. A., & Fleck, M. W. (2015). Dopamine directly modulates GABA$_A$ receptors. *The Journal of Neuroscience*, *35*(8), 3525–3536. http://dx.doi.org/10.1523/jneurosci.4390-14.2015.

Hoestgaard-Jensen, K., Dalby, N. O., Krall, J., Hammer, H., Krogsgaard-Larsen, P., Frølund, B., et al. (2014). Probing α4βδ GABA$_A$ receptor heterogeneity: Differential regional effects of a functionally selective α4β1δ/α4β3δ receptor agonist on tonic and phasic inhibition in rat brain. *The Journal of Neuroscience*, *34*(49), 16256–16272. http://dx.doi.org/10.1523/jneurosci.1495-14.2014.

Hoestgaard-Jensen, K., Dalby, N. O., Wolinsky, T. D., Murphey, C., Jones, K. A., Rottländer, M., et al. (2010). Pharmacological characterization of a novel positive modulator at α4β3δ-containing extrasynaptic GABA$_A$ receptors. *Neuropharmacology*, *58*(4–5), 702–711. http://dx.doi.org/10.1016/j.neuropharm.2009.12.023.

Homanics, G. E., DeLorey, T. M., Firestone, L. L., Quinlan, J. J., Handforth, A., Harrison, N. L., et al. (1997). Mice devoid of γ-aminobutyrate type a receptor β3 subunit have epilepsy, cleft palate, and hypersensitive behavior. *Proceedings of the National Academy of Sciences of the United States of America*, *94*(8), 4143–4148.

Hosie, A. M., Wilkins, M. E., da Silva, H. M. A., & Smart, T. G. (2006). Endogenous neurosteroids regulate GABA$_A$ receptors through two discrete transmembrane sites. *Nature*, *444*(7118), 486–489. http://dx.doi.org/10.1038/nature05324.

Hosie, A. M., Wilkins, M. E., & Smart, T. G. (2007). Neurosteroid binding sites on GABA$_A$ receptors. *Pharmacology & Therapeutics*, *116*(1), 7–19. http://dx.doi.org/10.1016/j.pharmthera.2007.03.011.

Im, W. B., Pregenzer, J. F., Binder, J. A., Dillon, G. H., & Alberts, G. L. (1995). Chloride channel expression with the tandem construct of α6-β2 GABA$_A$ receptor subunit requires a monomeric subunit of α6 or γ2. *Journal of Biological Chemistry*, *270*(44), 26063–26066. http://dx.doi.org/10.1074/jbc.270.44.26063.

Jacob, T. C., Moss, S. J., & Jurd, R. (2008). GABA$_A$ receptor trafficking and its role in the dynamic modulation of neuronal inhibition. *Nature Reviews Neuroscience*, *9*(5), 331–343.

Jayakar, S. S., Zhou, X., Chiara, D. C., Dostalova, Z., Savechenkov, P. Y., Bruzik, K. S., et al. (2014). Multiple propofol-binding sites in a γ-aminobutyric acid type a receptor (GABA$_A$R) identified using a photoreactive propofol analog. *Journal of Biological Chemistry*, *289*(40), 27456–27468. http://dx.doi.org/10.1074/jbc.M114.581728.

Jayakar, S. S., Zhou, X., Savechenkov, P. Y., Chiara, D. C., Desai, R., Bruzik, K. S., et al. (2015). Positive and negative allosteric modulation of an α1β3γ2 γ-aminobutyric acid type a (GABA$_A$) receptor by binding to a site in the transmembrane domain at the γ^+-β^- interface. *Journal of Biological Chemistry*, *290*(38), 23432–23446. http://dx.doi.org/10.1074/jbc.M115.672006.

Jensen, M. L., Wafford, K. A., Brown, A. R., Belelli, D., Lambert, J. J., & Mirza, N. R. (2013). A study of subunit selectivity, mechanism and site of action of the delta selective compound 2 (DS2) at human recombinant and rodent native GABA$_A$ receptors. *British Journal of Pharmacology*, *168*(5), 1118–1132. http://dx.doi.org/10.1111/bph.12001.

Johnston, G. A., Hanrahan, J. R., Chebib, M., Duke, R. K., & Mewett, K. N. (2006). Modulation of ionotropic GABA receptors by natural products of plant origin. *Advances in Pharmacology*, *54*, 285–316.

Jurd, R., Arras, M., Lambert, S., Drexler, B., Siegwart, R., Crestani, F., et al. (2003). General anesthetic actions in vivo strongly attenuated by a point mutation in the GABA$_A$ receptor β3 subunit. *The FASEB Journal*, *17*(2), 250–252. http://dx.doi.org/10.1096/fj.02-0611fje.

Karim, N., Wellendorph, P., Absalom, N., Bang, L. H., Jensen, M. L., Hansen, M. M., et al. (2012). Low nanomolar GABA effects at extrasynaptic α4β1/β3δ GABA$_A$ receptor subtypes indicate a different binding mode for GABA at these receptors. *Biochemical Pharmacology*, *84*(4), 549–557. http://dx.doi.org/10.1016/j.bcp.2012.05.017.

Kaur, K. H., Baur, R., & Sigel, E. (2009). Unanticipated structural and functional properties of δ-subunit-containing $GABA_A$ receptors. *Journal of Biological Chemistry*, *284*(12), 7889–7896. http://dx.doi.org/10.1074/jbc.M806484200.

Khom, S., Baburin, I., Timin, E., Hohaus, A., Trauner, G., Kopp, B., et al. (2007). Valerenic acid potentiates and inhibits $GABA_A$ receptors: Molecular mechanism and subunit specificity. *Neuropharmacology*, *53*(1), 178–187. http://dx.doi.org/10.1016/j.neuropharm.2007.04.018.

Khom, S., Strommer, B., Ramharter, J., Schwarz, T., Schwarzer, C., Erker, T., et al. (2010). Valerenic acid derivatives as novel subunit-selective $GABA_A$ receptor ligands—*In vitro* and *in vivo* characterization. *British Journal of Pharmacology*, *161*(1), 65–78. http://dx.doi.org/10.1111/j.1476-5381.2010.00865.x.

Krasowski, M. D., Koltchine, V. V., Rick, C. E., Ye, Q., Finn, S. E., & Harrison, N. L. (1998). Propofol and other intravenous anesthetics have sites of action on the γ-aminobutyric acid type a receptor distinct from that for isoflurane. *Molecular Pharmacology*, *53*(3), 530–538.

Laha, K. T., & Tran, P. N. (2013). Multiple tyrosine residues at the GABA binding pocket influence surface expression and mediate kinetics of the $GABA_A$ receptor. *Journal of Neurochemistry*, *124*(2), 200–209. http://dx.doi.org/10.1111/jnc.12083.

Lee, H. J., Absalom, N. L., Hanrahan, J. R., van Nieuwenhuijzen, P., Ahring, P. K., & Chebib, M. (2016). A pharmacological characterization of GABA, THIP and DS2 at binary α4β3 and β3δ receptors: GABA activates β3δ receptors via the β3(+)δ(−) interface. *Brain Research*, *1644*, 222–230. http://dx.doi.org/10.1016/j.brainres.2016.05.019.

Li, P., & Akk, G. (2015). Synaptic-type α1β2γ2L $GABA_A$ receptors produce large persistent currents in the presence of ambient GABA and anesthetic drugs. *Molecular Pharmacology*, *87*(5), 776–781. http://dx.doi.org/10.1124/mol.114.096453.

Li, P., Bandyopadhyaya, A. K., Covey, D. F., Steinbach, J. H., & Akk, G. (2009a). Hydrogen bonding between the 17β-substituent of a neurosteroid and the $GABA_A$ receptor is not obligatory for channel potentiation. *British Journal of Pharmacology*, *158*(5), 1322–1329. http://dx.doi.org/10.1111/j.1476-5381.2009.00390.x.

Li, G.-D., Chiara, D. C., Cohen, J. B., & Olsen, R. W. (2009b). Neurosteroids allosterically modulate binding of the anesthetic etomidate to γ-aminobutyric acid type a receptors. *The Journal of Biological Chemistry*, *284*(18), 11771–11775. http://dx.doi.org/10.1074/jbc.C900016200.

Li, G.-D., Chiara, D. C., Cohen, J. B., & Olsen, R. W. (2010). Numerous classes of general anesthetics inhibit etomidate binding to γ-aminobutyric acid type a ($GABA_A$) receptors. *Journal of Biological Chemistry*, *285*(12), 8615–8620. http://dx.doi.org/10.1074/jbc.M109.074708.

Li, G.-D., Chiara, D. C., Sawyer, G. W., Husain, S. S., Olsen, R. W., & Cohen, J. B. (2006). Identification of a $GABA_A$ receptor anesthetic binding site at subunit interfaces by photolabeling with an etomidate analog. *The Journal of Neuroscience*, *26*(45), 11599–11605. http://dx.doi.org/10.1523/jneurosci.3467-06.2006.

Li, D., Sulovari, A., Cheng, C., Zhao, H., Kranzler, H. R., & Gelernter, J. (2014). Association of Gamma-Aminobutyric Acid a Receptor [alpha]2 Gene (GABRA2) with alcohol use disorder. *Neuropsychopharmacology*, *39*(4), 907–918. http://dx.doi.org/10.1038/npp.2013.291.

Lummis, S. C. (2009). Locating GABA in GABA receptor binding sites. *Biochemical Society Transactions*, *37*(Pt 6), 1343–1346. http://dx.doi.org/10.1042/bst0371343.

Lynagh, T., & Pless, S. A. (2014). Principles of agonist recognition in Cys-loop receptors. *Frontiers in Physiology*, *5*. http://dx.doi.org/10.3389/fphys.2014.00160.

Ma, D. Q., Whitehead, P. L., Menold, M. M., Martin, E. R., Ashley-Koch, A. E., Mei, H., et al. (2005). Identification of significant association and gene-gene interaction of GABA receptor subunit genes in autism. *American Journal of Human Genetics*, 77(3), 377–388.

Macdonald, R. L., Rogers, C. J., & Twyman, R. E. (1989). Kinetic properties of the GABA$_A$ receptor main conductance state of mouse spinal cord neurones in culture. *The Journal of Physiology*, *410*, 479–499.

Miller, P. S., & Aricescu, A. R. (2014). Crystal structure of a human GABA$_A$ receptor. *Nature*, *512*(7514), 270–275. http://dx.doi.org/10.1038/nature13293.

Mortensen, M., Ebert, B., Wafford, K., & Smart, T. G. (2010). Distinct activities of GABA agonists at synaptic- and extrasynaptic-type GABA$_A$ receptors. *The Journal of Physiology*, *588*(Pt 8), 1251–1268. http://dx.doi.org/10.1113/jphysiol.2009.182444.

Mortensen, M., Patel, B., & Smart, T. (2012). GABA potency at GABA$_A$ receptors found in synaptic and extrasynaptic zones. *Frontiers in Cellular Neuroscience*, *6*(1). http://dx.doi.org/10.3389/fncel.2012.00001.

Mortensen, M., & Smart, T. G. (2006). Extrasynaptic αβ subunit GABA$_A$ receptors on rat hippocampal pyramidal neurons. *The Journal of Physiology*, *577*(3), 841–856. http://dx.doi.org/10.1113/jphysiol.2006.117952.

Mozrzymas, J. W., Barberis, A., Michalak, K., & Cherubini, E. (1999). Chlorpromazine inhibits miniature GABAergic currents by reducing the binding and by increasing the unbinding rate of GABA$_A$ receptors. *The Journal of Neuroscience*, *19*(7), 2474–2488.

Mozrzymas, J. W., Żarmowska, E. D., Pytel, M., & Mercik, K. (2003). Modulation of GABA$_A$ receptors by hydrogen ions reveals synaptic GABA transient and a crucial role of the desensitization process. *The Journal of Neuroscience*, *23*(22), 7981–7992.

Mueller, T. M., Haroutunian, V., & Meador-Woodruff, J. H. (2014). *N*-glycosylation of GABA$_A$ receptor subunits is altered in schizophrenia. *Neuropsychopharmacology*, *39*(3), 528–537. http://dx.doi.org/10.1038/npp.2013.190.

Nusser, Z., Sieghart, W., & Somogyi, P. (1998). Segregation of different GABA$_A$ receptors to synaptic and extrasynaptic membranes of cerebellar granule cells. *The Journal of Neuroscience*, *18*(5), 1693–1703.

Ogris, W., Lehner, R., Fuchs, K., Furtmüller, B., Höger, H., Homanics, G. E., et al. (2006). Investigation of the abundance and subunit composition of GABA$_A$ receptor subtypes in the cerebellum of α1-subunit-deficient mice. *Journal of Neurochemistry*, *96*(1), 136–147. http://dx.doi.org/10.1111/j.1471-4159.2005.03509.x.

Olsen, R. W., & Sieghart, W. (2008). International Union of Pharmacology. LXX. Subtypes of γ-aminobutyric acid$_A$ receptors: Classification on the basis of subunit composition, pharmacology, and function. Update. *Pharmacological Reviews*, *60*(3), 243–260. http://dx.doi.org/10.1124/pr.108.00505.

Patel, B., Mortensen, M., & Smart, T. G. (2014). Stoichiometry of δ subunit containing GABA$_A$ receptors. *British Journal of Pharmacology*, *171*(4), 985–994. http://dx.doi.org/10.1111/bph.12514.

Peng, Z., Hauer, B., Mihalek, R. M., Homanics, G. E., Sieghart, W., Olsen, R. W., et al. (2002). GABA$_A$ receptor changes in δ subunit-deficient mice: Altered expression of α4 and γ2 subunits in the forebrain. *The Journal of Comparative Neurology*, *446*(2), 179–197.

Pym, L. J., Cook, S. M., Rosahl, T., McKernan, R. M., & Atack, J. R. (2005). Selective labelling of diazepam-insensitive GABA$_A$ receptors *in vivo* using [^{3}H]Ro 15-4513. *British Journal of Pharmacology*, *146*(6), 817–825. http://dx.doi.org/10.1038/sj.bjp.0706392.

Ralvenius, W. T., Benke, D., Acuna, M. A., Rudolph, U., & Zeilhofer, H. U. (2015). Analgesia and unwanted benzodiazepine effects in point-mutated mice expressing only one benzodiazepine-sensitive GABA$_A$ receptor subtype. *Nature Communications*, *6*, 6803. http://dx.doi.org/10.1038/ncomms7803.

Ramerstorfer, J., Furtmüller, R., Sarto-Jackson, I., Varagic, Z., Sieghart, W., & Ernst, M. (2011). The GABA$_A$ receptor α+β-interface: A novel target forsubtype selective drugs. *The Journal of Neuroscience*, *31*(3), 870–877. http://dx.doi.org/10.1523/jneurosci.5012-10.2011.

Rudolph, U., Crestani, F., Benke, D., Brunig, I., Benson, J. A., Fritschy, J.-M., et al. (1999). Benzodiazepine actions mediated by specific γ-aminobutyric $acid_A$ receptor subtypes. *Nature*, *401*(6755), 796–800. http://dx.doi.org/10.1038/44579.

Rudolph, U., Crestani, F., & Möhler, H. (2001). GABAA receptor subtypes: Dissecting their pharmacological functions. *Trends in Pharmacological Sciences*, *22*(4), 188–194. http://dx.doi.org/10.1016/S0165-6147(00)01646-1.

Rudolph, U., & Knoflach, F. (2011). Beyond classical benzodiazepines: Novel therapeutic potential of $GABA_A$ receptor subtypes. *Nature Reviews Drug Discovery*, *10*(9), 685–697. http://dx.doi.org/10.1038/nrd3502.

Rudolph, U., & Möhler, H. (2004). Analysis of $GABA_A$ receptor function and dissection of the pharmacology of benzodiazepines and general anesthetics through mouse genetics. *Annual Review of Pharmacology and Toxicology*, *44*(1), 475–498. http://dx.doi.org/10.1146/annurev.pharmtox.44.101802.121429.

Sancar, F., & Czajkowski, C. (2004). A $GABA_A$ receptor mutation linked to human epilepsy (γ2R43Q) impairs cell surface expression of αβγ receptors. *Journal of Biological Chemistry*, *279*(45), 47034–47039. http://dx.doi.org/10.1074/jbc.M403388200.

Sanna, E., Motzo, C., Usala, M., Serra, M., Dazzi, L., Maciocco, E., et al. (1999). Characterization of the electrophysiological and pharmacological effects of 4-iodo-2,6-diisopropylphenol, a propofol analogue devoid of sedative-anaesthetic properties. *British Journal of Pharmacology*, *126*(6), 1444–1454. http://dx.doi.org/10.1038/sj.bjp.0702449.

Sarto, I., Klausberger, T., Ehya, N., Mayer, B., Fuchs, K., & Sieghart, W. (2002). A novel site on γ3 subunits important for assembly of $GABA_A$ receptors. *Journal of Biological Chemistry*, *277*(34), 30656–30664. http://dx.doi.org/10.1074/jbc.M203597200.

Sarto-Jackson, I., & Sieghart, W. (2008). Assembly of $GABA_A$ receptors (review). *Molecular Membrane Biology*, *25*(4), 302–310. http://dx.doi.org/10.1080/09687680801914516.

Seljeset, S., Laverty, D., & Smart, T. G. (2015). Inhibitory neurosteroids and the $GABA_A$ receptor. *Advances in Pharmacology*, *72*, 165–187. http://dx.doi.org/10.1016/bs.apha.2014.10.006.

Shu, H.-J., Bracamontes, J., Taylor, A., Wu, K., Eaton, M. M., Akk, G., et al. (2012). Characteristics of concatemeric $GABA_A$ receptors containing α4/δ subunits expressed in Xenopus oocytes. *British Journal of Pharmacology*, *165*(7), 2228–2243. http://dx.doi.org/10.1111/j.1476-5381.2011.01690.x.

Sieghart, W. (2015). Chapter three—Allosteric modulation of GABAA receptors via multiple drug-binding sites. In R. Uwe (Ed.), *Advances in Pharmacology: Vol. 72* (pp. 53–96). Amsterdam, The Netherlands: Elsevier B.V.

Sieghart, W., Ramerstorfer, J., Sarto-Jackson, I., Varagic, Z., & Ernst, M. (2012). A novel $GABA_A$ receptor pharmacology: Drugs interacting with the α+β-interface. *British Journal of Pharmacology*, *166*(2), 476–485. http://dx.doi.org/10.1111/j.1476-5381.2011.01779.x.

Siegwart, R., Krähenbühl, K., Lambert, S., & Rudolph, U. (2003). Mutational analysis of molecular requirements for the actions of general anaesthetics at the γ-aminobutyric $acid_A$ receptor subtype, α1β2γ2. *BMC Pharmacology*, *3*(1), 1–9. http://dx.doi.org/10.1186/1471-2210-3-13.

Skolnick, P. (2012). Anxioselective anxiolytics: On a quest for the holy grail. *Trends in Pharmacological Sciences*, *33*(11), 611–620. http://dx.doi.org/10.1016/j.tips.2012.08.003.

Smith, G. B., & Olsen, R. W. (1995). Functional domains of $GABA_A$ receptors. *Trends in Pharmacological Sciences*, *16*(5), 162–168. http://dx.doi.org/10.1016/S0165-6147(00)89009-4.

Spurny, R., Ramerstorfer, J., Price, K., Brams, M., Ernst, M., Nury, H., et al. (2012). Pentameric ligand-gated ion channel ELIC is activated by GABA and modulated by benzodiazepines. *Proceedings of the National Academy of Sciences*, *109*(44), E3028–E3034. http://dx.doi.org/10.1073/pnas.1208208109.

Steiger, J. L., & Russek, S. J. (2004). GABA$_A$ receptors: Building the bridge between subunit mRNAs, their promoters, and cognate transcription factors. *Pharmacology & Therapeutics*, *101*(3), 259–281. http://dx.doi.org/10.1016/j.pharmthera.2003.12.002.

Stewart, D. S., Desai, R., Cheng, Q., Liu, A., & Forman, S. A. (2008). Tryptophan mutations at azi-etomidate photo-incorporation sites on α1 or β2 subunits enhance GABA$_A$ receptor gating and reduce etomidate modulation. *Molecular Pharmacology*, *74*(6), 1687–1695. http://dx.doi.org/10.1124/mol.108.050500.

Stewart, D. S., Hotta, M., Desai, R., & Forman, S. A. (2013b). State-dependent etomidate occupancy of its allosteric agonist sites measured in a cysteine-substituted GABA$_A$ receptor. *Molecular Pharmacology*, *83*(6), 1200–1208. http://dx.doi.org/10.1124/mol.112.084558.

Stewart, D. S., Hotta, M., Li, G. D., Desai, R., Chiara, D. C., Olsen, R. W., et al. (2013a). Cysteine substitutions define etomidate binding and gating linkages in the α-M1 domain of γ-aminobutyric acid type a (GABA$_A$) receptors. *The Journal of Biological Chemistry*, *288*(42), 30373–30386. http://dx.doi.org/10.1074/jbc.M113.494583.

Stewart, D. S., Pierce, D. W., Hotta, M., Stern, A. T., & Forman, S. A. (2014). Mutations at beta N265 in γ-aminobutyric acid type a receptors alter both binding affinity and efficacy of potent anesthetics. *PLoS One*, *9*(10). e111470. http://dx.doi.org/10.1371/journal.pone.0111470.

Stórustovu, S. í., & Ebert, B. (2006). Pharmacological characterization of agonists at δ-containing GABA$_A$ receptors: Functional selectivity for extrasynaptic receptors is dependent on the absence of γ2. *Journal of Pharmacology and Experimental Therapeutics*, *316*(3), 1351–1359. http://dx.doi.org/10.1124/jpet.105.092403.

Taferner, B., Schuehly, W., Huefner, A., Baburin, I., Wiesner, K., Ecker, G. F., et al. (2011). Modulation of GABA$_A$-receptors by honokiol and derivatives: Subtype selectivity and structure-activity relationship. *Journal of Medicinal Chemistry*, *54*(15), 5349–5361. http://dx.doi.org/10.1021/jm200186n.

Taylor, P. M., Thomas, P., Gorrie, G. H., Connolly, C. N., Smart, T. G., & Moss, S. J. (1999). Identification of amino acid residues within GABA$_A$ receptor β subunits that mediate both homomeric and heteromeric receptor expression. *The Journal of Neuroscience*, *19*(15), 6360–6371.

Tretter, V., Ehya, N., Fuchs, K., & Sieghart, W. (1997). Stoichiometry and assembly of a recombinant GABA$_A$ receptor subtype. *The Journal of Neuroscience*, *17*(8), 2728–2737.

Tretter, V., Hauer, B., Nusser, Z., Mihalek, R. M., Höger, H., Homanics, G. E., et al. (2001). Targeted disruption of the GABA$_A$ receptor δ subunit gene leads to an up-regulation of γ2 subunit-containing receptors in cerebellar granule cells. *Journal of Biological Chemistry*, *276*(13), 10532–10538. http://dx.doi.org/10.1074/jbc.M011054200.

Twyman, R. E., Rogers, C. J., & Macdonald, R. L. (1990). Intraburst kinetic properties of the GABA$_A$ receptor main conductance state of mouse spinal cord neurones in culture. *The Journal of Physiology*, *423*(1), 193–220. http://dx.doi.org/10.1113/jphysiol.1990.sp018018.

Varagic, Z., Ramerstorfer, J., Huang, S., Rallapalli, S., Sarto-Jackson, I., Cook, J., et al. (2013a). Subtype selectivity of α+β-site ligands of GABA$_A$ receptors: Identification of the first highly specific positive modulators at α6β2/3γ2 receptors. *British Journal of Pharmacology*, *169*(2), 384–399. http://dx.doi.org/10.1111/bph.12153.

Varagic, Z., Wimmer, L., Schnürch, M., Mihovilovic, M. D., Huang, S., Rallapalli, S., et al. (2013b). Identification of novel positive allosteric modulators and null modulators at the GABA$_A$ receptor α+β-interface. *British Journal of Pharmacology*, *169*(2), 371–383. http://dx.doi.org/10.1111/bph.12151.

Vien, T. N., Modgil, A., Abramian, A. M., Jurd, R., Walker, J., Brandon, N. J., et al. (2015). Compromising the phosphodependent regulation of the GABA$_A$R β3 subunit reproduces the core phenotypes of autism spectrum disorders. *Proceedings of the National Academy of Sciences of the United States of America*, *112*(48), 14805–14810. http://dx.doi.org/10.1073/pnas.1514657112.

Wagoner, K. R., & Czajkowski, C. (2010). Stoichiometry of expressed α4β2δ γ-aminobutyric acid type a receptors depends on the ratio of subunit cDNA transfected. *Journal of Biological Chemistry*, *285*(19), 14187–14194. http://dx.doi.org/10.1074/jbc.M110.104257.

Walters, R. J., Hadley, S. H., Morris, K. D., & Amin, J. (2000). Benzodiazepines act on $GABA_A$ receptors via two distinct and separable mechanisms. *Nature Neuroscience*, *3*(12), 1274–1281. http://dx.doi.org/10.1038/81800.

Whittemore, E. R., Yang, W., Drewe, J. A., & Woodward, R. M. (1996). Pharmacology of the human gamma-aminobutyric $acid_A$ receptor α4 subunit expressed in *Xenopus laevis* oocytes. *Molecular Pharmacology*, *50*(5), 1364–1375.

Wieland, H. A., & Luddens, H. (1994). Four amino acid exchanges convert a diazepam-insensitive, inverse agonist-preferring $GABA_A$ receptor into a diazepam-preferring $GABA_A$ receptor. *Journal of Medicinal Chemistry*, *37*(26), 4576–4580.

Wieland, H. A., Lüddens, H., & Seeburg, P. H. (1992). A single histidine in $GABA_A$ receptors is essential for benzodiazepine agonist binding. *Journal of Biological Chemistry*, *267*(3), 1426–1429.

Wong, L.-W., Tae, H.-S., & Cromer, B. A. (2015). Assembly, trafficking and function of α1β2γ2 $GABA_A$ receptors are regulated by N-terminal regions, in a subunit-specific manner. *Journal of Neurochemistry*, *134*(5), 819–832. http://dx.doi.org/10.1111/jnc.13175.

Wongsamitkul, N., Baur, R., & Sigel, E. (2016). Toward understanding functional properties and subunit arrangement of α4β2δ γ-aminobutyric acid, type a ($GABA_A$) receptors. *Journal of Biological Chemistry*, *291*(35), 18474–18483. http://dx.doi.org/10.1074/jbc.M116.738906.

Wooltorton, J. R., Moss, S. J., & Smart, T. G. (1997). Pharmacological and physiological characterization of murine homomeric β3 $GABA_A$ receptors. *European Journal of Neuroscience*, *9*(11), 2225–2235.

Yamaura, K., Kiyonaka, S., Numata, T., Inoue, R., & Hamachi, I. (2016). Discovery of allosteric modulators for $GABA_A$ receptors by ligand-directed chemistry. *Nature Chemical Biology*, *12*(10), 822–830. http://dx.doi.org/10.1038/nchembio.2150.

Yeung, J. Y. T., Canning, K. J., Zhu, G., Pennefather, P., MacDonald, J. F., & Orser, B. A. (2003). Tonically activated $GABA_A$ receptors in hippocampal neurons are high-affinity, low-conductance sensors for extracellular GABA. *Molecular Pharmacology*, *63*(1), 2–8. http://dx.doi.org/10.1124/mol.63.1.2.

Yip, G. M. S., Chen, Z.-W., Edge, C. J., Smith, E. H., Dickinson, R., Hohenester, E., et al. (2013). A propofol binding site on mammalian $GABA_A$ receptors identified by photolabeling. *Nature Chemical Biology*, *9*(11), 715–720. http://dx.doi.org/10.1038/nchembio.1340.

CHAPTER TWO

Acid-Sensing Ion Channel Pharmacology, Past, Present, and Future …

Lachlan D. Rash[1]

School of Biomedical Sciences, The University of Queensland, St Lucia, QLD, Australia
[1]Corresponding author: e-mail address: l.rash@uq.edu.au

Contents

Abstract

pH is one of the most strictly controlled parameters in mammalian physiology. An extracellular pH of ~7.4 is crucial for normal physiological processes, and perturbations to this have profound effects on cell function. Acidic microenvironments occur in many physiological and pathological conditions, including inflammation, bone remodeling, ischemia, trauma, and intense synaptic activity. Cells exposed to these conditions respond in different ways, from tumor cells that thrive to neurons that are either suppressed or hyperactivated, often fatally. Acid-sensing ion channels (ASICs) are primary pH sensors in mammals and are expressed widely in neuronal and nonneuronal

Advances in Pharmacology, Volume 79
ISSN 1054-3589
http://dx.doi.org/10.1016/bs.apha.2017.02.001

cells. There are six main subtypes of ASICs in rodents that can form homo- or heteromeric channels resulting in many potential combinations. ASICs are present and activated under all of the conditions mentioned earlier, suggesting that they play an important role in how cells respond to acidosis. Compared to many other ion channel families, ASICs were relatively recently discovered—1997—and there is a substantial lack of potent, subtype-selective ligands that can be used to elucidate their structural and functional properties. In this chapter I cover the history of ASIC channel pharmacology, which began before the proteins were even identified, and describe the current arsenal of tools available, their limitations, and take a glance into the future to predict from where new tools are likely to emerge.

ABBREVIATIONS

ASIC acid-sensing ion channel
ECD extracellular domain
GMQ 2-guanidine-4-methylquinazoline
LPC lysophosphatidylcholine
NSAIDs nonsteroidal antiinflammatory drugs

1. INTRODUCTION

The pH or concentration of protons (actually hydronium ions, H_3O^+) in the extracellular and intracellular fluids are very tightly controlled physiological parameters and are maintained at around 7.4 and 6.9–7.3 (depending on cell type), respectively (Roos & Boron, 1981). There are several circumstances in normal physiology when the local pH deviates from these values, such as bone remodeling, synaptic transmission, lactate build-up in exercising muscle. However, sustained decreases in the extracellular pH are invariably associated with an underlying pathology (Dube, Elagoz, & Mangat, 2009; Reeh & Steen, 1996). Pathological extracellular acidosis occurs following ischemia and cellular damage (i.e., traumatic injury such as incisions or fractures), during inflammation (sterile and infective), and in tumorous tissue. The acidosis can arise from a mismatch in tissue perfusion and metabolism resulting in the accumulation of lactic acid and CO_2 and an increase in ATP hydrolysis. Alternatively, protons may be released by lysed cells, the activation of resident and infiltrating immune cells, the activation of nearby voltage-gated proton channels, and via excessive synaptic vesicle release as occurs in seizures or the resulting depolarization from CNS tissue damage (Reeh & Steen, 1996; Wang & Xu, 2011; Zeng et al., 2015).

Given the almost ubiquitous occurrence of acidosis (and pain) in pathological situations, it would seem logical that there is a rapid signaling system to detect increases in local proton concentration.

Just over 35 years ago Krishtal and Pidoplichko (1980) made the accidental discovery that rapidly applying an acidic solution to neurons elicited a robust and transient inward sodium current and proposed the idea of a receptor for protons (see Krishtal, 2015, for a detailed and entertaining account of the accidental discovery). As they observed this current in several types of sensory neurons, and low tissue pH is highly correlated with pain, they proposed that the "receptor for protons" should play a key role in nociception (this is now fairly well established). Some 15 years later, during the gold rush of cloning, the protein family responsible for acid-induced currents was identified. Two groups concurrently cloned rat and human isoforms of a novel neuronal sodium channel (BNC1 or MDEG) closely related to the epithelial Na^+ channels and the *Caenorhabditis elegans* degenerin channel (Price, Snyder, & Welsh, 1996; Waldmann, Champigny, Voilley, Lauritzen, & Lazdunski, 1996). However, it was not until the following year, and the discovery of a second member, that this new family of channels was discovered to be robustly activated by protonation resulting in a Na^+-selective current (Waldmann, Champigny, Bassilana, Heurteaux, & Lazdunski, 1997), thus matching the sensory neuron currents observed in the early 1980s. The new channel was aptly named acid-sensing ion channel (or ASIC) and was detected in rat dorsal root ganglion neurons and brain. The sequence of the human isoform of ASIC was actually reported 1 month earlier but no function was identified (Garcia-Anoveros, Derfler, Neville-Golden, Hyman, & Corey, 1997). Within a few years of the discovery of BNC1/MDEG (which became ASIC2a) and ASIC (now ASIC1a) essentially all of the other main ASIC isoforms were identified (Akopian, Chen, Ding, Cesare, & Wood, 2000; Chen, England, Akopian, & Wood, 1998; Gründer, Geissler, Bassler, & Ruppersberg, 2000; Lingueglia et al., 1997; Waldmann, Bassilana, et al., 1997).

Since then, a substantial amount of work has been carried out on the ASIC family and there are now multiple crystal structures, many genetic knockout mouse lines and a substantial suite of pharmacological tools with which to study them. Despite the rapid progress made in our understanding of ASIC structure and function, there are some key questions that remain unanswered, and I will point these out as I go. In this chapter I will specifically focus on the current state of the pharmacological toolbox we have at our disposal, and identify some key gaps in the toolbox, and what we most need to answer some of the big outstanding questions. Finally, I will make some predictions as to where the desired tools might be found.

1.1 The ASIC Family

ASICs appear to be vertebrate-specific members of the degenerin/epithelial sodium channel (ENaC) family. There are six main ASIC subunits in rodents (ASIC1a/b, ASIC2a/b, ASIC3, and ASIC4) with ASIC1a/b and ASIC2a/b being splice variants that differ in the first third of the protein. The different subunits can combine to form homo- (ASIC1a, 1b, 2a, and 3 only) or heteromeric channels with ASIC2b and ASIC4 standing out in that they do not form proton-activated homomers. ASIC2b combines with other subunits to form functional heteromers, while the role of ASIC4 is still somewhat mysterious, although recent work using conditional knockout of this channel suggests a role in modulating fear and anxiety in rodents (Lin, Chien, et al., 2015). The subunit composition of each channel determines its pH sensitivity, kinetics, and pharmacology with the formation of heteromeric channels modifying the dynamic pH-sensing range and level of channel expression (Cristofori-Armstrong et al., 2015; Hesselager, Timmermann, & Ahring, 2004; Kellenberger & Schild, 2015). There appears to be no stoichiometric preference for heteromer formation of functional ASICs, at least when assessed in a heterologous expression system (Bartoi, Augustinowski, Polleichtner, Grunder, & Ulbrich, 2014), a property that has hindered attempts to advance the pharmacology of ASICs and is a major challenge to understanding their physiological and pathological roles. Theoretically there are hundreds of possible heteromeric combinations of functional ASIC channels; however, the number of combinations that exist physiologically will be limited by the cell-specific expression of the channel subtypes. For example, ASIC1a and ASIC2a are the major subtypes in rat hippocampal CA1 neurons (Gao, Wu, Xu, & Xu, 2004), while ASIC1a appears to be the only subtype functionally expressed in human cortical neurons (Li, Inoue, et al., 2010), and ASIC1, ASIC2a, and ASIC3 are all expressed in rodent sensory neurons (Benson et al., 2002). Even then, not all the ASIC subunits present in a cell are surface expressed at the same time or under the same conditions. For example, one study using both immunofluorescence and Western blotting showed that ASICs in CNS neurons were mainly distributed in the cell membrane/cytoplasm, while in astrocytes most of the ASICs were expressed in the nucleus (Huang et al., 2010). This may suggest a substantial level of dynamic capacity to quickly regulate the make-up of cell surface-expressed (therefore presumably functional) ASICs under various conditions, such as inflammation (Mamet, Baron, Lazdunski, & Voilley, 2002). Furthermore, it raises the possibility that ASICs may also be functional and play as yet unknown roles in intracellular organelles. Indeed, an intracellular functional role for ASIC1a in mitochondria has been suggested (Wang et al., 2013). It seems that even at a very basic cellular level we still have a lot to learn about ASICs.

1.2 ASIC Distribution

At the whole animal level, ASICs are very widely distributed throughout the body, and although most often described as neuronal ion channels they are also very well represented in nonneuronal cells. In the central nervous system, ASIC1a, ASIC2, and ASIC4 are the dominant isoforms and widely expressed throughout the brain and spinal cord. ASIC3, originally thought to be restricted to peripheral sensory neurons in rodents (Waldmann, Bassilana, et al., 1997), is also present in both rodent and human brain (Babinski, Le, & Seguela, 1999; Wang, Yan, Zhang, Liu, & Zhang, 2014; Wu, Lin, Min, & Chen, 2010), making ASIC1b the only ASIC subtype apparently absent from the CNS. Despite the expression of multiple ASIC subtypes and therefore heteromeric channels in the CNS, ASIC1a is generally considered the most abundant and the primary acid sensor in the mammalian brain. Central roles of ASIC1a include learning, memory, and anxiety via effects on synaptic plasticity and transmission (Wemmie, Taugher, & Kreple, 2013). ASIC1a is also a CNS chemoreceptor for CO_2 and can elicit fear via its activation in the amygdala (Ziemann et al., 2009) or control respiration via activation in the brain stem (Huda et al., 2012). In the periphery, neurons and other excitable cells of the sensory system, such as dorsal root and trigeminal ganglia, retina, cochlear hair cells, taste receptors, and vagal afferents, can express all subtypes of ASICs with the exception of ASIC4. Outside the nervous system, ASICs are expressed in central and peripheral immune cells (e.g., astrocytes, microglia, macrophages, leukocytes, etc.), bone cells (osteoclasts and osteoblasts), adipose cells, and vascular endothelial cells. The role that ASICs play in many of these cells is still not well understood (Kellenberger & Schild, 2015). For a detailed summary of the distribution of ASICs in mice, see Lin, Sun, and Chen (2015).

The relative expression and distribution of ASICs between rodents and human seem to be largely quite similar (Deval & Lingueglia, 2015), yet some subtle differences do occur. For example, rodent sensory neurons express nearly all ASIC subtypes with ASIC1b and ASIC3 seeming to be the dominant isoforms. However, rat DRG neurons express substantially lower levels of ASIC2 mRNA than those from mice (Price et al., 2001; Voilley, de Weille, Mamet, & Lazdunski, 2001), a finding that has been supported by functional studies comparing the acid-evoked responses of rat and mouse DRGs (Leffler, Monter, & Koltzenburg, 2006). Furthermore, in human DRGs, ASIC1a and ASIC3 are dominant (Deval & Lingueglia, 2015) with only relatively low levels of ASIC1b (Hoagland, Sherwood, Lee, Walker, & Askwith, 2010). Likewise, ASIC2 is expressed in the rodent spinal cord (Chen, Zimmer, Sun, Hall, & Brownstein, 2002) but has not yet been detected in human spinal cord. In addition to several differences in ASIC expression patterns, humans also have three functional splice variants of ASIC3 (a, b, and c), which do not appear to be present in rodents (Delaunay et al., 2012). Although seemingly subtle differences, these can have profound effects on translating the results of rodent studies to humans and the clinic.

1.3 ASIC Function and Structure

As the name suggests, ASICs are cation channels activated by protonation. Upon abrupt application of a low pH solution, ASICs rapidly activate carrying an inward current that is ~10-fold selective for Na^+ over K^+. ASIC1a and human ASIC1b are also mildly permeable to Ca^{2+} (Hoagland et al., 2010; Waldmann, Champigny, et al., 1997) and an often-overlooked fact is that ASIC1a is also highly permeable to protons (Waldmann, Champigny, et al., 1997). In the continued presence of low pH, ASICs desensitize leaving little or no sustained current, the exceptions being ASIC3 and ASIC3 containing heteromers, and to a lesser degree human ASIC1b, which display varying and substantial degrees of sustained current (Hesselager et al., 2004; Hoagland et al., 2010). Activation of ASICs in excitable cells can result in sufficient depolarization to trigger action potentials (Vukicevic & Kellenberger, 2004). The consequence of ASIC activation in nonneuronal cells is less clear and a very interesting new area in the field. Upon sustained application of mild acidic pH, ASICs enter a steady state of desensitization (SSD), the pH sensitivity of which is likely to represent the true proton affinity of ASICs (Gründer & Pusch, 2015).

The first structure of an ASIC channel was solved in 2007 using a truncated, nonfunctional construct of chicken ASIC1 (cASIC1) (Jasti, Furukawa, Gonzales, & Gouaux, 2007). Shortly after, the structure of a less truncated and functional ASIC was obtained (Gonzales, Kawate, & Gouaux, 2009). These structures revealed that three ASIC subunits combine to form a trimer with a large extracellular domain (ECD), a small transmembrane region comprised of two helices from each subunit, and intracellular N- and C-termini. The overall structure was described as resembling a hand holding a ball, and the various regions of the ECD have been named as follows: the transmembrane (TM), wrist, thumb, finger, knuckle, β-ball, and palm domains (Fig. 1A). A dominant feature of the surface of the ECD is an acidic pocket at the subunit interface (formed between the thumb, finger, and β-ball on one subunit and the palm of the adjacent subunit), so-called due to the high density and close proximity of acidic residues. The short distance between several of these carboxyl–carboxylate pairs suggested the binding of protons at these sites and a role in gating of the

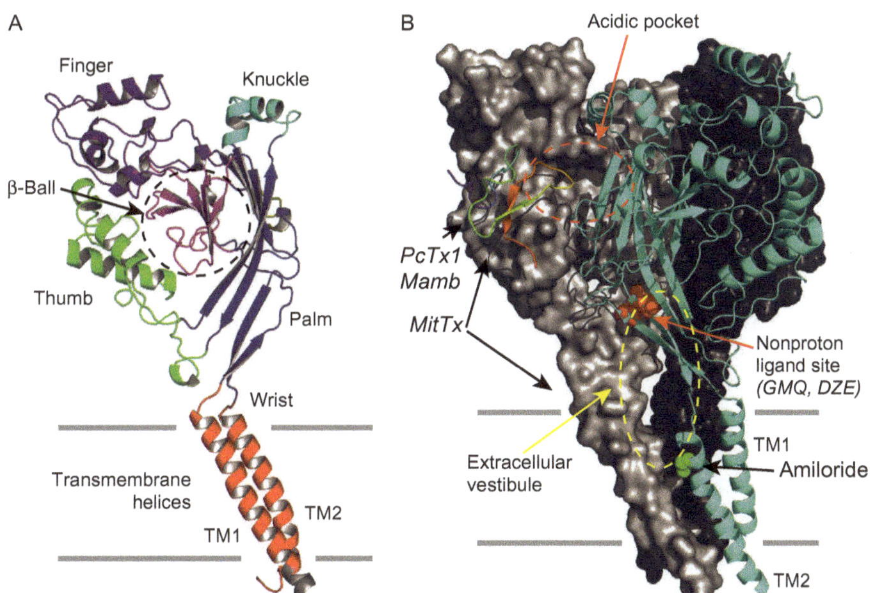

Fig. 1 Acid-sensing ion channel structure and known modulatory sites. (A) Ribbon representation of a single ASIC1 subunit illustrating the domains named for its resemblance of a hand clasping a β-ball. (B). A hybrid surface/ribbon representation illustrating the timeric nature of ASICs and the location of the currently known ligand-binding sites. The figure was made using the cocrystal complex of PcTx1:cASIC1 (PDB: 4FZ0).

channel. This was verified using mutagenesis of residues at the proposed protonation sites (Asp238Ala and Glu239Ala), which resulted in a significant shift in the pH-dependence of activation of ASIC1a to higher proton concentrations (pH_{50} 6.42 for wild type compared to pH_{50} 3.92 for the double mutant). Thus, the acidic pocket appears to play a central role in pH sensing. However, proton gating of ASICs appears to be highly complex with multiple studies highlighting a role in proton sensing for residues away from the acidic pocket (reviewed in detail in Gründer & Pusch, 2015; Kellenberger & Schild, 2015). In the last 4–5 years several more structures of cASIC1, either cocrystalized with the venom peptides Psalmotoxin 1 (PcTx1) and MitTx or soaked with the small molecule inhibitor amiloride, have been reported (Baconguis, Bohlen, Goehring, Julius, & Gouaux, 2014; Baconguis & Gouaux, 2012; Dawson et al., 2012). All of the ASIC structures solved to date are of cASIC1 and represent either the desensitized or open state of the channel, which differ rather subtly in the ECD (the major difference being in the palm domain) with more pronounced differences in the transmembrane helices, together these conformational differences reveal in a substantial change in the size of the extracellular vestibule in going from the open to desensitized state (Baconguis et al., 2014). Despite the groundbreaking work of Eric Gouaux's group in revealing the desensitized and open structures of cASIC1, nothing is known about the conformation of the closed/resting state of the channel. *This remains one of the biggest questions in the ASIC field.*

Our current knowledge of ASICs strongly suggests that they are the primary acid sensors in mammals. Due to the rapid nature of ASIC signaling, they may in fact be some of the first responders to biochemical changes that occur in pathological conditions. Having the appropriate selective molecular tools should allow us to more definitively identify the subtype compositions, physiological and pathological roles of ASICs in acidosis-induced cell signalling. With prudent use, they will also help reveal the missing structural pieces of the ASIC puzzle.

2. A BRIEF HISTORY OF ASIC PHARMACOLOGY

Even before the ion channel protein was identified, the "receptor for protons" was known to be inhibited by amiloride, a clinically used diuretic (Korkushko & Kryshtal, 1984), making it the first pharmacological tool to study ASICs. Likewise, amiloride was shown to inhibit MDEG before it was identified as ASIC2 (Waldmann et al., 1996). Divalent and trivalent ions (including but not limited to zinc, calcium, and gadolinium) were also found to have mostly inhibitory effects on ASICs early on in their history, and zinc has been a particularly useful tool due to its selective potentiation of ASIC2a containing channels (Baron & Lingueglia, 2015; Baron, Schaefer, Lingueglia, Champigny, & Lazdunski, 2001). ASICs are related to the FMRFamide-gated FaNaC channel from molluscs (Lingueglia, Champigny, Lazdunski, & Barbry, 1995). This fact and the role of related mammalian neuropeptides in pain and inflammation (e.g., neuropeptide FF and RFamide-related peptides), a predicted role for ASICs, prompted the study that identified the RFamide family as positive modulators of ASIC1 and ASIC3 (Table 1) (Askwith et al., 2000; Vick & Askwith, 2015). The first highly selective and potent pharmacological tool to study ASICs came in the form of a tarantula venom peptide, PcTx1 (Fig. 1 and Table 2), within a few years of the identification of ASICs (Escoubas et al., 2000). PcTx1 was discovered in the same group that identified and named the ASIC family (the group of Michel Lazdunski at the IPMC-CNRS, where I had the good fortune to carry out my postdoctoral training in ASIC pharmacology). Not surprisingly, this team has been a dominant force in the field of ASIC pharmacology, discovering and characterizing many of the key research tools available (e.g., NSAIDs, APETx2, and Mambalgins).

Several nonsteroidal antiinflammatory drugs (NSAIDs) were the next agents found to affect ASICs, directly inhibiting ASIC1a and ASIC3 currents as well as inhibiting the inflammation-induced increase in ASIC expression (Voilley et al., 2001). At around the same time in the early 2000s, and quite fittingly given the discovery that antiinflammatory/analgesic drugs could inhibit ASICs, the proinflammatory and algesic endogenous mediators, spermine and lactate, were shown to potentiate the activity of ASIC1 and ASIC3, respectively (Babini, Paukert, Geisler, & Gründer, 2002; Immke & McCleskey, 2001b). The ASIC enhancing activity of these mediators has now been substantially linked to ischemia-related pain in the heart (angina) (Immke & McCleskey, 2001a), and neuronal damage in the CNS (Duan et al., 2011). In a study assessing the effect of several ischemia-related mediators on ASIC function in cerebellar Purkinje cells, arachidonic acid was found to be a moderately potent potentiator (Allen & Attwell, 2002). This period of ASIC modulator discovery really highlighted a main pathological role for ASICs (at least ASIC1a and ASIC3), the detection of acidosis-mediated pain. Another, more serious, consequence of ischemia-related ASIC activation came to light in 2004 when Xiong et al. reported that

ASIC1a plays a key role in the neuronal damage following ischemic stroke (Xiong et al., 2004), which we have also demonstrated using pure PcTx1 as opposed to PcTx1 venom (McCarthy, Rash, Chassagnon, King, & Widdop, 2015).

In the same year as Xiong's seminal publication on ASICs in stroke, the first ASIC3-selective inhibitor, APETx2, was reported (Diochot et al., 2004). This 42-amino acid, sea anemone peptide selectively inhibits the fast, transient ASIC3 current with no effect on the sustained current, and although the peptide was not readily available for many years (Jensen et al., 2009), it has since become a key tool to study the role of ASIC3. The Abbott laboratories compound, A-317567 was the first non-guanidine, non-NSAID small molecule inhibitor of ASICs identified, and unlike APETx2, it inhibits both the transient and sustained components of ASIC3 (Dube et al., 2005). Although the pharmacology of ASICs developed slowly over the first 10 years of their known existence, with only five inhibitors and a few endogenous modulators reported, the last decade has seen the pharmacological toolbox for ASICs grow considerably as detailed in Section 3.

3. THE CURRENT ASIC TOOL BOX

3.1 Nonselective Inhibitors of ASICs (Table 1)

Amiloride is a potassium-sparing diuretic that targets ENaC with 100 nM potency and has been used clinically since the late 1960s. Amiloride, and its derivatives benzamil and EIPA, have essentially no selectivity, inhibiting all ASIC homomeric channels with IC_{50}s in the 10–30 μM range (Table 1) (Waldmann, Bassilana, et al., 1997; Waldmann, Champigny, et al., 1997; Waldmann et al., 1996) in a voltage-dependent manner (Adams, Price, Snyder, & Welsh, 1999). Amiloride also "paradoxically" activates ASIC3 at high concentrations (Waldmann, Bassilana, et al., 1997). Amiloride is a very promiscuous drug and has a wide variety of non-ASIC/non-ENaC targets (including sodium/hydrogen antiporters, sodium/calcium exchangers, and GPCRs) (Howard, Hughes, Motulsky, Mullen, & Insel, 1987; Xiong, Pignataro, Li, Chang, & Simon, 2008). Despite this, amiloride has been used as a primary tool to study the role of ASICs in isolated cells and in vivo. The binding site for amiloride is at the bottom of the extracellular vestibule (lined by TM2) (Fig. 1B), which is the entry for ions to cross the membrane and is consistent with recent cocrystal structures and its known pore-blocking

Table 1 Summary of the Activity of the Nonselective ASIC Modulators at Homomeric Channels

Inhibitors	ASIC1a	ASIC1b	ASIC2a	ASIC3
Amiloride[a] (EIPA, Benzamil)	12	20	28	16
Nafamostat	13	?	70	2.5
Diminazene [a]	0.32	0.2	0.86	0.32
A-317567 [a]	2	?	30	10
A-317567(10b) [a]	0.45	?	?	0.356
4-Aminopyridine	760	~800	~800	30% @ 10 mM
Benzothiophene methylamine		?	?	
Tetracaine	80% @ 3 mM	?	?	10 mM
Propofol (inhib. @ 30 μM)	~28%	—	—	~15%
Potentiators				
Arachidonic acid	~5		~5	~5
RFamides	10–50	10–50		10–50

[a]Indicates multiple known off-targets.
All values are IC_{50} or EC_{50}s in μM unless otherwise indicated.

activity (Baconguis et al., 2014; Champigny, Voilley, Waldmann, & Lazdunski, 1998).

Nafamostat is a serine protease inhibitor used as an anticoagulant and to treat acute pancreatitis. Based on the observation that nafamostat also inhibited ENaCs (Muto, Imai, & Asano, 1993), Ugawa et al. reasoned that it might also inhibit ASICs. Using *Xenopus* oocyte electrophysiology, they found that micromolar concentrations of nafamostat did indeed inhibit ASICs when coapplied with low pH with a rank order potency of ASIC3 > ASIC1a > ASIC2a (Ugawa et al., 2007). The efficacy of coapplication with the low pH stimulus suggests that nafamostat might be an open channel blocker and its structural similarity to the diarylamidines (see Baron & Lingueglia, 2015) suggests it could share their binding site; however, this hypothesis requires experimental validation.

The *diarylamidines* (4′,6-diamidino-2-phenylindole [DAPI], *diminazene*, hydroxystilbamidine [HSB], and pentamidine) are veterinary antiprotozoal drugs that were part of a systematic study to determine if bi- or polycharged ions have modulatory effects on ASICs. All four diarylamidines tested had potent inhibitory activity on the native ASIC current in mouse hippocampal neurons. DAPI, HSB, and pentamidine had IC_{50}s of 2.8, 1.5, and 38 μM, respectively, whereas diminazene was the most potent at 0.3 μM and had a rank order potency of ASIC1b > ASIC3 > ASIC2a ≥ ASIC1a (Chen et al., 2010). The binding site of nafamostat and the diarylamidines was proposed, based on blind, rigid body docking studies, to be a hydrophobic groove between the palm and β-ball next to the acidic pocket (Chen et al., 2010). However, a recent study using channel mutants showed that the two key residues involved in the "nonproton ligand site," E79 and E416 (see Fig. 1B), in the inner vestibule contribute to diminazene's ability to inhibit channel function (Carattino & Krauson, 2016) making the proposed "diarylamidine groove" highly unlikely as a binding site. The mechanism of action of these drugs has not yet been well studied. Despite the higher potency and slightly different subtype selectivity of nafamostat and diminazene in comparison to amiloride, neither appear to have been widely adopted as pharmacological tools to study ASICs.

A potent novel inhibitor of ASIC1-, 2-, and 3-like currents in rat DRG neurons, *A-317567*, was discovered by Abbott laboratories and shown to provide effective analgesia in both inflammatory and postoperative pain (Dube et al., 2005). A-317567 was subsequently used as a tool to study the role of ASIC1a in the brain and highlighted the potential for ASIC1a inhibition to reduce depression and anxiety (Coryell et al., 2009; Dwyer et al., 2009). Some years later, the medicinal chemistry team at Merck carried out a structure–activity study on A-317567 (IC_{50} at hASIC3 ~1 μM) and developed a more potent alkyne-analog (named 10b; IC_{50} ASIC3 ~356 nM, ASIC1a ~450 nM) that also had promising analgesic activity. However, both compounds were found to have substantial off-target activity (~39 targets with <10 μM binding) and caused sedation and analgesia in both wild-type and ASIC3 KO mice, thus destroying its prospects as a drug lead and limiting its use as an ASIC tool in vivo (Kuduk et al., 2010). The binding site and mechanism of action of A-317567 and its analogs are currently unknown. As a result of further SAR studies based on A-317567(10b), the same group at Merck successfully developed a very potent, nonamidine, and brain penetrant ASIC3 inhibitor (a *benzothiophene methylamine, 7d*; IC_{50} ~220 nM); however, this molecule was also equipotent at ASIC1a and had a similar undesirable off-target profile as the lead compound (Kuduk et al., 2011).

4-Aminopyridine (4-AP) is a well known and nonselective, voltage-gated potassium channel blocker (IC_{50}s in the high μM to mM range) that is used to manage the symptoms of multiple sclerosis. Boiko et al. recently found that this molecule can also completely inhibit ASIC1a with an IC_{50} of ~760 μM (and similar potency at ASIC1b and ASIC2a) while having little effect on ASIC3 (Boiko, Kucher, Eaton, & Stockand, 2013). The local anesthetics *tetracaine* and *propofol* were also found to have either relatively weak (3–10 mM) or only partial inhibitory effects on ASIC1a and ASIC3 (Lei et al., 2014; Leng, Lin, Cottrell, & Xiong, 2013). The ASIC activity of these drugs occurs at a similar concentration to the clinically used doses and the authors in both cases suggest this novel activity may contribute to the clinical efficacy of these drugs.

3.2 Nonselective Potentiators of ASICs (Table 1)

Arachidonic acid (AA) is a major inflammatory intermediate that is converted to prostaglandins and thromboxane via the action of cyclooxygenase enzymes and is also a mediator of inflammation and ischemia in its own right. AA (5–10 μM) was first observed to enhance ASIC signaling in rat cerebellar Purkinje cells where it potentiated peak current and increased the proportion of cells displaying sustained current from 30% to 77% (Allen & Attwell, 2002). It was subsequently found that the effect of AA is direct and nonselective, potentiating ASIC1a, ASIC2a, and ASIC3 (Smith, Cadiou, & McNaughton, 2007) and does so by sensitizing the channels to proton activation (i.e., shifts the pH activation curve toward 7.4) (Deval et al., 2008).

The inflammation-related neuropeptides known collectively as *RF-amides* (named after their C-terminal Arg-Phe-amide motif) were briefly introduced in Section 2. They are nonselective potentiators of ASICs that decrease the pH sensitivity of channel steady-state desensitization with EC_{50}s in the 10–50 μM range. In addition to making ASICs more resistant to desensitization they enhance peak current and slow inactivation, which can result in a sustained current. *Big dynorphin* and *Dynorphin A* are also endogenous neuropeptides that, although unrelated to the RFamides, share the ability to enhance ASIC currents (29 nM and 32 μM, respectively). Unlike the RFamides, the effects of the dynorphins appear to be restricted to ASIC1a and ASIC1b and may share their binding site with PcTx1 (Sherwood & Askwith, 2009; reviewed in Vick & Askwith, 2015).

3.3 Selective Modulators: ASIC1a Agonists/Potentiators (Table 2)

MitTx is a noncovalent heterodimeric peptide isolated from the venom of the Texas coral snake (*Micrurus tener tener*) which is renowned for its painful

Table 2 ASIC Modulators With Relative Selectivity for One Subtype (*Tau, Time Constant*)

ASIC1a	**Activators**	**EC_{50}**	**Inhibitors**	**IC_{50}**
$pH_{50\ act}$ 6.2–6.8	MitTx	9 nM	PcTx1	0.4–4 nM
$pH_{50\ SSD}$ ~7.2			Flurbiprofen, ibuprofen	350 μM
	Potentiators		Mambalgins	10–50 nM
Tau_{act} 6–13 ms	Spermine	500 μM	Chloroquine	600 μM
Tau_{desen} 1–4 s	Dynorphins	30 μM	Lidocaine	12 mM
	Histamine	30 μM	PPC-5650	500 nM
			Sinomenine	1 μM
			NS383 (1a > 3)	440 nM
			Sevanol (3 > 1a)	2 μM
ASIC1b	**Activators**	**EC_{50}**	**Inhibitors**	**IC_{50}**
$pH_{50\ act}$ 5.9–6.3	MitTx	23 nM	Mambalgins	100 nM
$pH_{50\ SSD}$ ~6.7	PcTx1	100 nM		
	Potentiators			
Tau_{act} ~10 ms	Spermine	500 μM		
Tau_{desen} 1–2 s	Dynorphins	30 μM		
ASIC2a	**Activators**	**EC_{50}**	**Inhibitors**	**@500 μM**
$pH_{50\ act}$ 4.0–4.9	—	—	Diclofenac (partial)	40%
$pH_{50\ SSD}$ ~5.6	**Potentiators**			
Tau_{act} n/d	MitTx	75 nM		
Tau_{desen} 3–6 s	Zn^{2+}	120 μM		
ASIC3	**Activators**	**EC_{50}**	**Inhibitors**	**IC_{50}**
$pH_{50\ act}$ 6.4–6.7	MitTx	800 nM	APETx2 (trans.)	37–80 nM
$pH_{50\ SSD}$ ~7.1	GMQ	1 mM	Salicylic acid (sust.)	260 μM
	LysoPC	4.3 μM	Aspirin (sust.)	500 nM
Tau_{act} <5 ms	Chloroquine	~3 mM	Diclofenac (sust.)	92 μM
Tau_{desen} 0.3 s	**Potentiators**		UGR-9-1	10 μM
	Serotonin (5-HT)	41 μM	Sevanol	353 μM
	Agmatine	~5 mM	NS383 (1a > 3)	2.1 μM
	Chloroquine (sust)	462 μM		

bite. The individual components (a Kunitz-like α-subunit and phospholipase A_2-like β-subunit) are inactive on their own, but when applied together directly activate ASIC1a and ASIC1b with 88- and 35-fold selectivity over ASIC3. At 75 nM, instead of direct activation, MitTx strongly potentiates acid-induced currents through ASIC2a (Bohlen et al., 2011). Moreover, MitTx induces robust pain behavior in rodents, providing some of the most compelling evidence so far for a role of ASICs in peripheral nociceptive pathways. This is likely to be due primarily to its action on ASIC1b and ASIC3 containing channels based on the observations that these subtypes appear to be the main ASIC subunits involved in peripheral pain in rodents (Deval et al., 2008; Diochot et al., 2012; Yu et al., 2010). MitTx has been cocrystalized with cASIC1 and binds almost exclusively to the thumb domain, with a small amount of contact between the α-subunit and the top of transmembrane helix 1, locking the channel in an open state (Baconguis et al., 2014).

Spermine is an endogenous cationic polyamine that is abundant in the brain. Two independent studies found that extracellular spermine (250–500 μM) enhances ASIC1a and ASIC1b currents by decreasing the pH sensitivity of channel steady-state desensitization (similar to the RFamides) (Babini et al., 2002; Duan et al., 2011). Duan et al. showed that, via its effect on ASIC1a, increased extracellular spermine could exacerbate the neuronal damage following ischemic stroke. Another endogenous mediator, *histamine* (~30 μM), was also found to directly and selectively potentiate ASIC1a homomers, most effectively when applied at modest levels of acidification (Nagaeva, Tikhonova, Magazanik, & Tikhonov, 2016), an effect which may contribute to its proinflammatory role.

3.4 Selective Modulators: ASIC1a Inhibitors (Table 2)

PcTx1 is a 40-amino acid, inhibitor-cystine knot peptide isolated from tarantula venom and was the first highly potent and selective ASIC1a inhibitor discovered (Escoubas et al., 2000). Although used as a selective inhibitor of ASIC1a homomers, it also inhibits heteromeric ASIC1a/ASIC2 channels (Joeres, Augustinowski, Neuhof, Assmann, & Grunder, 2016; Sherwood, Lee, Gormley, & Askwith, 2011) and potentiates homomeric ASIC1b currents (Chen, Kalbacher, & Grunder, 2006). Given that ASIC1b does not appear to be expressed in the brain or spinal cord, PcTx1 remains a highly useful tool for studying the contribution of ASIC1a in the CNS. PcTx1 has been cocrystalized with cASIC1

(Baconguis & Gouaux, 2012), and several structure–activity studies carried out using rat ASIC1a (Saez et al., 2011, 2015). These studies demonstrate that PcTx1 binds predominantly to α-helix 5 in the thumb domain with its positively charged β-hairpin loop poking into the acidic pocket (Fig. 1B), thereby stabilizing ASIC1a in its desensitized state (Chen, Kalbacher, & Gründer, 2005).

The *mambalgins* are a family of three-finger peptides isolated from the venom of several mamba snake (*Dendroaspis*) species. They are selective for ASIC1, with highest potency (~10 nM) and 100% efficacy at inhibiting ASIC1a (Diochot et al., 2012). The mambalgin-binding site overlaps that of PcTx1 at the acidic pocket (Salinas et al., 2014; Schroeder et al., 2014); however, unlike PcTx1 (which induces desensitization) they appear to inhibit ASIC channel activation by stabilizing the closed state (Salinas et al., 2014). The substantial difference in mechanism and subtype selectivity, relative to PcTx1, makes the *mambalgins* invaluable tools for structure–function studies of ASIC1.

Of the five NSAIDs found to modulate ASIC function, *flurbiprofen* and *ibuprofen* are not particularly potent (IC_{50} ~350 μM) but appear to be quite selective for ASIC1a (Voilley et al., 2001). The NSAIDs probably inhibit ASICs via open channel block but do not compete with amiloride (Dorofeeva, Barygin, Staruschenko, Bolshakov, & Magazanik, 2008), thus may define a novel modulatory site in the channel pore making them useful tools to understand new regulatory-binding sites. The antimalarial drug *chloroquine* (also used in rheumatoid arthritis) is toxic to the retina, a fact that led to the discovery of its ASIC1a inhibitory activity (IC_{50} ~600 μM) (Li et al., 2014). *Sinomenine* is an alkaloid from a climbing plant (*Sinomenium acutum*) used in Chinese medicine to treat arthritis and neuralgia. Its traditional therapeutic use in pain and inflammation and the discovery that sinomenine is a potent blocker of ASIC1a (~1 μM IC_{50}), as well as having substantial neuroprotective effects in cerebral ischemia (Wu et al., 2011), makes it a very interesting tool for further study. It appears that chloroquine and sinomenine have so far only been tested on ASIC1a; therefore, their subtype selectivity and mechanism of action are unknown. Unlike the local anesthetics tetracaine and propofol, which are largely nonselective in their effects on ASICs, *lidocaine* inhibited heterologously expressed ASIC1a (IC_{50} ~12 mM) without affecting ASIC2a currents, however, was not tested on ASIC3 (Lin et al., 2011).

PPC-5650 is claimed to be a selective ASIC1a inhibitor (IC_{50} ~500 nM) and was a novel drug candidate for a small biotech company called

Painceptor. This drug was tested in a small human trial for analgesic activity (UV sunburn model) and showed promising effects (Dube et al., 2009); however, there is not much available data demonstrating its ASIC subtype selectivity, binding site, or mechanism of action. PPC-5650 has recently resurfaced, being tested in two more experimental human pain models (rectal and esophageal pain), where it was reasonably well tolerated but only mildly efficacious in the esophageal model but not in the rectal model (Nielsen et al., 2015; Olesen, Nielsen, Larsen, & Drewes, 2015). Until more is reported on the ASIC activity of this compound, its value as a research tool is unclear.

NS383 is a small molecule drug lead from the Danish company NeuroSearch and was identified using a fluorescence-based screen against human ASIC1a (Munro et al., 2016). It has potent and relatively selective ASIC1a inhibitory activity (IC_{50} 0.44 μM vs 2.1 μM for ASIC3 homomers) and also potently blocks currents in cells coexpressing ASIC1a and ASIC3 with little apparent effect on ASIC2a, and unknown activity at ASIC1b. The inhibitory activity of NS383 is apparent during coapplication with low pH and is strongly pH-dependent suggesting competition with protons, thus it may have a novel mechanism of action. NS383 had effective analgesic activity in both inflammatory and neuropathic rodent pain models with no obvious motor impairment when delivered intraperitoneally. Consistent with this, NS383 was found to be very selective for ASICs in an off-target screen making this a promising new therapeutic lead and valuable tool to study ASICs in vivo.

3.5 Selective Modulators: ASIC1b and ASIC2a (Table 2)

ASIC1b is a splice variant of ASIC1a and differs only in the first third of the protein encompassing the N-terminus, the first transmembrane helix and first third of the ECD. There are currently no known selective modulators of ASIC1b. As it is identical to ASIC1a in the thumb domain, which seems to be a relative hotspot at least for venom peptide interactions, some of the above-mentioned ASIC1a modulators also affect ASIC1b, but often with lower potency (for example, MitTx, spermine, dynorphins). The *mambalgins* are incomplete blockers and around 10-fold less potent on ASIC1b than ASIC1a. Nevertheless they are still the first known and only potent inhibitors of ASIC1b. Thanks to this property, use of the mambalgins in ASIC1a −/− mice has suggested a key role for ASIC1b in peripheral pain (at least in rodents) (Diochot et al., 2012).

ASIC2a is an odd one out among the pH-activated homomeric ASICs, in that it is not particularly sensitive, its pH_{50} of activation is a full log unit lower than its relatives (Table 2). There are no selective inhibitors of ASIC2a. Although *diclofenac* was found to be a partial inhibitor at ~500 μM, it is more potent at ASIC3 but has little activity at ASIC1. Despite inhibiting other ASICs, zinc uniquely potentiates ASIC2a and ASIC2a-containing channels and has proven to be very useful as a diagnostic tool to study whether the native channels do or do not contain ASIC2 subunits (Baron & Lingueglia, 2015; Baron et al., 2001).

3.6 Selective Modulators: ASIC3 Agonists/Potentiators (Table 2)

Given its now well-established role in peripheral nociceptive pathways (Deval et al., 2008; Marra et al., 2016; Walder et al., 2010; Yen et al., 2009), ASIC3 has been the subject of many studies to identify novel modulators. One such study identified *GMQ* (*2-guanidine-4-methylquinazoline*) as the first nonproton agonist of ASICs (Yu et al., 2010). GMQ selectively activates ASIC3 with an EC_{50} of ~1 mM when applied at pH 7.4 and 1–2 mM $[Ca^{2+}]_e$, which drops to <100 μM when coapplied with low pH or low extracellular [Ca]. The discovery of GMQ's stimulatory effects revealed a "nonproton ligand site" defined by E79 and E423 at the top of the large extracellular vestibule (Fig. 1). The activation of ASIC3 by GMQ is due to an alkaline shift in the pH of activation and concurrent acidic shift of steady-state desensitization, creating substantial overlap of the curves and a large window current at neutral pH (Alijevic & Kellenberger, 2012). *Agmatine*, an endogenous inhibitor of NMDA receptors, is structurally related to GMQ and has similar effects to its synthetic relative, although is slightly less potent (Li, Yu, Zhang, Cao, & Xu, 2010), suggesting that the nonproton ligand site has physiological significance. The nonproton ligand site also appears to be responsible for the "paradoxical" and ASIC3 selective activating effect of amiloride (Li, Yu, Huang, Cao, & Xu, 2011). The antimalarial drug *chloroquine* is also structurally similar to GMQ and was recently found to interact with the nonproton ligand site to potentiate/activate ASIC3 but not ASIC1a (Lei et al., 2016). Unlike GMQ, which enhances both peak and sustained ASIC3 currents, chloroquine appears to preferentially potentiate the sustained ASIC3 current (EC_{50} of 426 μM), thus provides a new tool to study the subtleties of ASIC3 activation.

As the result of studying the effects of human inflammatory exudates on ASICs, *lysophosphatidylcholine (LPC)* was recently found to be another direct, but endogenous and potent (EC_{50} ~4.3 μM), activator of ASIC3 (Marra et al., 2016). LPC, like AA, activates ASIC3 by sensitizing the channels to proton activation with little apparent effect on channel desensitization, thus distinguishing its agonistic mechanism slightly from GMQ. LPCs effects are more pronounced on human ASIC3 as compared to rat ASIC3, fitting with a primary role for this lipid in clinical inflammatory states.

3.7 Selective Modulators: ASIC3 Inhibitors (Table 2)

APETx2 is a peptide isolated from extracts of the sea anemone *Anthopleura elagantissima* and is still the most potent inhibitor of ASIC3 and ASIC3-containing heteromers (IC_{50} 37–2000 nM) (Diochot et al., 2004). Despite being discovered over 10 years ago, the binding site and mechanism of action of APETx2 are still unknown. Although now widely used as a "selective" tool to study ASIC3 function in vitro and in vivo, we and others have shown that APETx2 also inhibits several voltage-gated channels (Na_V1.2, Na_V1.8, and hERG) (Blanchard, Rash, & Kellenberger, 2012; Jensen et al., 2014; Peigneur et al., 2012) of which Na_V1.8 is also involved in inflammatory pain. Thus, caution is advised when interpreting data on nociceptor signaling when using APETx2 (Rash, 2013). A main focus of my own research is to understand and improve the properties and selectivity of APETx2 in order to provide cleaner research tools (Anangi, Rash, Mobli, & King, 2012; Jensen et al., 2014, 2012).

UGR-9-1 is another sea anemone peptide that selectively inhibits ASIC3, although substantially less potent than APETx2, UGR-9-1 appears to be more selective than the prototypical ASIC3 blocker and retains analgesic activity in rodent models of inflammatory pain (Osmakov et al., 2013). UGR-9-1 (29 a.a.) is smaller than AEPTx2 and has a β-hairpin structure as opposed to a defensin-like fold, but as for APETx2, the mechanism of action and binding site are still unknown.

From the study that first identified their ASIC inhibitory activity, *salicylic acid* and *diclofenac* appeared to be the most potent ASIC inhibitors and are selective for ASIC3 (IC_{50}s of 260 and 92 μM, respectively, vs ~500 μM for *aspirin*) (Voilley et al., 2001). A subsequent mechanistic study confirmed the relative selectivity (at least for diclofenac) and demonstrated an open channel mode of action that results in enhanced channel desensitization (Dorofeeva et al., 2008).

The aromatic herb thyme (*Thymus armeniacus*) has been used extensively in herbal medicine, and in 2012, an analgesic ASIC3 inhibitor called *sevanol* was identified from extracts of this plant (Dubinnyi et al., 2012). Sevanol is sixfold selective for ASIC3 (IC_{50} ~350 nM) over ASIC1a (IC_{50} ~2 μM) and has no effect on either ASIC1b or ASIC2a up to low millimolar concentrations. Determined as epiphyllic acid 9,10-diisocitryl ester, sevanol is structurally unrelated to other known ASIC inhibitors and has a pH-independent action, thus represents another novel tool to help define modulatory sites on ASIC channels.

3.8 As yet Uncharacterized Modulators (Tested Only on Native ASIC Currents) (Table 3)

CHF5074 (also called CSP-1103) is a potential drug for the treatment of Alzheimer's disease that passed Phase 2 clinical trials. As a derivative of flurbiprofen, CHF5074 was also tested for activity against ASIC1a (using the native current in rat hippocampal neurons) and found to induce very potent inhibition of acid-induced currents (IC_{50} ~50 nM) when pre-incubated with cells for 1 h (Mango et al., 2014). Furthermore, CHF5074 provided substantial neuroprotection in an in vitro model of ischemic stroke (oxygen glucose deprivation). All this suggests that

Table 3 ASIC Modulators so far Only Tested on Native Currents (i.e., Subtype Selectivity Unknown)

Compound	Source	IC_{50} (μM)	Cell Tested
CHF5074	NSAID-derived (flurbiprofen analog)	0.05	Hippocampal neurons
Gastrodin	Plant: *Gastrodia elata*	0.2	Rat sensory neurons
Chlorogenic acid	Plants: many (e.g., hibiscus, bamboo, eggplant, etc.)	0.2	Rat sensory neurons
Thalassiolin B	Plant: *Thalassia testudinum*	27	Rat sensory neurons
Puerarin	Plant: *Pueraria lobata*	9.3	Hippocampal neurons
Paeoniflorin	Plant: *Paeonia lactiflora*	5	PC12 cells (ASIC1a)
PhcrTx1	Sea anemone: *Phymanthus crucifer*	0.1	Rat DRG neurons
α-Dendrotoxin	Snake venom: (*Dendroaspis*)	0.8	Rat DRG neurons

CHF5074 is potentially useful ASIC tool as well as another promising therapeutic lead; however, further work to determine its subtype selectivity and mechanism is required.

Thousands of years of traditional medicines the world over have relied on the myriad of pharmacologically active compounds in plants, many of them possessing analgesic and/or antiinflammatory properties. So it is no surprise that handful of interesting ASIC modulators, in addition to sevanol, have been identified from plant sources. *Gastrodin, chlorogenic acid, thalassiolin B, puerarin,* and *paeoniflorin* are all plant-derived molecules that have been shown to have substantial inhibitory activity on native, acid-induced currents in a variety of cell types often with impressive potency (IC_{50}s from 200 nM to 27 μM, see Table 3 for details) (Garateix et al., 2011; Gu, Yang, Sun, & Zheng, 2010; Qiu et al., 2014; Qu, Liu, Qiu, Li, & Hu, 2014; Sun et al., 2011). Not much work has yet been carried out to determine subtype selectivity, mechanism, or binding site of these compounds; however, given the low micromolar to nanomolar potency and the fact that the herbal medicines that yielded these compounds have been used for centuries in humans, further studies on them are highly warranted.

In addition to the well-characterized venom-derived ASIC modulators described earlier, two more have recently been identified but not yet well studied. *PhcrTx1* is the third ASIC modulator isolated from sea anemones (in this case, *Phymanthus crucifer*) and partially inhibits native ASIC currents in sensory neurons with an IC_{50} ~100 nM (Rodriguez et al., 2014). *α-Dendrotoxin*, an already well-known $K_V1.x$ family potassium channel blocker from Mamba snake venom, was recently found to also inhibit ASICs in rat sensory neurons in the sub-micromolar range (IC_{50} ~800 nM) (Baez et al., 2015). The binding site and mechanism of action of both of these peptides are yet to be determined.

4. THE FUTURE: WHAT DO WE NEED AND WHERE WILL IT COME FROM

From the above overview of pharmacological tools currently available to study ASICs, several things are clear: (1) We do not sufficiently understand the majority of the tools we already have in terms of their selectivity, mechanism, binding site, and off-target effects. (2) Of the tools that have been studied in substantial detail, many of them are not as selective as we had originally and perhaps naïvely, hoped. (3) ASIC1b and ASIC2a homomers may be somewhat difficult to target selectively. As there are still many questions to answer about the structure, gating, distribution, and role of ASICs from both physiological and pathological perspectives, we definitely need better characterized and more selective tools. So, from where are these tools likely to come? The obvious first step is to properly characterize the most promising compounds we already have identified with a focus on those with novel mechanisms and selectivity profiles. Some other suggestions as to where new pharmacological agents might come from are discussed below.

The classical medicinal chemistry approach (based on the well-published efforts of Merck) has so far been applied to four different starting scaffolds. All resulted in more potent molecules against ASIC3 (and often ASIC1a), which is encouraging. However, they also all had significant off-target effects (>30 targets with <10 μM binding) and resulted in substantial sedation in animal studies which may explain their analgesic activity in both wild-type and ASIC3 KO mice (Kuduk et al., 2011, 2010; Kuduk, Chang, et al., 2009; Kuduk, Di Marco, et al., 2009). This suggests it may be quite difficult to develop selective small molecule ASIC inhibitors as therapeutic leads. Some of the recently discovered natural compounds from plants (in particular, gastrodin, sevanol, and chlorogenic acid) as well as the clinical/preclinical candidates CHF5074 and NS383 may offer novel scaffolds with lower off-target liabilities as starting points for future medchem studies.

NS383 and PPC5650 (along with A317567) are the only reported examples of ASIC modulators discovered using targeted screens of chemical libraries. This may suggest that standard screening approaches on ASICs are not easy and may explain the relative dearth of selective compounds from Pharma companies. However, as illustrated by the fact that amiloride, the NSAIDs and the flurbiprofen analogue CHF5074 (all already approved drugs or drugs in clinical testing) also inhibit ASICs, perhaps screening panels of existing well-tolerated drugs may reveal new classes of ASIC modulators with novel mechanisms and binding sites. A downside of screening known drugs is that they will certainly have protein targets other than ASICs, which may not be a problem for therapeutic development but is not ideal for use as tools to demonstrate the role of ASICs, particularly in in vivo studies.

Another possible (dare I say likely ...) source of new tools with improved subtype selectivity is of course, animal venoms. From Section 3 and Table 2, it is evident that animal venoms have so far been the most consistent source of potent and subtype-selective ASIC modulators. Some of these appear to be incredibly selective for ASIC3 (e.g., UGR-9-1), while three (PcTx1, MitTx, and the mambalgins) preferentially target ASIC1a with subtly or substantially different effects on ASIC1b. Understanding the molecular basis of these differences, in terms of both selectivity and mechanism, and from both the channel and the peptide side, will give us valuable information on how to engineer these peptides for enhanced selectivity. The mambalgins appear to be the only modulator so far to inhibit the activation of ASIC1 and thus may be our best chance to capture an ASIC channel in the closed state to help answer outstanding structural questions in the field. Unfortunately the mambalgins have a very rapid off rate, whether this is an issue for structural studies remains to be seen.

The total lack of selective tools for ASIC1b and ASIC2a could be due to them being inherently more difficult to target than ASIC1a or ASIC3, but has more likely resulted from a lack of focused attention. ASIC1a and ASIC3 were demonstrated early on to be involved in two very large and unmet medical needs: ischemic stroke (1a) and pain (3 and possibly also 1a), consequently they have attracted most of the research attention. The identification or design/development of more selective tools for ASIC1b and ASIC2a is an important goal for ongoing and future research. This is an area where I think venom peptides have a distinct advantage as two cocrystal structures of peptides that modulate ASIC1 have already been solved. This allows us to carry out very targeted mutagenesis work to exploit known subtype sequence differences and attempt the rational design of novel, more selective modulators.

5. CONCLUSION

ASICs were identified and reported as such in 1997, the same year that saw the discovery of the first mammalian transient receptor potential channel (the capsaicin receptor, TRPV1) (Caterina et al., 1997). In the intervening 20 years, the intensity of research on the ASICs has been dwarfed by the efforts poured into understanding TRP channels (according to Scopus there are ~1200 papers on or related to ASICs compared to >13,000 for TRPs). Despite this, our knowledge on many aspects of ASICs have come a very long way, due in no small part to the use of the pharmacological tools described here. Nevertheless, there are still many questions to answer. In addition to those mentioned already, some other important questions are:

– *How does our pharmacological data in rodent models translate to the clinic?* ASIC modulators largely interact with both rodent and human isoforms of ASICs, yet there are some species-dependent differences in efficacy and mechanism of action, not to mention relative tissue distributions of the ASIC subtypes, raising the possibility that some subtypes may have different roles in humans vs rodents.

- *What are the nonneuronal roles of ASICs?* The majority of research on ASICs so far has focused on them being "neuronal ion channels"; however, as pointed out in Section 1, they are also widely expressed in many types of nonneuronal cells. Thus, an interesting question is what are they doing there? Some roles have been established (see next question); however, many are still completely unknown. Both of these questions bring us to another major question in the field;
- *What is the therapeutic potential of selective ASIC modulators?* ASICs have been implicated to play roles in a very wide variety of processes, both physiological (e.g., sour taste, breathing control, neurotransmission/synaptic plasticity, fear, learning, sensing muscle lactate/acidosis, bone turnover, etc.) and pathophysiological (peripheral and central nociception, migraine, depression, seizure termination, neurodegeneration associated with either ischemia or inflammation, tumor growth and migration, retinal ischemic damage, etc.) with varying degrees of evidence. Thus, selective and biologically stable ASIC modulators are not only excellent tools to further validate (or refute) these roles, they are potential therapeutic leads to treat perhaps a multitude of medical conditions. So far, the therapeutic areas for which ASIC inhibitors appear to show the most promise are as analgesics (including migraine; Dussor, 2015) and as neuroprotective agents for ischemia-, trauma-, or autoinflammation induced nerve damage (i.e., stroke, traumatic spinal/brain injury, and multiple sclerosis, respectively) (Huang et al., 2015). This is strongly reflected by the current suite of patents on ASIC modulators with 7 of 15 covering pain and four on neuroprotection (Santos et al., 2015). This is a very extensive topic, and readers are directed to the series of excellent reviews in a special ASIC edition of *Neuropharmacology* (Vol. 94, 2015) for more thorough coverage of this area.

Although a relatively young ion channel family (in terms of when they were discovered), ASICs have proven to be very interesting from a biophysical and medical point of view. Obtaining a thorough understanding of the mechanisms, selectivity and species-dependent pharmacology of the existing tools, and the imminent discovery of novel tools will no doubt help to answer many of the outstanding questions and hopefully provide some promising therapeutic lead molecules.

CONFLICT OF INTEREST

The author declares no conflict of interest.

ACKNOWLEDGMENTS

I would like to thank Mr. Ben Cristofori-Armstrong for critical reading of this work. L.D.R.'s work on ASIC pharmacology has been supported by NHMRC project Grant APP1067940.

REFERENCES

Adams, C. M., Price, M. P., Snyder, P. M., & Welsh, M. J. (1999). Tetraethylammonium block of the BNC1 channel. *Biophysical Journal*, *76*(3), 1377–1383.

Akopian, A. N., Chen, C. C., Ding, Y., Cesare, P., & Wood, J. N. (2000). A new member of the acid-sensing ion channel family. *Neuroreport*, *11*(10), 2217–2222.

Alijevic, O., & Kellenberger, S. (2012). Subtype-specific modulation of acid-sensing ion channel (ASIC) function by 2-guanidine-4-methylquinazoline. *The Journal of Biological Chemistry*, *287*(43), 36059–36070.

Allen, N. J., & Attwell, D. (2002). Modulation of ASIC channels in rat cerebellar Purkinje neurons by ischaemia-related signals. *The Journal of Physiology*, *543*(Pt. 2), 521–529.

Anangi, R., Rash, L. D., Mobli, M., & King, G. F. (2012). Functional expression in *Escherichia coli* of the disulfide-rich sea anemone peptide APETx2, a potent blocker of acid-sensing ion channel 3. *Marine Drugs*, *10*(7), 1605–1618.

Askwith, C. C., Cheng, C., Ikuma, M., Benson, C., Price, M. P., & Welsh, M. J. (2000). Neuropeptide FF and FMRFamide potentiate acid-evoked currents from sensory neurons and proton-gated DEG/ENaC channels. *Neuron*, *26*(1), 133–141.

Babini, E., Paukert, M., Geisler, H. S., & Gründer, S. (2002). Alternative splicing and interaction with di- and polyvalent cations control the dynamic range of acid-sensing ion channel 1 (ASIC1). *The Journal of Biological Chemistry*, *277*(44), 41597–41603.

Babinski, K., Le, K. T., & Seguela, P. (1999). Molecular cloning and regional distribution of a human proton receptor subunit with biphasic functional properties. *Journal of Neurochemistry*, *72*(1), 51–57.

Baconguis, I., Bohlen, C. J., Goehring, A., Julius, D., & Gouaux, E. (2014). X-ray structure of acid-sensing ion channel 1-snake toxin complex reveals open state of a Na(+)-selective channel. *Cell*, *156*(4), 717–729.

Baconguis, I., & Gouaux, E. (2012). Structural plasticity and dynamic selectivity of acid-sensing ion channel-spider toxin complexes. *Nature*, *489*(7416), 400–405.

Baez, A., Salceda, E., Flo, M., Grana, M., Fernandez, C., Vega, R., & Soto, E. (2015). alpha-Dendrotoxin inhibits the ASIC current in dorsal root ganglion neurons from rat. *Neuroscience Letters*, *606*, 42–47.

Baron, A., & Lingueglia, E. (2015). Pharmacology of acid-sensing ion channels—Physiological and therapeutical perspectives. *Neuropharmacology*, *94*, 19–35.

Baron, A., Schaefer, L., Lingueglia, E., Champigny, G., & Lazdunski, M. (2001). Zn2+ and H+ are coactivators of acid-sensing ion channels. *The Journal of Biological Chemistry*, *276*(38), 35361–35367.

Bartoi, T., Augustinowski, K., Polleichtner, G., Grunder, S., & Ulbrich, M. H. (2014). Acid-sensing ion channel (ASIC) 1a/2a heteromers have a flexible 2:1/1:2 stoichiometry. *Proceedings of the National Academy of Sciences of the United States of America*, *111*(22), 8281–8286.

Benson, C. J., Xie, J., Wemmie, J. A., Price, M. P., Henss, J. M., Welsh, M. J., & Snyder, P. M. (2002). Heteromultimers of DEG/ENaC subunits form H+-gated channels in mouse sensory neurons. *Proceedings of the National Academy of Sciences of the United States of America*, *99*(4), 2338–2343.

Blanchard, M. G., Rash, L. D., & Kellenberger, S. (2012). Inhibition of voltage-gated Na^+ currents in sensory neurones by the sea anemone toxin APETx2. *British Journal of Pharmacology*, *165*(7), 2167–2177.

Bohlen, C. J., Chesler, A. T., Sharif-Naeini, R., Medzihradszky, K. F., Zhou, S., King, D., ...Julius, D. (2011). A heteromeric Texas coral snake toxin targets acid-sensing ion channels to produce pain. *Nature*, *479*(7373), 410–414.

Boiko, N., Kucher, V., Eaton, B. A., & Stockand, J. D. (2013). Inhibition of neuronal degenerin/epithelial Na+ channels by the multiple sclerosis drug 4-aminopyridine. *The Journal of Biological Chemistry*, *288*(13), 9418–9427.

Carattino, M. D., & Krauson, A. J. (2016). Molecular basis of inhibition of acid sensing ion channels by diminazene. *The FASEB Journal*, *30*(Suppl. 1), 1224–1243.

Caterina, M. J., Schumacher, M. A., Tominaga, M., Rosen, T. A., Levine, J. D., & Julius, D. (1997). The capsaicin receptor: A heat-activated ion channel in the pain pathway. *Nature*, *389*(6653), 816–824.

Champigny, G., Voilley, N., Waldmann, R., & Lazdunski, M. (1998). Mutations causing neurodegeneration in Caenorhabditis elegans drastically alter the pH sensitivity and inactivation of the mammalian H+-gated Na+ channel MDEG1. *The Journal of Biological Chemistry*, *273*(25), 15418–15422.

Chen, C. C., England, S., Akopian, A. N., & Wood, J. N. (1998). A sensory neuron-specific, proton-gated ion channel. *Proceedings of the National Academy of Sciences of the United States of America*, *95*(17), 10240–10245.

Chen, X., Kalbacher, H., & Gründer, S. (2005). The tarantula toxin psalmotoxin 1 inhibits acid-sensing ion channel (ASIC) 1a by increasing its apparent H^+ affinity. *The Journal of General Physiology*, *126*(1), 71–79.

Chen, X., Kalbacher, H., & Grunder, S. (2006). Interaction of acid-sensing ion channel (ASIC) 1 with the tarantula toxin psalmotoxin 1 is state dependent. *The Journal of General Physiology*, *127*(3), 267–276.

Chen, X., Qiu, L., Li, M., Durrnagel, S., Orser, B. A., Xiong, Z. G., & MacDonald, J. F. (2010). Diarylamidines: High potency inhibitors of acid-sensing ion channels. *Neuropharmacology*, *58*(7), 1045–1053.

Chen, C. C., Zimmer, A., Sun, W. H., Hall, J., & Brownstein, M. J. (2002). A role for ASIC3 in the modulation of high-intensity pain stimuli. *Proceedings of the National Academy of Sciences of the United States of America*, *99*(13), 8992–8997.

Coryell, M. W., Wunsch, A. M., Haenfler, J. M., Allen, J. E., Schnizler, M., Ziemann, A. E., ... Wemmie, J. A. (2009). Acid-sensing ion channel-1a in the amygdala, a novel therapeutic target in depression-related behavior. *The Journal of Neuroscience*, *29*(17), 5381–5388.

Cristofori-Armstrong, B., Soh, M. S., Talwar, S., Brown, D. L., Griffin, J. D., Dekan, Z., ... Rash, L. D. (2015). Xenopus borealis as an alternative source of oocytes for biophysical and pharmacological studies of neuronal ion channels. *Scientific Reports*, *5*, 14763.

Dawson, R. J., Benz, J., Stohler, P., Tetaz, T., Joseph, C., Huber, S., ... Ruf, A. (2012). Structure of the acid-sensing ion channel 1 in complex with the gating modifier Psalmotoxin 1. *Nature Communications*, *3*, 936.

Delaunay, A., Gasull, X., Salinas, M., Noel, J., Friend, V., Lingueglia, E., & Deval, E. (2012). Human ASIC3 channel dynamically adapts its activity to sense the extracellular pH in both acidic and alkaline directions. *Proceedings of the National Academy of Sciences of the United States of America*, *109*(32), 13124–13129.

Deval, E., & Lingueglia, E. (2015). Acid-sensing ion channels and nociception in the peripheral and central nervous systems. *Neuropharmacology*, *94*, 49–57.

Deval, E., Noel, J., Lay, N., Alloui, A., Diochot, S., Friend, V., ... Lingueglia, E. (2008). ASIC3, a sensor of acidic and primary inflammatory pain. *The EMBO Journal*, *27*(22), 3047–3055.

Diochot, S., Baron, A., Rash, L. D., Deval, E., Escoubas, P., Scarzello, S., ... Lazdunski, M. (2004). A new sea anemone peptide, APETx2, inhibits ASIC3, a major acid-sensitive channel in sensory neurons. *The EMBO Journal*, *23*(7), 1516–1525.

Diochot, S., Baron, A., Salinas, M., Douguet, D., Scarzello, S., Dabert-Gay, A. S., … Lingueglia, E. (2012). Black mamba venom peptides target acid-sensing ion channels to abolish pain. *Nature*, *490*(7421), 552–555.
Dorofeeva, N. A., Barygin, O. I., Staruschenko, A., Bolshakov, K. V., & Magazanik, L. G. (2008). Mechanisms of non-steroid anti-inflammatory drugs action on ASICs expressed in hippocampal interneurons. *Journal of Neurochemistry*, *106*(1), 429–441.
Duan, B., Wang, Y. Z., Yang, T., Chu, X. P., Yu, Y., Huang, Y., … Xu, T. L. (2011). Extracellular spermine exacerbates ischemic neuronal injury through sensitization of ASIC1a channels to extracellular acidosis. *The Journal of Neuroscience*, *31*(6), 2101–2112.
Dube, G. R., Elagoz, A., & Mangat, H. (2009). Acid sensing ion channels and acid nociception. *Current Pharmaceutical Design*, *15*(15), 1750–1766.
Dube, G. R., Lehto, S. G., Breese, N. M., Baker, S. J., Wang, X., Matulenko, M. A., … Brioni, J. D. (2005). Electrophysiological and in vivo characterization of A-317567, a novel blocker of acid sensing ion channels. *Pain*, *117*(1–2), 88–96.
Dubinnyi, M. A., Osmakov, D. I., Koshelev, S. G., Kozlov, S. A., Andreev, Y. A., Zakaryan, N. A., … Grishin, E. V. (2012). Lignan from thyme possesses inhibitory effect on ASIC3 channel current. *The Journal of Biological Chemistry*, *287*(39), 32993–33000.
Dussor, G. (2015). ASICs as therapeutic targets for migraine. *Neuropharmacology*, *94*, 64–71.
Dwyer, J. M., Rizzo, S. J., Neal, S. J., Lin, Q., Jow, F., Arias, R. L., … Beyer, C. E. (2009). Acid sensing ion channel (ASIC) inhibitors exhibit anxiolytic-like activity in preclinical pharmacological models. *Psychopharmacology*, *203*(1), 41–52.
Escoubas, P., De Weille, J. R., Lecoq, A., Diochot, S., Waldmann, R., Champigny, G., … Lazdunski, M. (2000). Isolation of a tarantula toxin specific for a class of proton-gated Na^+ channels. *The Journal of Biological Chemistry*, *275*(33), 25116–25121.
Gao, J., Wu, L. J., Xu, L., & Xu, T. L. (2004). Properties of the proton-evoked currents and their modulation by Ca2+ and Zn2+ in the acutely dissociated hippocampus CA1 neurons. *Brain Research*, *1017*(1–2), 197–207.
Garateix, A., Salceda, E., Menendez, R., Regalado, E. L., Lopez, O., Garcia, T., … Soto, E. (2011). Antinociception produced by Thalassia testudinum extract BM-21 is mediated by the inhibition of acid sensing ionic channels by the phenolic compound thalassiolin B. *Molecular Pain*, 7, 10.
Garcia-Anoveros, J., Derfler, B., Neville-Golden, J., Hyman, B. T., & Corey, D. P. (1997). BNaC1 and BNaC2 constitute a new family of human neuronal sodium channels related to degenerins and epithelial sodium channels. *Proceedings of the National Academy of Sciences of the United States of America*, *94*(4), 1459–1464.
Gonzales, E. B., Kawate, T., & Gouaux, E. (2009). Pore architecture and ion sites in acid-sensing ion channels and P2X receptors. *Nature*, *460*(7255), 599–604.
Gründer, S., Geissler, H. S., Bassler, E. L., & Ruppersberg, J. P. (2000). A new member of acid-sensing ion channels from pituitary gland. *Neuroreport*, *11*(8), 1607–1611.
Gründer, S., & Pusch, M. (2015). Biophysical properties of acid-sensing ion channels (ASICs). *Neuropharmacology*, *94*, 9–18.
Gu, L., Yang, Y., Sun, Y., & Zheng, X. (2010). Puerarin inhibits acid-sensing ion channels and protects against neuron death induced by acidosis. *Planta Medica*, *76*(6), 583–588.
Hesselager, M., Timmermann, D. B., & Ahring, P. K. (2004). pH Dependency and desensitization kinetics of heterologously expressed combinations of acid-sensing ion channel subunits. *The Journal of Biological Chemistry*, *279*(12), 11006–11015.
Hoagland, E. N., Sherwood, T. W., Lee, K. G., Walker, C. J., & Askwith, C. C. (2010). Identification of a calcium permeable human acid-sensing ion channel 1 transcript variant. *The Journal of Biological Chemistry*, *285*(53), 41852–41862.
Howard, M. J., Hughes, R. J., Motulsky, H. J., Mullen, M. D., & Insel, P. A. (1987). Interactions of amiloride with alpha- and beta-adrenergic receptors: Amiloride reveals an allosteric site on alpha 2-adrenergic receptors. *Molecular Pharmacology*, *32*(1), 53–58.

Huang, C., Hu, Z. L., Wu, W. N., Yu, D. F., Xiong, Q. J., Song, J. R., … Chen, J. G. (2010). Existence and distinction of acid-evoked currents in rat astrocytes. *Glia, 58*(12), 1415–1424.

Huang, Y., Jiang, N., Li, J., Ji, Y. H., Xiong, Z. G., & Zha, X. M. (2015). Two aspects of ASIC function: Synaptic plasticity and neuronal injury. *Neuropharmacology, 94*, 42–48.

Huda, R., Pollema-Mays, S. L., Chang, Z., Alheid, G. F., McCrimmon, D. R., & Martina, M. (2012). Acid-sensing ion channels contribute to chemosensitivity of breathing-related neurons of the nucleus of the solitary tract. *The Journal of Physiology, 590*(19), 4761–4775.

Immke, D. C., & McCleskey, E. W. (2001a). ASIC3: A lactic acid sensor for cardiac pain. *ScientificWorldJournal, 1*, 510–512.

Immke, D. C., & McCleskey, E. W. (2001b). Lactate enhances the acid-sensing Na^+ channel on ischemia-sensing neurons. *Nature Neuroscience, 4*(9), 869–870.

Jasti, J., Furukawa, H., Gonzales, E. B., & Gouaux, E. (2007). Structure of acid-sensing ion channel 1 at 1.9 Å resolution and low pH. *Nature, 449*(7160), 316–323.

Jensen, J. E., Cristofori-Armstrong, B., Anangi, R., Rosengren, K. J., Lau, C. H., Mobli, M., … Rash, L. D. (2014). Understanding the molecular basis of toxin promiscuity: The analgesic sea anemone peptide APETx2 interacts with acid-sensing ion channel 3 and hERG channels via overlapping pharmacophores. *Journal of Medicinal Chemistry, 57*(21), 9195–9203.

Jensen, J. E., Durek, T., Alewood, P. F., Adams, D. J., King, G. F., & Rash, L. D. (2009). Chemical synthesis and folding of APETx2, a potent and selective inhibitor of acid sensing ion channel 3. *Toxicon, 54*(1), 56–61.

Jensen, J. E., Mobli, M., Brust, A., Alewood, P. F., King, G. F., & Rash, L. D. (2012). Cyclisation increases the stability of the sea anemone peptide APETx2 but decreases its activity at acid-sensing ion channel 3. *Marine Drugs, 10*(7), 1511–1527.

Joeres, N., Augustinowski, K., Neuhof, A., Assmann, M., & Grunder, S. (2016). Functional and pharmacological characterization of two different ASIC1a/2a heteromers reveals their sensitivity to the spider toxin PcTx1. *Scientific Reports, 6*, 27647.

Kellenberger, S., & Schild, L. (2015). International Union of Basic and Clinical Pharmacology. XCI. Structure, function, and pharmacology of acid-sensing ion channels and the epithelial Na+ channel. *Pharmacological Reviews, 67*(1), 1–35.

Korkushko, A. O., & Kryshtal, O. A. (1984). Blocking of proton-activated sodium permeability of the membranes of trigeminal ganglion neurons in the rat by organic cations. *Neĭrofiziologiia, 16*(4), 557–561.

Krishtal, O. (2015). Receptor for protons: First observations on acid sensing ion channels. *Neuropharmacology, 94*, 4–8.

Krishtal, O. A., & Pidoplichko, V. I. (1980). A receptor for protons in the nerve cell membrane. *Neuroscience, 5*(12), 2325–2327.

Kuduk, S. D., Chang, R. K., Di Marco, C. N., Dipardo, R. M., Cook, S. P., Cato, M. J., … Bilodeau, M. T. (2011). Identification of non-amidine inhibitors of acid-sensing ion channel-3 (ASIC3). *Bioorganic & Medicinal Chemistry Letters, 21*(14), 4255–4258.

Kuduk, S. D., Chang, R. K., Wai, J. M., Di Marco, C. N., Cofre, V., DiPardo, R. M., … Bilodeau, M. T. (2009). Amidine derived inhibitors of acid-sensing ion channel-3 (ASIC3). *Bioorganic & Medicinal Chemistry Letters, 19*(15), 4059–4063.

Kuduk, S. D., Di Marco, C. N., Bodmer-Narkevitch, V., Cook, S. P., Cato, M. J., Jovanovska, A., … Bilodeau, M. T. (2010). Synthesis, structure-activity relationship, and pharmacological profile of analogs of the ASIC-3 inhibitor A-317567. *ACS Chemical Neuroscience, 1*(1), 19–24.

Kuduk, S. D., Di Marco, C. N., Chang, R. K., Dipardo, R. M., Cook, S. P., Cato, M. J., … Bock, M. G. (2009). Amiloride derived inhibitors of acid-sensing ion channel-3 (ASIC3). *Bioorganic & Medicinal Chemistry Letters, 19*(9), 2514–2518.

Leffler, A., Monter, B., & Koltzenburg, M. (2006). The role of the capsaicin receptor TRPV1 and acid-sensing ion channels (ASICS) in proton sensitivity of subpopulations of primary nociceptive neurons in rats and mice. *Neuroscience, 139*(2), 699–709.

Lei, Z., Li, X., Wang, G., Fei, J., Meng, T., Zhang, X., ... Li, J. (2014). Inhibition of acid-sensing ion channel currents by propofol in rat dorsal root ganglion neurons. *Clinical and Experimental Pharmacology & Physiology, 41*(4), 295–300.

Lei, Z., Sami Shaikh, A., Zheng, W., Yu, X., Yu, J., & Li, J. (2016). Non-proton ligand-sensing domain of acid-sensing ion channel 3 is required for itch sensation. *Journal of Neurochemistry, 139*(6), 1093–1101.

Leng, T., Lin, J., Cottrell, J. E., & Xiong, Z. G. (2013). Subunit and frequency-dependent inhibition of acid sensing ion channels by local anesthetic tetracaine. *Molecular Pain, 9*, 27.

Li, X., Fei, J., Lei, Z., Liu, K., Wu, J., Meng, T., ... Li, J. (2014). Chloroquine impairs visual transduction via modulation of acid sensing ion channel 1a. *Toxicology Letters, 228*(3), 200–206.

Li, M., Inoue, K., Branigan, D., Kratzer, E., Hansen, J. C., Chen, J. W., ... Xiong, Z. G. (2010). Acid-sensing ion channels in acidosis-induced injury of human brain neurons. *Journal of Cerebral Blood Flow and Metabolism, 30*(6), 1247–1260.

Li, W. G., Yu, Y., Huang, C., Cao, H., & Xu, T. L. (2011). Nonproton ligand sensing domain is required for paradoxical stimulation of acid-sensing ion channel 3 (ASIC3) channels by amiloride. *The Journal of Biological Chemistry, 286*(49), 42635–42646.

Li, W. G., Yu, Y., Zhang, Z. D., Cao, H., & Xu, T. L. (2010). ASIC3 channels integrate agmatine and multiple inflammatory signals through the nonproton ligand sensing domain. *Molecular Pain, 6*, 88.

Lin, S. H., Chien, Y. C., Chiang, W. W., Liu, Y. Z., Lien, C. C., & Chen, C. C. (2015). Genetic mapping of ASIC4 and contrasting phenotype to ASIC1a in modulating innate fear and anxiety. *The European Journal of Neuroscience, 41*(12), 1553–1568.

Lin, J., Chu, X., Maysami, S., Li, M., Si, H., Cottrell, J. E., ... Xiong, Z. (2011). Inhibition of acid sensing ion channel currents by lidocaine in cultured mouse cortical neurons. *Anesthésie et Analgésie, 112*(4), 977–981.

Lin, S. H., Sun, W. H., & Chen, C. C. (2015). Genetic exploration of the role of acid-sensing ion channels. *Neuropharmacology, 94*, 99–118.

Lingueglia, E., Champigny, G., Lazdunski, M., & Barbry, P. (1995). Cloning of the amiloride-sensitive FMRFamide peptide-gated sodium channel. *Nature, 378*(6558), 730–733.

Lingueglia, E., de Weille, J. R., Bassilana, F., Heurteaux, C., Sakai, H., Waldmann, R., & Lazdunski, M. (1997). A modulatory subunit of acid sensing ion channels in brain and dorsal root ganglion cells. *The Journal of Biological Chemistry, 272*(47), 29778–29783.

Mamet, J., Baron, A., Lazdunski, M., & Voilley, N. (2002). Proinflammatory mediators, stimulators of sensory neuron excitability via the expression of acid-sensing ion channels. *The Journal of Neuroscience, 22*(24), 10662–10670.

Mango, D., Barbato, G., Piccirilli, S., Panico, M. B., Feligioni, M., Schepisi, C., ... Nistico, R. (2014). Electrophysiological and metabolic effects of CHF5074 in the hippocampus: Protection against in vitro ischemia. *Pharmacological Research, 81*, 83–90.

Marra, S., Ferru-Clement, R., Breuil, V., Delaunay, A., Christin, M., Friend, V., ... Deval, E. (2016). Non-acidic activation of pain-related acid-sensing ion channel 3 by lipids. *The EMBO Journal, 35*(4), 414–428.

McCarthy, C. A., Rash, L. D., Chassagnon, I. R., King, G. F., & Widdop, R. E. (2015). PcTx1 affords neuroprotection in a conscious model of stroke in hypertensive rats via selective inhibition of ASIC1a. *Neuropharmacology, 99*, 650–657.

Munro, G., Christensen, J. K., Erichsen, H. K., Dyhring, T., Demnitz, J., Dam, E., & Ahring, P. K. (2016). NS383 selectively inhibits acid-sensing ion channels containing

1a and 3 subunits to reverse inflammatory and neuropathic hyperalgesia in rats. *CNS Neuroscience & Therapeutics*, *22*(2), 135–145.
Muto, S., Imai, M., & Asano, Y. (1993). Effect of nafamostat mesilate on Na + and K + transport properties in the rabbit cortical collecting duct. *British Journal of Pharmacology*, *109*(3), 673–678.
Nagaeva, E. I., Tikhonova, T. B., Magazanik, L. G., & Tikhonov, D. B. (2016). Histamine selectively potentiates acid-sensing ion channel 1a. *Neuroscience Letters*, *632*, 136–140.
Nielsen, L. M., Olesen, A. E., Andresen, T., Simren, M., Tornblom, H., & Drewes, A. M. (2015). Efficacy and safety of PPC-5650 on experimental rectal pain in patients with irritable bowel syndrome. *Basic & Clinical Pharmacology & Toxicology*, *116*(2), 140–145.
Olesen, A. E., Nielsen, L. M., Larsen, I. M., & Drewes, A. M. (2015). Randomized clinical trial: Efficacy and safety of PPC-5650 on experimental esophageal pain and hyperalgesia in healthy volunteers. *Scandinavian Journal of Gastroenterology*, *50*(2), 138–144.
Osmakov, D. I., Kozlov, S. A., Andreev, Y. A., Koshelev, S. G., Sanamyan, N. P., Sanamyan, K. E., … Grishin, E. V. (2013). Sea anemone peptide with uncommon beta-hairpin structure inhibits acid-sensing ion channel 3 (ASIC3) and reveals analgesic activity. *The Journal of Biological Chemistry*, *288*(32), 23116–23127.
Peigneur, S., Beress, L., Moller, C., Mari, F., Forssmann, W. G., & Tytgat, J. (2012). A natural point mutation changes both target selectivity and mechanism of action of sea anemone toxins. *The FASEB Journal*, *26*(12), 5141–5151.
Price, M. P., McIlwrath, S. L., Xie, J., Cheng, C., Qiao, J., Tarr, D. E., … Welsh, M. J. (2001). The DRASIC cation channel contributes to the detection of cutaneous touch and acid stimuli in mice. *Neuron*, *32*(6), 1071–1083.
Price, M. P., Snyder, P. M., & Welsh, M. J. (1996). Cloning and expression of a novel human brain Na^+ channel. *The Journal of Biological Chemistry*, *271*(14), 7879–7882.
Qiu, F., Liu, T. T., Qu, Z. W., Qiu, C. Y., Yang, Z., & Hu, W. P. (2014). Gastrodin inhibits the activity of acid-sensing ion channels in rat primary sensory neurons. *European Journal of Pharmacology*, *731*, 50–57.
Qu, Z. W., Liu, T. T., Qiu, C. Y., Li, J. D., & Hu, W. P. (2014). Inhibition of acid-sensing ion channels by chlorogenic acid in rat dorsal root ganglion neurons. *Neuroscience Letters*, *567*, 35–39.
Rash, L. D. (2013). ASIC3: First the heartache, now a migraine!. *Headache*, *53*(8), 1204–1206.
Reeh, P. W., & Steen, K. H. (1996). Tissue acidosis in nociception and pain. *Progress in Brain Research*, *113*, 143–151.
Rodriguez, A. A., Salceda, E., Garateix, A. G., Zaharenko, A. J., Peigneur, S., Lopez, O., … Soto, E. (2014). A novel sea anemone peptide that inhibits acid-sensing ion channels. *Peptides*, *53*, 3–12.
Roos, A., & Boron, W. F. (1981). Intracellular pH. *Physiological Reviews*, *61*(2), 296–434.
Saez, N. J., Deplazes, E., Cristofori-Armstrong, B., Chassagnon, I. R., Lin, X., Mobli, M., … King, G. F. (2015). Molecular dynamics and functional studies define a hot spot of crystal contacts essential for PcTx1 inhibition of acid-sensing ion channel 1a. *British Journal of Pharmacology*, *172*(20), 4985–4995.
Saez, N. J., Mobli, M., Bieri, M., Chassagnon, I. R., Malde, A. K., Gamsjaeger, R., … King, G. F. (2011). A dynamic pharmacophore drives the interaction between psalmotoxin-1 and the putative drug target acid-sensing ion channel 1a. *Molecular Pharmacology*, *80*, 796–808.
Salinas, M., Besson, T., Delettre, Q., Diochot, S., Boulakirba, S., Douguet, D., & Lingueglia, E. (2014). Binding site and inhibitory mechanism of the mambalgin-2 pain-relieving peptide on acid-sensing ion channel 1a. *The Journal of Biological Chemistry*, *289*(19), 13363–13373.

Santos, P. L., Guimaraes, A. G., Barreto, R. S., Serafini, M. R., Quintans, J. S., & Quintans-Junior, L. J. (2015). A review of recent patents on the ASICs as a key drug target. *Recent Patents on Biotechnology*, *9*(1), 30–41.

Schroeder, C. I., Rash, L. D., Vila-Farres, X., Rosengren, K. J., Mobli, M., King, G. F., … Durek, T. (2014). Chemical synthesis, 3D structure, and ASIC binding site of the toxin mambalgin-2. *Angewandte Chemie (International Ed in English)*, *53*(4), 1017–1020.

Sherwood, T. W., & Askwith, C. C. (2009). Dynorphin opioid peptides enhance acid-sensing ion channel 1a activity and acidosis-induced neuronal death. *The Journal of Neuroscience*, *29*(45), 14371–14380.

Sherwood, T. W., Lee, K. G., Gormley, M. G., & Askwith, C. C. (2011). Heteromeric acid-sensing ion channels (ASICs) composed of ASIC2b and ASIC1a display novel channel properties and contribute to acidosis-induced neuronal death. *The Journal of Neuroscience*, *31*(26), 9723–9734.

Smith, E. S., Cadiou, H., & McNaughton, P. A. (2007). Arachidonic acid potentiates acid-sensing ion channels in rat sensory neurons by a direct action. *Neuroscience*, *145*(2), 686–698.

Sun, X., Cao, Y. B., Hu, L. F., Yang, Y. P., Li, J., Wang, F., & Liu, C. F. (2011). ASICs mediate the modulatory effect by paeoniflorin on alpha-synuclein autophagic degradation. *Brain Research*, *1396*, 77–87.

Ugawa, S., Ishida, Y., Ueda, T., Inoue, K., Nagao, M., & Shimada, S. (2007). Nafamostat mesilate reversibly blocks acid-sensing ion channel currents. *Biochemical and Biophysical Research Communications*, *363*(1), 203–208.

Vick, J. S., & Askwith, C. C. (2015). ASICs and neuropeptides. *Neuropharmacology*, *94*, 36–41.

Voilley, N., de Weille, J., Mamet, J., & Lazdunski, M. (2001). Nonsteroid anti-inflammatory drugs inhibit both the activity and the inflammation-induced expression of acid-sensing ion channels in nociceptors. *The Journal of Neuroscience*, *21*(20), 8026–8033.

Vukicevic, M., & Kellenberger, S. (2004). Modulatory effects of acid-sensing ion channels on action potential generation in hippocampal neurons. *American Journal of Physiology Cell Physiology*, *287*(3), C682–C690.

Walder, R. Y., Rasmussen, L. A., Rainier, J. D., Light, A. R., Wemmie, J. A., & Sluka, K. A. (2010). ASIC1 and ASIC3 play different roles in the development of hyperalgesia after inflammatory muscle injury. *The Journal of Pain*, *11*(3), 210–218.

Waldmann, R., Bassilana, F., de Weille, J., Champigny, G., Heurteaux, C., & Lazdunski, M. (1997). Molecular cloning of a non-inactivating proton-gated Na^+ channel specific for sensory neurons. *The Journal of Biological Chemistry*, *272*(34), 20975–20978.

Waldmann, R., Champigny, G., Bassilana, F., Heurteaux, C., & Lazdunski, M. (1997). A proton-gated cation channel involved in acid-sensing. *Nature*, *386*(6621), 173–177.

Waldmann, R., Champigny, G., Voilley, N., Lauritzen, I., & Lazdunski, M. (1996). The mammalian degenerin MDEG, an amiloride-sensitive cation channel activated by mutations causing neurodegeneration in Caenorhabditis elegans. *The Journal of Biological Chemistry*, *271*(18), 10433–10436.

Wang, Y. Z., & Xu, T. L. (2011). Acidosis, acid-sensing ion channels, and neuronal cell death. *Molecular Neurobiology*, *44*(3), 350–358.

Wang, X. Y., Yan, W. W., Zhang, X. L., Liu, H., & Zhang, L. C. (2014). ASIC3 in the cerebrospinal fluid-contacting nucleus of brain parenchyma contributes to inflammatory pain in rats. *Neurological Research*, *36*(3), 270–275.

Wang, Y. Z., Zeng, W. Z., Xiao, X., Huang, Y., Song, X. L., Yu, Z., … Xu, T. L. (2013). Intracellular ASIC1a regulates mitochondrial permeability transition-dependent neuronal death. *Cell Death and Differentiation*, *20*(10), 1359–1369.

Wemmie, J. A., Taugher, R. J., & Kreple, C. J. (2013). Acid-sensing ion channels in pain and disease. *Nature Reviews Neuroscience*, *14*(7), 461–471.

Wu, W. L., Lin, Y. W., Min, M. Y., & Chen, C. C. (2010). Mice lacking Asic3 show reduced anxiety-like behavior on the elevated plus maze and reduced aggression. *Genes, Brain, and Behavior*, *9*(6), 603–614.

Wu, W. N., Wu, P. F., Chen, X. L., Zhang, Z., Gu, J., Yang, Y. J., … Chen, J. G. (2011). Sinomenine protects against ischaemic brain injury: Involvement of co-inhibition of acid-sensing ion channel 1a and L-type calcium channels. *British Journal of Pharmacology*, *164*(5), 1445–1459.

Xiong, Z. G., Pignataro, G., Li, M., Chang, S. Y., & Simon, R. P. (2008). Acid-sensing ion channels (ASICs) as pharmacological targets for neurodegenerative diseases. *Current Opinion in Pharmacology*, *8*(1), 25–32.

Xiong, Z. G., Zhu, X. M., Chu, X. P., Minami, M., Hey, J., Wei, W. L., … Simon, R. P. (2004). Neuroprotection in ischemia: Blocking calcium-permeable acid-sensing ion channels. *Cell*, *118*(6), 687–698.

Yen, Y. T., Tu, P. H., Chen, C. J., Lin, Y. W., Hsieh, S. T., & Chen, C. C. (2009). Role of acid-sensing ion channel 3 in sub-acute-phase inflammation. *Molecular Pain*, *5*, 1.

Yu, Y., Chen, Z., Li, W. G., Cao, H., Feng, E. G., Yu, F., … Xu, T. L. (2010). A nonproton ligand sensor in the acid-sensing ion channel. *Neuron*, *68*(1), 61–72.

Zeng, W. Z., Liu, D. S., Liu, L., She, L., Wu, L. J., & Xu, T. L. (2015). Activation of acid-sensing ion channels by localized proton transient reveals their role in proton signaling. *Scientific Reports*, *5*, 14125.

Ziemann, A. E., Allen, J. E., Dahdaleh, N. S., Drebot, I. I., Coryell, M. W., Wunsch, A. M., … Wemmie, J. A. (2009). The amygdala is a chemosensor that detects carbon dioxide and acidosis to elicit fear behavior. *Cell*, *139*(5), 1012–1021.

CHAPTER THREE

Sodium Channels and Venom Peptide Pharmacology

Mathilde R. Israel*, Bryan Tay*, Jennifer R. Deuis*[,1], Irina Vetter*[,†,1]
*Centre for Pain Research, Institute for Molecular Bioscience, The University of Queensland, Brisbane, QLD, Australia
†School of Pharmacy, The University of Queensland, Brisbane, QLD, Australia
[1]Corresponding authors: e-mail address: j.deuis@uq.edu.au; i.vetter@uq.edu.au

Contents

Abstract

Venomous animals including cone snails, spiders, scorpions, anemones, and snakes have evolved a myriad of components in their venoms that target the opening and/or closing of voltage-gated sodium channels to cause devastating effects on the neuromuscular systems of predators and prey. These venom peptides, through design and serendipity, have not only contributed significantly to our understanding of sodium channel pharmacology and structure, but they also represent some of the most phyla- and isoform-selective molecules that are useful as valuable tool compounds and drug leads. Here, we review our understanding of the basic function of mammalian voltage-gated sodium channel isoforms as well as the pharmacology of venom peptides that act at these key transmembrane proteins.

Advances in Pharmacology, Volume 79
ISSN 1054-3589
http://dx.doi.org/10.1016/bs.apha.2017.01.004

ABBREVIATIONS

aa amino acid
CCI chronic constriction injury
CNS central nervous system
hNE human neuroendocrine
Na^+ sodium ion
NaN novel Na channel
Na_V voltage-gated sodium channel
PN1 peripheral nerve type 1
PN3 peripheral nerve type 3
PNS peripheral nervous system
SNS sensory nerve specific
SNS2 sensory nerve specific 2
TRTX theraphotoxin
TTX tetrodotoxin

1. INTRODUCTION

1.1 Nerve Excitability: An Historical Perspective

The nervous system's ability to carry electrical currents was discovered in 1780 by Luigi Galvani in seminal work showing that the muscles of a dead frog's leg could be made to twitch upon stimulation by an electrical spark. Further experiments, without the presence of electrical sparks, demonstrated that nerve cells possess an intrinsic electrical force which he coined "animal electricity" (Piccolino, 2006). However, the precise mechanism of neuronal conduction was not understood until the 20th century, when experiments on squid giant axons—published in a series of highly influential papers by Hodgkin and Huxley (1952a, 1952b, 1952c, 1952d)—revealed the crucial contribution of the inward sodium (Na^+) current to action potential generation. It is now understood that large transmembrane channels that open and close in response to changes in the electrical potential—the voltage-gated sodium channels or Na_V—mediate this selective influx of Na^+ ions. These channels are thus crucial for the function of excitable cells, with catastrophic physiological consequences arising from either enhanced or reduced channel gating. Accordingly, many animal venoms and peptidic venom components specifically interfere with the processes of Na_V gating or ionic conductance, facilitating capture of prey, and deterring predators. Moreover, despite significant advances in our understanding of Na_V function at the molecular and structural level, venom peptides remain crucial pharmacological probes, tool compounds, and drug leads.

1.2 Voltage-Gated Sodium Channel Structure

Early studies on the structure and function of Na_V channels were greatly facilitated by toxins, leading to the purification of the 260-kDa pore-forming α subunit from electrical tissue of *Electrophorus electricus* and later mammalian Na_V isoforms (Beneski & Catterall, 1980; Catterall, 1979, 1980; Catterall & Beress, 1978). Later it was found that the pore-forming α subunit associates with one or more 30–40 kDa auxiliary β subunits (β1–β4), which can modulate cell surface expression and functional properties of the α subunit, as well as the pharmacology of toxins (Chahine & O'Leary, 2011; Zhang et al., 2013).

Structurally, Na_V channels consist of four homologous domains (I, II, III, and IV) each containing 6 alpha helical transmembrane spanning segments (S1–S6) connected by large intra- and extracellular loops (Hartshorne & Catterall, 1984; Noda et al., 1984). In functional channels, the four domains are arranged in a concentric manner surrounding the ion-conducting pore of the channel which in turn is formed by the S5–S6 helices as well as their connecting, membrane reentrant pore loop (Noda, Suzuki, Numa, & Stuhmer, 1989). Notably, the arrangement of the voltage-sensing (S1–S4) and pore-forming (S5–S6) segments are offset so that in functional channels, the voltage sensor of each domain is closest to the pore-forming segment of the following domain (Payandeh, Scheuer, Zheng, & Catterall, 2011). The selectivity filter consists of a four-glutamate-residue motif in the pore of the channel which allows the passage of Na^+, but not K^+ and Ca^{2+} ions and thus imparts the high Na^+ selectivity characteristic of these channels (Heinemann, Terlau, Stuhmer, Imoto, & Numa, 1992). This structural arrangement was recently confirmed by crystal structures of the homotetrameric bacterial Na_V channel which have provided a better understanding of ion selectivity, channel gating, and drug interactions (Payandeh, Gamal El-Din, Scheuer, Zheng, & Catterall, 2012; Payandeh et al., 2011), albeit a high-resolution structure of mammalian Na_V channels remains to be determined.

1.3 Voltage-Gated Sodium Channel Gating

Na_V channels exist, at a minimum, in three discrete states: resting (closed), open (active), and inactive (Fig. 1). In both the closed and inactive state, the

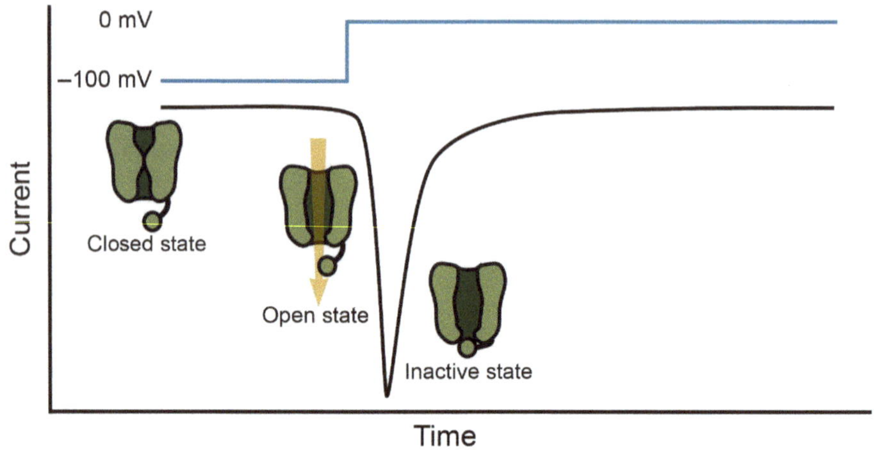

Fig. 1 Na_V gating. During a depolarizing voltage step, Na_V channels transition from the closed or resting to open state, where permeation of Na^+ ions through the pore occurs. The process of fast inactivation leads to closure of the channel via occlusion of the pore by the inactivation particle, preceding the return to the closed state once membrane potentials returns to resting levels.

channels are impermeable to Na^+ ions, with ion conduction only possible in the open state. In a simplified model of Na_V gating, depolarization of the membrane causes the channel to transition from the resting to the active state, allowing the flow of Na^+ ions along their concentration gradient (Hille, 2001; Hodgkin & Huxley, 1952b). Following depolarization and subsequent ion influx, channel inactivation halts ion conductance, a necessary prerequisite for return of the membrane potential to resting levels. Recovery from inactivation describes the—relatively poorly understood—process of returning inactivated channels to the resting state and completes channel gating transitions (Hille, 2001). Importantly, venom peptides can not only modulate ion permeability but also affect transition of Na_V between these states, leading to diverse functional effects as discussed later.

1.3.1 Channel Activation

The voltage-dependent activation of Na_V channels depends crucially on the S4 transmembrane segments of domains I–III, which each contain a repeated motif consisting of positively charged amino acid residues uniformly separated by nonpolar amino acids (Catterall, 1986; Guy & Seetharamulu, 1986; Noda et al., 1984; Stuhmer et al., 1989). During membrane depolarization, these "gating charges" move toward the extracellular surface as ion pair interactions between the positive charges of the S4 segment and the negative charges of adjacent transmembrane regions are released (DeCaen, Yarov-Yarovoy, Sharp, Scheuer, & Catterall, 2009; DeCaen, Yarov-Yarovoy, Zhao, Scheuer, & Catterall, 2008). The resultant conformational rearrangement leads to opening of the pore and subsequent influx of Na^+ ions. During repolarization of the membrane, the activation gate is released in a process known as deactivation that is separate from, and not to be confused with, the process of inactivation described later.

1.3.2 Channel Inactivation

The process of inactivation ultimately results in the channel no longer conducting ions and can occur from the open state (fast inactivation) or from the closed state (closed state inactivation) (Ahern, 2013). Fast inactivation is the result of the occlusion of the pore by the cytosolic inactivation particle, which consists of the intracellular loop linking domains III and IV (Armstrong, Bezanilla, & Rojas, 1973; Goldin, 2003). During the activation process, movement of the voltage sensors, in particular of domain IV, exposes the inactivation particle binding site and leads to a physical block of the movement of ions into the cell (Armstrong et al., 1973). As the voltage sensors of domains I–III respond more rapidly to membrane depolarization than the domain IV voltage sensors (Chanda & Bezanilla, 2002), inactivation typically occurs subsequent to channel activation. Accordingly, the process of inactivation is intricately linked to activation, albeit the experimentally observed membrane potential-dependent characteristics of inactivation are likely largely derived from the intrinsic coupling to activation, with movement of the DIV voltage-sensing domain a necessary prerequisite for inactivation.

However, as movement of two of the voltage-sensing domains may be sufficient for the inactivation particle to bind (Armstrong, 2006), it is possible for Na_V channels to proceed directly from the closed (in these studies often called preopen) to the inactivated state (Bähring & Covarrubias, 2011; Horn, Patlak, & Stevens, 1981) under conditions that kinetically favor the development of inactivation. In this way, the channel does not have to fully open before being blocked by the inactivation particle leading to a closed channel block.

In contrast to fast inactivation, "slow inactivation" is a distinct type of inactivation that does not involve movement of the inactivation particle

(Armstrong & Bezanilla, 1977). Slow inactivation occurs after prolonged depolarization of the membrane or a long period of high frequency firing (Ong, Tomaselli, & Balser, 2000). Unlike fast inactivation, channels that are in the slow inactivation state require longer periods (100 ms–10 s) of time to recover. Slow inactivation is thought to arise from a conformational change in the channel, most likely associated with the domain IV S4 region and S6 pore-forming segments, whereby the pore is not fully blocked (Mitrovic, George, Horn, & Horn, 2000; Ong et al., 2000; Payandeh et al., 2012). Unfortunately, the effects of toxins on slow inactivation are rarely studied, and thus not discussed in this review.

1.4 Na_V Isoforms

At present, nine mammalian Na_V subtypes (isoforms) have been identified, which can be distinguished according to their expression pattern, biophysical characteristics, and pharmacology. To eliminate confusion arising from the inconsistent naming conventions for these isoforms (Table 1), a standardized nomenclature based on a numerical system to define subtypes was introduced (Goldin et al., 2000). According to their highly selective permeability to Na^+ ions, gating by membrane voltage, and similar sequence and functional characteristics, the accepted naming convention for these α subunits is $Na_V1.1$–1.9 (Goldin et al., 2000).

Table 1 Naming Convention for the Nine Known Subtypes of the Mammalian Voltage-Gated Sodium Channels

Channel	Previous Name(s)	Genes
$Na_V1.1$	Brain type I	*SCN1A*
$Na_V1.2$	Brain type II	*SCN2A*
$Na_V1.3$	Brain type III	*SCN3A*
$Na_V1.4$	SkM1, μ1	*SCN4A*
$Na_V1.5$	h1, SkM2	*SCN5A*
$Na_V1.6$	Brain type VI, Na6	*SCN8A*
$Na_V1.7$	PN1, hNE, NaS	*SCN9A*
$Na_V1.8$	SNS, PN3	*SCN10A*
$Na_V1.9$	SNS2, NaN	*SCN11A*

hNE, human neuroendocrine; *NaN*, novel Na channel; *PN1*, peripheral nerve type 1; *PN3*, peripheral nerve type 3; *SNS*, sensory nerve specific; *SNS2*, sensory nerve specific 2.

Early functional classification based on the sensitivity to block by tetrodotoxin (TTX), a neurotoxin isolated from puffer-fish, has been retained (Narahashi, 1972, 1977). Specifically, Na_V isoforms that respond to low nanomolar concentrations of TTX (Na_V1.1, 1.2, 1.3, 1.4, 1.6, and 1.7) are characterized as TTX-sensitive (TTX-S), while those that require micromolar concentrations of TTX for significant inhibition (Na_V1.5, 1.8, and 1.9) are classified as TTX-resistant (TTX-R) (Kostyuk, Veselovsky, & Tsyndrenko, 1981; Roy & Narahashi, 1992). Importantly, Na_V isoforms are present in distinct populations across different tissues, including both excitable and nonexcitable cells (Table 2), where they perform critical roles in mammalian physiology. In nonexcitable cells and tissue that are not capable of producing an action potential, such as in astrocytes (Barres, Chun, & Corey, 1989;

Table 2 Distribution of Na_V Subtypes in Excitable and Nonexcitable Cells

Type	TTX Sensitivity	Primary Tissue	Nonexcitable Tissue	Channelopathies
Na_V1.1	**S**	CNS neurons	Microglia	Epilepsy, migraine
Na_V1.2	**S**	CNS neurons	Islet β-cells osteoblasts Schwann cells	Epilepsy
Na_V1.3	**S**	CNS neurons	Islet β-cells	Epilepsy
Na_V1.4	**S**	Skeletal muscle	Cancer cells	Myotonia, periodic paralysis
Na_V1.5	**R**	Uninnervated skeletal muscle, Heart	Macrophages Microglia Astrocytes Cancer cells	Cardiac arrhythmias
Na_V1.6	**S**	CNS neurons	Macrophages Astrocytes Cancer cells	Epilepsy, movement disorders
Na_V1.7	**S**	PNS neurons	Dendritic cell Cancer cells	Altered pain sensitivity
Na_V1.8	**R**	PNS neurons	Keratinocytes	Altered pain sensitivity
Na_V1.9	**R**	PNS neurons	Müller glia	Altered pain sensitivity

CNS, central nervous system; PNS, peripheral nervous system.

Barres, Chun, & Corey, 1988; Sontheimer, Black, Ransom, & Waxman, 1992; Sontheimer & Waxman, 1992), microglia (Black, Liu, & Waxman, 2009; Korotzer & Cotman, 1992; Nicholson & Randall, 2009), islet β-cells (Barnett, Pressel, & Misler, 1995; Donatsch, Lowe, Richardson, & Taylor, 1977; Eberhardson & Grapengiesser, 1999), Müller glia (Linnertz et al., 2011; O'Brien et al., 2008), osteoblasts (Black, Westenbroek, Catterall, & Waxman, 1995), Schwann cells (Chiu, Schrager, & Ritchie, 1984; Schaller, Krzemien, Yarowsky, Krueger, & Caldwell, 1995), cancer cells (Brackenbury & Djamgoz, 2006; Diss, Archer, Hirano, Fraser, & Djamgoz, 2001), macrophages (Carrithers et al., 2009, 2007), dendritic cells (Zsiros et al., 2009), and keratinocytes (Zhao et al., 2008), Na_Vs play a role in cell migration, proliferation (Yang et al., 2012), and metastasis (Fraser et al., 2005; Martin, Ufodiama, Watt, Bland, & Brackenbury, 2015). In contrast, in excitable cells, Na_Vs are crucial for regulating excitability and action potential firing. Accordingly, gain- and loss-of-function mutations in individual Na_V isoforms are causally associated with a number of diseases or "channelopathies," including epilepsy, migraine, myotonia, periodic paralysis, cardiac arrhythmias, and altered pain sensitivity (Table 2).

1.4.1 Na_V1.1

Na_V1.1, formerly known as the brain type I channel, which is encoded by the SCN1A gene, is highly expressed throughout the central and peripheral nervous system (PNS), including in predominantly large dorsal root ganglion neurons from which myelinated peripheral fibers arise. In the central nervous system, Na_V1.1 is expressed in both cell bodies and projections of retinal ganglion cells, dentate granule cells, cerebellar Purkinje cells, and pyramidal cells in the hippocampus (Van Wart, Trimmer, & Matthews, 2007). Na_V1.1 is also expressed in spinal cord neurons, including 80% of motor neurons, where its subcellular location complements Na_V1.6 expression more proximally to the axon initial segment. Notably, Na_V1.1 is also highly expressed in inhibitory GABAergic interneurons, causing seemingly paradoxical global hyperexcitability as a result of Na_V1.1 loss-of-function mutations (Cheah et al., 2012). Accordingly, Na_V1.1 channelopathies lead to seizures, which range from a spectrum of mild familial febrile epilepsy with partial loss-of-function mutations to devastating epileptic conditions such as Dravet syndrome or generalized epilepsy with febrile seizures with more serious phenotypes (Claes et al., 2001; Escayg et al., 2000; Mantegazza et al., 2005).

1.4.2 $Na_V1.2$

$Na_V1.2$, previously known as the brain type II channel, is the most abundantly expressed Na_V isoform in the brain, where it is located predominantly in axons of neurons in the cortex, thalamus, global pallidus, hippocampus, and cerebellar Purkinje, as well as granule cells (Westenbroek, Merrick, & Catterall, 1989). During development, $Na_V1.2$ is progressively replaced by $Na_V1.6$ in myelinated neurons and in particular at the nodes of Ranvier, with $Na_V1.2$ expression in adults seen predominantly in unmyelinated neurons (Boiko et al., 2001; Kaplan et al., 2001). Like $Na_V1.1$, mutations in $Na_V1.2$ are associated with seizures, albeit the correlation between functional effects on channel gating with clinical phenotypes is less clear than for $Na_V1.1$ (Heron et al., 2002; Misra, Kahlig, & George, 2008; Sugawara et al., 2001).

1.4.3 $Na_V1.3$

$Na_V1.3$ is present at high levels in embryonic rodent primary sensory neurons, but only at low levels in adults (Waxman, Kocsis, & Black, 1994). Interestingly, expression of $Na_V1.3$ returns in adult primary sensory neurons after axotomy, suggesting that the channel contributes to the pathogenesis of neuropathic pain (Berta et al., 2008; Dib-Hajj et al., 1999; Fukuoka et al., 2008; Waxman et al., 1994). Knockdown of $Na_V1.3$ by antisense oligodeoxynucleotide attenuates mechanical allodynia in the chronic constriction injury (CCI) model but not in the spared nerve injury model (Hains, Saab, Klein, Craner, & Waxman, 2004; Lindia, Kohler, Martin, & Abbadie, 2005). Similar results are seen in global $Na_V1.3^{-/-}$ mice, which develop neuropathic pain normally following spinal nerve transection, but development of cold and mechanical allodynia is attenuated in CCI (Minett et al., 2014; Nassar et al., 2006). Thus, there are conflicting results regarding the role of $Na_V1.3$ in neuropathic pain, and selective $Na_V1.3$ inhibitors are required to further examine contribution of the channel in different pathological pain states.

1.4.4 $Na_V1.4$

$Na_V1.4$ is highly expressed in skeletal muscle, representing more than 90% of Na_V channels in adult muscle tissue, and is a key for initiation and propagation of action potentials that regulate skeletal muscle contractility. Specifically, $Na_V1.4$, encoded by SCN4A, mediates sarcolemmal action potentials arising from endplate potentials and also contributes to the spread of depolarizations along the membranes of the T-tubules (Simkin & Bendahhou, 2011). Consistent with its important physiological role in skeletal muscle contraction, mutations in $Na_V1.4$ are associated with at least five hereditary channelopathies, including hyperkalemic periodic paralysis, hypokalemic periodic paralysis, paramyotonia congenita, potassium-aggravated myotonia, and congenital myasthenic syndrome (Jurkat-Rott, Holzherr, Fauler, & Lehmann-Horn, 2010).

1.4.5 $Na_V1.5$

$Na_V1.5$, encoded by SCN5A, is typically considered a cardiac-specific isoform and represents the majority of channels in adult cardiomyocytes. Consistent with a key role in surface conduction and intermyocyte transmission, $Na_V1.5$ is expressed at the cell surface including, in particular, high-density expression at intercalated discs, but not in the transverse tubular system (Westenbroek et al., 2013). Befitting this expression pattern, $Na_V1.5$ is intimately involved in cardiac action potential conduction and accordingly, mutations are associated with cardiac arrhythmias including Long QT syndrome type 3, Brugada syndrome, cardiac conduction disease, dilated cardiomyopathy, and sick sinus node syndrome (Liu, Yang, & Dudley, 2016). The diversity of these conditions is attributable to the varied effects on the biophysical characteristics of mutant $Na_V1.5$ channels, which may lead to altered conduction velocity, impulse propagation, and action potential duration. However, as comorbidities and factors such as age, gender, and temperature can influence the clinical presentation, genotype–phenotype associations are not always clear.

1.4.6 $Na_V1.6$

The $Na_V1.6$ isoform, encoded by SCN8A, was originally discovered in the rat central and peripheral nervous systems where it is widely expressed in different cell types including Purkinje cells, motor neurons, pyramidal, and granule neurons, as well as glial and Schwann cells (Schaller et al., 1995). Moreover, $Na_V1.6$ is highly localized at the nodes of Ranvier, the gaps between the myelin sheath which allow for saltatory conduction (Hille, 2001). Therefore, in the PNS, the highest level of expression of $Na_V1.6$ is in myelinated A-fibers (Fukuoka et al., 2008), although emerging evidence indicates that $Na_V1.6$ is also expressed in peripherin-positive unmyelinated fibers (Black, Renganathan, & Waxman, 2002). Several human conditions associated with $Na_V1.6$ mutations have been described, including cases presenting with cerebellar atrophy, ataxia, intellectual disability, dyskinesia, epileptic encephalopathy; as well as trigeminal neuralgia (Fung, Kwok, & Tsui, 2015; Gardella et al., 2016; Tanaka et al., 2016;

Trudeau, Dalton, Day, Ranum, & Meisler, 2006; Veeramah et al., 2012). In mice, a naturally occurring $Na_V1.6$ splice variant leading to nonfunctional protein expression leads to a neurological disorder known as "motor endplate disease" (Burgess et al., 1995), which has provided crucial insight into the physiological role of $Na_V1.6$. The phenotype of these animals characterized by cerebellar ataxia and muscle atrophy due to the loss of excitatory innervation to the muscle leading to juvenile death (Kohrman et al., 1995), has in particular highlighted an important contribution to the resurgent current of Purkinje neurons (Raman, Sprunger, Meisler, & Bean, 1997).

1.4.7 $Na_V1.7$

$Na_V1.7$ (SCN9A) is preferentially expressed in the PNS, specifically in sympathetic ganglia and in both small and large sensory neurons (Sangameswaran et al., 1997; Toledo-Aral et al., 1997). Human genetic data provide compelling evidence for a role of $Na_V1.7$ in pain. Loss-of-function mutations of SCN9A, the gene encoding $Na_V1.7$, have been identified as the cause of congenital insensitivity to pain, a rare condition characterized by the inability to sense pain in otherwise normal individuals (Cox et al., 2006; Goldberg et al., 2007). In contrast, gain-of-function mutations of SCN9A are the cause of two hereditary pain disorders, inherited erythromelalgia and paroxysmal extreme pain disorder, which are associated with redness, swelling, and burning pain (Drenth et al., 2001; Fertleman et al., 2006; Yang et al., 2004). Accordingly, subtype-selective $Na_V1.7$ inhibitors are highly sought after as particularly promising analgesics.

1.4.8 $Na_V1.8$

The TTX-R $Na_V1.8$ (SCN10A), like $Na_V1.7$, is primarily expressed on small, unmyelinated peripheral sensory neurons, most of which are nociceptors (Akopian, Sivilotti, & Wood, 1996; Amaya et al., 2000; Djouhri et al., 2003). Consistent with this expression pattern, as well as biophysical characteristics—including depolarized activation, slow inactivation, and rapid recovery from inactivation—that position $Na_V1.8$ as a mediator of rapid, sustained firing, this channel plays an important role in pain and nociception. In recent years, a number of $Na_V1.8$ gain-of-function mutations leading to painful small fiber neuropathy have been described (Dabby et al., 2016; Faber et al., 2012; Garrison, Weyer, Barabas, Beutler, & Stucky, 2014; Han et al., 2014). Accordingly, selective $Na_V1.8$ inhibitors are being investigated as analgesics.

1.4.9 $Na_V1.9$

$Na_V1.9$ (SCN11A), another sensory neuron-specific isoform, is among the least-studied Na_V isoforms, in part because difficulties with heterologous expression have limited studies in overexpressing cell lines (Goral, Leipold, Nematian-Ardestani, & Heinemann, 2015). $Na_V1.9$ is characterized by unique biophysical properties including ultraslow inactivation (>100 ms) compared to TTXs Na_V channels (<5 ms) and activation at hyperpolarized membrane potentials (Dib-Hajj, Yang, Black, & Waxman, 2013). The resulting TTX-R persistent current, while too slow to contribute significantly to the upstroke of an action potential, modulates membrane excitability and thus regulates neuronal firing. Despite a lack of selective $Na_V1.9$ inhibitors, genetic studies provide evidence for a clear role in nociception, with altered pain behaviors reported in $Na_V1.9$ knockout mice as well as humans with gain- and loss-of-function mutations (Huang et al., 2014; Leo, D'Hooge, & Meert, 2010).

1.5 Pharmacology of Venom Peptides Acting at Na_V Channels

The critical contribution of Na_V channels to cellular excitability underpins their role in many essential physiological processes including neuromuscular and cardiac function. As Na_V channels are conserved across many phyla, it is not surprising that evolution of Na_V-targeting venom peptides has occurred in many species, including scorpions, cone snails, spiders, anemones, and snakes.

Venom-derived peptides exert diverse effects on Na_V channel function, including inhibitory effects that are mediated via physical occlusion of the pore or impairing the movement of voltage sensors that occurs during activation; as well as excitatory effects resulting from enhanced activation or impaired inactivation (Table 3). The consequences of these effects on the biophysical properties of Na_V channels are summarized in Fig. 2. These effects invariably lead to a loss of coordinated membrane excitability, thus conferring a key defensive and predatory advantage to these venomous animals. Naming conventions for conotoxins, theraphotoxins, and hexatoxins use the μ-prefix to denote toxins that lead to functional channel inhibition, while the δ-prefix is associated with peptides that lead to a net "activator" effect. In contrast, scorpion toxins are typically denoted as α- or β-toxins depending on whether they predominantly affect channel inactivation or activation, respectively. Structurally, venom-derived Na_V modulators are highly diverse and include relatively small (~20 amino acid) conotoxins

Table 3 Na_V Channel Modulators, Their Binding Site, Structure, and Mechanism of Action

Molecule	Source	Site	Na_V Domain	Class	Mechanism	References
Inhibitors						
Tetrodotoxin, saxitoxin	Bacteria	1	Pore	Small molecule	Pore blocker	Terlau et al. (1991)
Local anesthetics	Synthetic	9	Pore	Small molecule	Pore blocker	Ragsdale, McPhee, Scheuer, and Catterall (1994)
μ-Conotoxins	Cone snails	1	Pore	Peptide (~20–25 aa)	Pore blocker	Stephan, Potts, and Agnew (1994) and Yanagawa, Abe, and Satake (1986)
μ/β-Therapho-/cteni-/thornitoxins toxins	Spiders	3 and/or 4	DIV S3–4 DII S3–4	Peptide (~30–35 aa)	Trap channel in closed state. Some toxins also shift voltage dependence of activation	Bosmans and Swartz (2010)
μO-conotoxins	Cone snails	4	DII S3–4	Peptide (31–32 aa)	Trap channel in closed state	Leipold et al. (2007)
μO§ GVIIJ	Cone snails	8	DII S5	Peptide (35 aa)	Inhibits peak current. Mechanism unknown	Gajewiak et al. (2014)
Activators						
Veratridine, grayanotoxin, aconitine	Plants	2	DI S6, DIV S6	Small molecule	Delayed inactivation, hyperpolarizing shift in voltage dependence of activation	Logan, Toma, Thomas-Tran, and Du Bois (2016) and Wang and Wang (2003)
δ-Conotoxins	Cone snails	6	DIV S3–4	Peptide (~30–35 aa)	Delayed inactivation	Fainzilber, Kofman, Zlotkin, and Gordon (1994)

Continued

Table 3 Na_V Channel Modulators, Their Binding Site, Structure, and Mechanism of Action—cont'd

Molecule	Source	Site	Na_V Domain	Class	Mechanism	References
α-Scorpion toxins	Scorpions	3	DI S5–6, DIV S1–2, DIV S3–4	Peptide (~60–70 aa)	Delayed inactivation	Rogers, Qu, Tanada, Scheuer, and Catterall (1996) and Wang et al. (2011)
Anemone toxins	Anemones	3	DIV S3–4	Peptide (~27–54 aa)	Delayed inactivation	Rogers et al. (1996)
β-Scorpion toxins	Scorpions	4	DII S1–2, DII S3–4, DIII S5–6	Peptide (~60–70 aa)	Hyperpolarizing shift in voltage dependence of activation	Cestele et al. (1998) and Cohen et al. (2007)
δ-Therapo-/hexatoxins	Spiders	3	DIV S1–2, DIV S3–4	Peptide (~30–42 aa)	Delayed inactivation	Bosmans and Swartz (2010) and Osteen et al. (2016)
Brevetoxin, ciguatoxin	Dinoflagellates	5	DI S6, DIV S5	Polyethers	Delayed inactivation, hyperpolarizing shift in voltage dependence of activation	Strachan, Lewis, and Nicholson (1999) and Trainer, Baden, and Catterall (1994)
Pyrethroids	Synthetic	7	DII S6, DIII S6	Small molecule	Delayed inactivation, hyperpolarizing shift in voltage dependence of activation	Tan et al. (2005)
Batrachotoxin	Frog	2	DI S6, DII S6, DIII S6, DIV S6	Small molecule	Delayed inactivation, hyperpolarizing shift in voltage dependence of activation	Linford, Cantrell, Qu, Scheuer, and Catterall (1998)
δ-Calliotoxin	Snake	?	?	Three-finger toxin (~80 aa)	Delayed inactivation, hyperpolarizing shift in voltage dependence of activation	Yang et al. (2016)

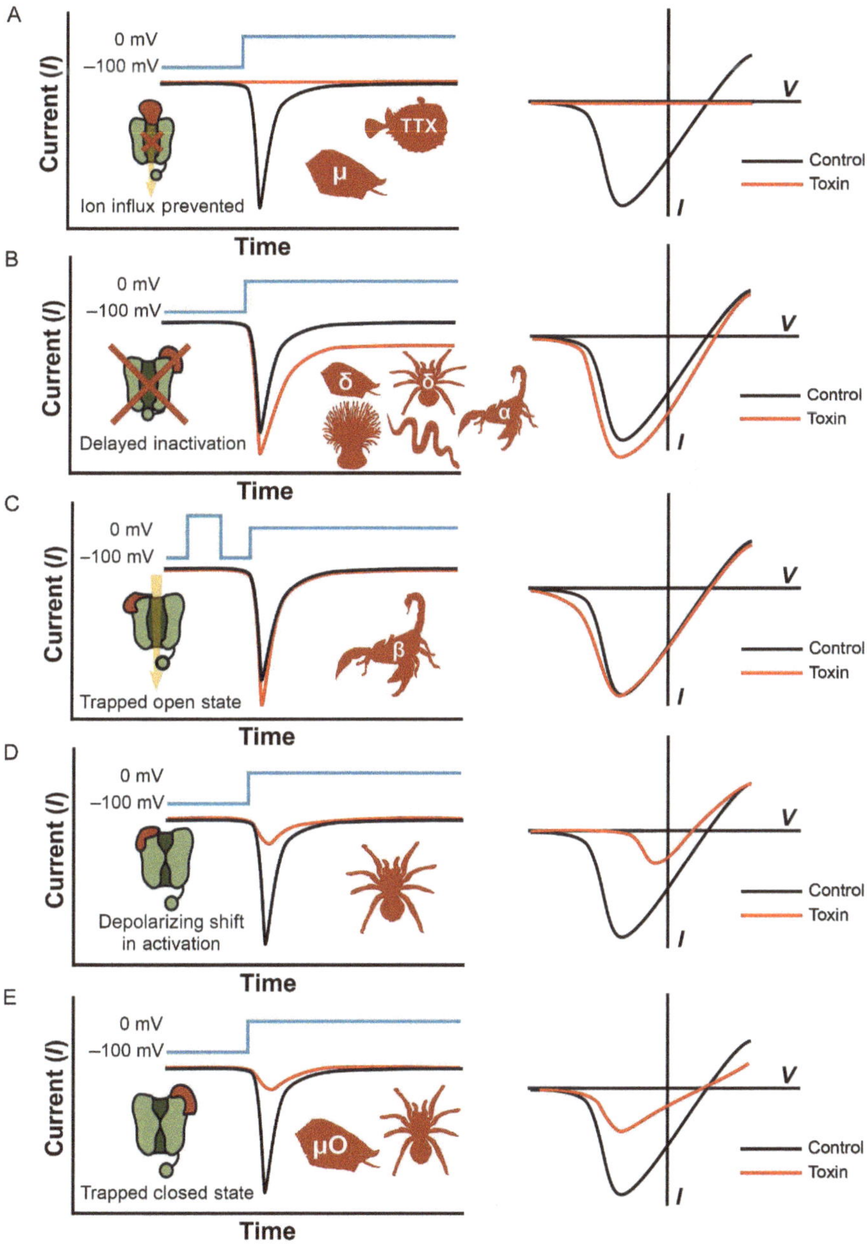

Fig. 2 Schematic diagrams representing the common effects toxins have on the biophysical properties of Na_V channels. *Left panels* represent current–time plots. *Right panels* represent current–voltage (*I*–*V*) curves. Toxin effects are representative of an EC_{100} concentration. (A) Pore blockers, including the guanidinium neurotoxin TTX and *(Continued)*

stabilized by 3 disulfide bonds, large (>50 amino acid) peptides stabilized by an inhibitory cysteine knot, and even three-finger toxins in the case of the newly described snake venom-derived δ-calliotoxin.

To define the pharmacological activity of these molecules, a steadily increasing number of defined binding sites—currently nine (Table 3)—have been proposed. However, it is becoming increasingly clear that there is significant overlap between sites and that the boundaries of these presumed distinct binding pockets are both poorly defined and can be occupied simultaneously by a single molecule. For example, toxins from the Agelenidae spider family, denoted β/δ-agatoxins, exert effects consistent with interaction with both sites 3 and 4, opposing the classical concept of single site binding (Billen, Vassilevski, et al., 2010). Similarly, although the binding site of δ-calliotoxin remains to be defined, pharmacologically it combines features of both α- and β-scorpion toxins as it affects Na_V activation as well as inactivation, as do some α/β-scorpion toxins such as OD1 (Durek et al., 2013; Yang et al., 2016). As an additional confounding factor, the effects of venom peptides on Na_V function can be subtype-specific (Durek et al., 2013), making distinction of binding sites, appropriate nomenclature, and generalization of functional effects difficult. There are also a number of Na_V modulators, including the μO-conotoxins, B-toxins from the ribbon worm *Cerebratulus lacteus*; meroditerpenoids from brown algae, clathrodin, and dibromosceptrin from sponges of the genus *Agelas*; jamaicamides from *Lyngbya majuscule*; and ostreotoxin-3 from *Ostreopsis lenticularis*, with poorly defined binding sites. For these reasons, we categorize all venom peptides based on their mechanism of action at Na_V channels rather than proposed binding sites in this review.

The diversity of the effects of venom peptides on Na_V function arises at least in part from their complex structures and comparatively large size,

Fig. 2—Cont'd the μ-conotoxins, inhibit Na^+ current by physically occluding the pore of Na_V channels. (B) Toxins that delay fast inactivation include δ-conotoxins, δ-spider toxins, sea anemone toxins, α-scorpion toxins, and the new described snake toxin δ-calliotoxin, all with differing effects on peak current. The schematic diagram illustrates the effect of the α-scorpion toxin OD1. (C) β-Scorpion toxins have different effects on peak current, but generally cause a hyperpolarizing shift in the voltage dependence of activation. The schematic diagram illustrates the effect of the β-scorpion toxin Css-IV. (D) Some spider peptides (including ProTx-II) inhibit peak current by shifting the voltage dependence of activation to more depolarized potentials, with some residual current at more depolarized potentials. (E) μO-conotoxins and some spider peptides are believed to trap the voltage sensors in the closed state, inhibiting peak current without shifting the voltage dependence of activation.

which leads to interaction with many more residues of the Na_V channel than is typically achievable by small molecules. Accordingly, venom peptides often achieve exquisite potency and selectivity, making them important tool compounds and drug leads. High subtype selectivity in particular has remained largely elusive for small molecules, making venom peptides crucial pharmacological tools to delineate the physiological and pathological role(s) of mammalian Na_V isoforms. While significant insights have been obtained from gain- and loss-of-function mutations and inherited channelopathies, the value of highly subtype-selective pharmacological tools is particularly apparent for isoforms where global gene deletion lead to premature death, such as $Na_V1.1$, $Na_V1.2$, $Na_V1.4$, $Na_V1.5$, and $Na_V1.6$ (Burgess et al., 1995; Cheah et al., 2012; Papadatos et al., 2002; Planells-Cases et al., 2000).

1.5.1 Pore Blockers

1.5.1.1 Guanidinium Neurotoxins

The guanidinium neurotoxin TTX has been an indispensable tool for the study of Na_V channel function for decades, and no review of Na_V toxin pharmacology would be complete without its inclusion. It is named for the *Tetraodontidae*, the puffer-fish family, in the flesh of which it can be found at high concentrations. However, TTX is not produced by these animals, but accumulates in organs including the ovaries, liver, skin, intestine, and muscle as a result of contamination of the food chain with this bacterial toxin (Simidu, Noguchi, Hwang, Shida, & Hashimoto, 1987). Accordingly, TTX can also be found in many other unrelated species including the blue ringed octopus, frogs, molluscs, and lizards (Chau, Kalaitzis, & Neilan, 2011). Similarly, the related nonpeptide marine toxin saxitoxin (STX), found in clams and mussels, is produced by microorganisms that are ingested by shellfish (Hackett et al., 2013).

TTX and STX both inhibit Na_V channels by binding to site 1, one of the most-studied and best-defined sites, which is formed by the two rings of amino acids that form the ion selectivity filter (Cestele & Catterall, 2000; Terlau et al., 1991). Specifically, mutation of one residue (analogous to Y371 in $Na_V1.6$)—a tyrosine or phenylalanine in $Na_V1.1$, 1.2, 1.3, 1.4, 1.6, and 1.7 and a cysteine in $Na_V1.5$—to the serine found in $Na_V1.8$ and $Na_V1.9$ recapitulates the TTX-R pharmacology of these subtypes (Kuo, Chen, & Yang, 2004; Leffler, Herzog, Dib-Hajj, Waxman, & Cummins, 2005). Binding of the guanidinium toxins to this site leads to pore block by physically occluding the intracellular influx of Na^+ ions (Fig. 2A). However, by taking advantage of interactions with additional residues, differential effects even on TTX-S isoforms are possible. For instance, STX is several hundred fold less potent at human $Na_V1.7$ than the rodent analog or human $Na_V1.4$, due to the presence of T1398 and I1399 in the pore loop of domain III of human $Na_V1.7$ (Table 4) (Walker et al., 2012). In contrast, an acetylated STX analog potently inhibits human $Na_V1.7$ (Thomas-Tran & Du Bois, 2016). Similarly improved pharmacology may also be achievable for TTX analogs, with 4,9-anhydro-TTX reported to be a $Na_V1.6$-selective inhibitor (Table 4) (Rosker et al., 2007).

1.5.1.2 μ-Conotoxins

μ-Conotoxins are able to inhibit the binding of TTX, suggesting that they also bind to site 1 and act as pore blockers (Yanagawa et al., 1986). However, the comparatively larger size of the μ-conotoxins—typically comprising 16–26 residues stabilized by three intramolecular disulfide bonds—significantly increases the points of interaction with the channel. Accordingly, the currently accepted view places the μ-conotoxin binding site in an overlapping but nonidentical area of site 1, with these larger toxins occluding the ion-conducting pore more superficially than TTX and STX (Stephan et al., 1994). Indeed, μ-conotoxins likely interact with the Na_V pore like an inverted pyramid that is tilted off-center, leading to incomplete steric occlusion of the pore (Hui, Lipkind, Fozzard, & French, 2002). Consistent with this view, residual Na^+ influx in the presence of bound μ-conotoxin has been observed, albeit not for all toxins (Korkosh, Zhorov, & Tikhonov, 2014; Zhang et al., 2010, 2009). Multiple charged residues of the μ-conotoxin facilitate interaction with key amino acids of the Na_V channel, including residues in the domain II pore loop, pore loop S6 linker, and S5 pore loop linker (Chang, French, Lipkind, Fozzard, & Dudley, 1998; Li et al., 2001, 2003). Interestingly, residues in the domain II S5–S6 linker also contribute to species selectivity observed with some μ-conotoxins, including the approximately 30-fold reduced affinity of GIIIA for human $Na_V1.4$ channels compared with the rat skeletal muscle isoform (Chahine, Bennett, George, & Horn, 1994; Cummins, Aglieco, & Dib-Hajj, 2002). The μ-conotoxins are typically most potent at either the neuronal isoform $Na_V1.2$ or the skeletal muscle isoform $Na_V1.4$ (Lewis, Dutertre, Vetter, & Christie, 2012; Wilson, Yoshikami, et al., 2011); however, the pharmacological activity at other mammalian Na_V isoforms has been systematically characterized for only a few peptides. These studies revealed additional surprising subtype selectivity—including differential activity at $Na_V1.1$, $Na_V1.3$, $Na_V1.6$, and $Na_V1.7$—for GIIIA, TIIIA, SIIIA, KIIIA, MIIIA,

Table 4 Potency of Selected Guanidinium Neurotoxins at $Na_V1.1–1.8$

Toxin	Mechanism of Action	$Na_V1.1$	$Na_V1.2$	$Na_V1.3$	$Na_V1.4$	$Na_V1.5$	$Na_V1.6$	$Na_V1.7$	$Na_V1.8$	References
TTX	Pore blocker	6 nM	8 nM	2 nM	5 nM	2 μM	4 nM	6 nM	60 μM	Akopian et al. (1996), Clare, Tate, Nobbs, and Romanos (2000), and Rosker et al. (2007)
4,9-Anhydro-TTX	Pore blocker	n.d	1 μM	341 nM	988 nM	79 μM	8 nM	1 μM	>30 μM	Rosker et al. (2007)
STX	Pore blocker	n.d	1 nM	n.d	3 nM	149 μM	n.d	702 nM	11 μM	Penzotti, Fozzard, Lipkind, and Dudley (1998), Terlau et al. (1991), Walker et al. (2012), and Wilson, Zhang, et al. (2011)
C13-OAc STX	Pore blocker	n.d	32 nM	n.d	83 nM	5 μM	n.d	19 nM	n.d	Thomas-Tran and Du Bois (2016)

The Na_V subtype that each toxin is most potent at and any subtype with less than 10-fold selectivity is highlighted in gray.

and BuIIIA, making these peptides suitable as tool compounds to dissect contribution of individual isoforms to neuronal excitability (Table 5) (Wilson, Yoshikami, et al., 2011). However, activity at $Na_V1.7$, one of the main isoforms contributing to excitability of nociceptive sensory neurons, is generally weak, making the μ-conotoxins relatively poor analgesic drug leads. Given the overlapping binding site with TTX, lack of activity at recombinantly expressed $Na_V1.8$ is perhaps not surprising, although some μ-conotoxins do act at TTX-R amphibian isoforms. Activity at $Na_V1.9$ has not been assessed, but given absence of effects on TTX-R currents in mammalian sensory neurons, μ-conotoxins likely have little activity at this isoform.

It is particularly noteworthy that when expressed in oocytes, binding affinities, and kinetics of the μ-conotoxins at Na_V isoforms is also affected by the presence of auxiliary β subunits (Zhang et al., 2013). In the most extreme case, coexpression of the β4 instead of the β1 or β3 subunit increased k_{on} of SmIIIA at $Na_V1.1$ several hundredfold (Zhang et al., 2013). While these complexities make interpretation of the effects of the μ-conotoxins in native cells difficult, they also offer the opportunity for pharmacological dissection of the native stoichiometry of Na_V as well as the contribution of individual isoforms to the physiology of excitable cells.

1.5.2 Gating Modifiers

1.5.2.1 α-Scorpion Toxins

Scorpion toxins acting at Na_V channels have been broadly categorized according to the biophysical effects on channel gating: the α-scorpion toxins, acting at site 3 which involves residues in the domain IV voltage sensor, predominantly affect inactivation, while the β-scorpion toxins, acting at site 4 which is located near the domain II voltage sensor, affect channel activation.

Classical α-scorpion toxins appear to stabilize an open configuration of the Na_V channel from which inactivation can only proceed slowly (Fig. 2B), presumably by preventing the full outward movement of the domain IV S4 voltage sensor, which is not required for channel activation, but which precedes channel inactivation (Campos, Chanda, Beirao, & Bezanilla, 2008). Accordingly, binding of α-scorpion toxins is voltage-dependent and can be displaced by strong depolarizations as well as mutations of residues in the domain IV S1–S2 and S3–S4 linkers and domain I S5–S6 linker (Catterall, 1977; Rogers et al., 1996; Wang et al., 2011). This results in persistent, noninactivating currents that prolong action potentials and impairs

Table 5 Affinities of Selected μ-Conotoxins (IC_{50} or K_d) at $Na_V1.1$–1.8

Toxin	Mechanism of Action	$Na_V1.1$	$Na_V1.2$	$Na_V1.3$	$Na_V1.4$	$Na_V1.5$	$Na_V1.6$	$Na_V1.7$	$Na_V1.8$	References
GIIIA	Pore blocker	0.26 μM	18 μM	>100 μM	0.02 μM	>100 μM	0.68 μM	>100 μM	>100 μM	Wilson, Yoshikami, et al. (2011)
TIIIA	Pore blocker	0.9 μM	0.045 μM	8 μM	0.005 μM	>100 μM	25 μM	>100 μM	>100 μM	Wilson, Yoshikami, et al. (2011)
SIIIA	Pore blocker	11 μM	0.05 μM	11 μM	0.13 μM	>100 μM	0.76 μM	65 μM	>100 μM	Wilson, Yoshikami, et al. (2011) and Yao et al. (2008)
KIIIA	Pore blocker	0.29 μM	0.003 μM	8 μM	0.09 μM	>100 μM	0.24 μM	0.29 μM	>100 μM	Wilson, Yoshikami, et al. (2011) and Zhang et al. (2007)
MIIIA	Pore blocker	23 μM	0.45 μM	8 μM	0.33 μM	>100 μM	22 μM	97 μM	>100 μM	Wilson, Yoshikami, et al. (2011)
BuIIIA	Pore blocker	0.35 μM	0.012 μM	0.35 μM	0.012 μM	14 μM	4 μM	>100 μM	>100 μM	Holford et al. (2009) and Wilson, Yoshikami, et al. (2011)

The Na_V subtype that each toxin is most potent at and any subtype with less than 10-fold selectivity is highlighted in gray.

coordinated neuronal activity, causing spastic paralysis and death of envenomed predators or prey.

However, α-scorpion toxins that also affect voltage dependence of activation in a concentration- and Na_V subtype-specific manner have been described, blurring the pharmacological distinction from β-scorpion toxins. For example, OD1 from the yellow Iranian scorpion *Odonthobuthus doriae* has predominant effects on inactivation at $Na_V1.7$ consistent with its classification as an α-scorpion toxin, but it also affects the voltage dependence of activation at $Na_V1.4$, $Na_V1.6$, and $Na_V1.7$ at higher concentrations (Deuis, Wingerd, et al., 2016; Durek et al., 2013). Nonetheless, the high subtype selectivity of OD1 for $Na_V1.7$ has been utilized to establish an in vivo target engagement assay for the development of putative analgesic $Na_V1.7$ inhibitors (Deuis, Wingerd, et al., 2016).

α-Scorpion toxins were additionally distinguished based on their activity at mammalian and insect Na_V channels, with classical Old World scorpion toxins such as AaHII and Lqh2 acting only at mammalian but not insect Na_V homologues, insect-selective toxins such as LqhαIT and Lqq3 exerting effects mainly on insect but not mammalian Na_V isoforms, and toxins such as BmKM1 and Lqh3 displaying effects at both insect and mammalian channels (Bosmans & Tytgat, 2007b). However, most early pharmacological studies were carried out using either rodent brain preparations or evaluated the effects of α-scorpion toxins after intracerebroventricular injection in rodents, with few studies systematically evaluating effects at heterologously expressed insect and mammalian Na_V isoforms (Table 6). Drawing these functional classifications into question are observations that some toxins, such as Lqh VI and Lqh VII, delay inactivation of muscular $rNa_V1.4$ and $hNa_V1.5$ but not neuronal $rNa_V1.2A$ channels expressed in *Xenopus* oocytes (Hamon et al., 2002).

In addition, differential effects of α-scorpion toxins at locust and cockroach Na_V homologues suggest that activity at "insect" channels may not be generalizable (Gilles et al., 2000) and that activity at specific insect and mammalian Na_V isoforms may represent a continuum of poorly understood subtype selectivity. Thus, we propose that classification based on species selectivity needs to be revisited once comprehensive pharmacological characterization at mammalian (including, where possible, rodent, and human isoforms) and different insect Na_V channels (including isoforms from drosophila, cockroach, housefly, and arachnids) has been carried out for a greater number of α-scorpion toxins. Comprehensive pharmacological profiling studies are particularly pertinent as differential effects at mammalian

Table 6 Potency of Selected α-Scorpion Toxins at $Na_V1.1–1.8$ and Insect $DmNa_V1$

Toxin	Mechanism of Action	$Na_V1.1$	$Na_V1.2$	$Na_V1.3$	$Na_V1.4$	$Na_V1.5$	$Na_V1.6$	$Na_V1.7$	$Na_V1.8$	$DmNa_V1$	References
OD1	Inhibits inactivation	n.d	5 μM	3 μM	10 nM	4 μM	47 nM	7 nM	>1 μM	n.d	Durek et al. (2013) and Maertens et al. (2006)
MeuNaTxα-1	Inhibits inactivation	n.d.	>1 μM	>1 μM	Inactive	Inactive	3.10 μM	>1 μM	Inactive	1.17 μM	Zhu et al. (2012)
MeuNaTxα-2	Inhibits inactivation	n.d.	Inactive	Inactive	2.2 μM	Inactive	Inactive	Inactive	Inactive	0.22 μM	Zhu et al. (2012)
MeuNaTxα-4	Inhibits inactivation	n.d.	Inactive	Inactive	Inactive	Inactive	Inactive	Inactive	Inactive	0.13 μM	Zhu et al. (2012)
MeuNaTxα-5	Inhibits inactivation	n.d.	Inactive	>2 μM	>2 μM	>2 μM	0.79 μM	>2 μM	Inactive	0.28 μM	Zhu et al. (2012)
CvIV4	Inhibits inactivation	n.d.	0.58 μM	1.31 μM	0.53 μM	23.3 μM	n.d.	1.34 μM	Inactive	n.d.	Rowe et al. (2011)
MeuNaTxα-12	Inhibits inactivation	0.91 μM	>10 μM	n.d.	>10 μM	>10 μM	>10 μM	n.d.	n.d.	19.95 μM	Zhu, Peigneur, Gao, Tytgat, and Zhu (2013)
MeuNaTxα-13	Inhibits inactivation	2.5 μM	>10 μM	n.d.	>10 μM	>10 μM	>10 μM	n.d.	n.d.	65.5 μM	Zhu et al. (2013)
Ts2	Inhibits inactivation	n.d.	Active (1 μM)	Active (1 μM)	Inactive	Active (1 μM)	Active (1 μM)	Active (1 μM)	Inactive	Inactive	Cologna et al. (2012)

The Na_V subtype that each toxin is most potent at and any subtype with less than 10-fold selectivity is highlighted in gray.

Na_V isoforms make the α-scorpion toxins useful tools to dissect the functional roles of these channels in native cells.

1.5.2.2 β-Scorpion Toxins

The family of β-scorpion toxins binds to site 4, formed by the S1–S2 and S3–S4 extracellular loops in domain II and the S5–S6 linker of domain III (Cestele et al., 1998; Cohen et al., 2007; Pedraza Escalona & Possani, 2013; Quintero-Hernandez, Jimenez-Vargas, Gurrola, Valdivia, & Possani, 2013). The binding of some β-scorpion toxins causes the voltage sensor to be trapped in the activated position—ultimately increasing channel opening probability (Campos, Chanda, Beirao, & Bezanilla, 2007; Cestele et al., 1998, 2006; Zhang et al., 2011). This experimentally manifests itself as a shift in the voltage dependence of activation of these channels, albeit complex effects on peak Na^+ conductance are also observed (Fig. 2C). Interestingly, a depolarizing prepulse is required to observe a hyperpolarizing shift in the voltage dependence of activation for some, but not all, β-scorpion toxins. The "voltage sensor trapping" model was developed using Css-IV, a β-scorpion toxin that requires a depolarizing prepulse to observe effects on channel gating. This model describes binding of β-scorpion toxins to site 4 in the resting state, with outward movement of the voltage-sensing domain during channel activation leading to high-affinity interaction with the toxin that prevents the subsequent inward movement on deactivation and effectively "traps" the voltage sensor in the activated state (Cestele et al., 1998, 2006). Cumulatively, this leads to enhancement of subsequent channel activation and repetitive action potential firing. Interestingly, experiments with Ts1 (Tsγ or Ts VII), which elicits a shift in the voltage dependence of activation independent of prepulse channel activation, confirmed that the β-scorpion toxins immobilize the domain II voltage sensor, facilitating allosteric activation of the remaining voltage sensors from domains I, III, and IV (Campos et al., 2007).

As for α-scorpion toxins, the affinity for mammalian or insect Na_V isoforms, as well as the resultant observed effects on channel gating permits hypothetical subclassification into "classical," "Tsγ-like," "excitatory insect-specific," and "depressant insect-specific" toxins (reviewed in de la Vega & Possani, 2007). However, as for the α-scorpion toxins, comprehensive pharmacological evaluation is lacking for the majority of β-scorpion toxins. Nonetheless, some interesting phylar and subtype-selective effects on Na_V function have been reported (Table 7). For example, Tf2 elicits $Na_V1.3$-selective shifts in the voltage dependence of activation (in the absence of prepulse), while Cn2, a β-scorpion toxin purified from the crude venom

Table 7 Potency of Selected β-Scorpion Toxins at $Na_V1.1–1.8$

Toxin	Mechanism of Action	$Na_V1.1$	$Na_V1.2$	$Na_V1.3$	$Na_V1.4$	$Na_V1.5$	$Na_V1.6$	$Na_V1.7$	$Na_V1.8$	References
Tf2	Causes a hyperpolarizing shift in the voltage dependence of activation	Inactive	Inactive	Active (1 μM)	Inactive	Inactive	Inactive	Inactive	Inactive	Camargos, Bosmans, Rego, Mourao, and Schwartz (2015)
Tz1	Causes a hyperpolarizing shift in the voltage dependence of activation	n.d	Inactive	n.d	active (10 μM)	Inactive	Active (10 μM)	Inactive	n.d	Leipold, Hansel, Borges, and Heinemann (2006)
Cn2	Causes a hyperpolarizing shift in the voltage dependence of activation	Inactive (300 nM)	Inactive (300 nM)	Inactive (300 nM)	Inactive (300 nM)	Inactive (300 nM)	40 nM	Inactive (300 nM)	n.d	Schiavon et al. (2006)

The Na_V subtype that each toxin is most potent at and any subtype with less than 10-fold selectivity is highlighted in gray.

of *Centruroides noxius* (Pintar, Possani, & Delepierre, 1999), causes selective effects on $Na_V1.6$, albeit only after prepulse activation (Schiavon et al., 2006). This activity has contributed to unraveling the contribution of $Na_V1.6$ to sensory neuron function, in particular relating to the development of oxaliplatin-induced cold allodynia (Deuis et al., 2013).

1.5.2.3 Sea Anemone Toxins

Toxins targeting Na_V channels are abundant in the venom of sea anemones, with more than 50 toxins identified to date (Bosmans & Tytgat, 2007a). Sea anemone toxins belong to at least two structurally distinct classes—the type I and II peptides, comprise 46–51 amino acids, have high sequence identity, and share identical disulfide connectivity, while type III peptides consist of only 27–30 amino acids with inflexible β and γ turns and are far fewer in number (Frazao, Vasconcelos, & Antunes, 2012; Moran, Gordon, & Gurevitz, 2009; Wanke, Zaharenko, Redaelli, & Schiavon, 2009). The remaining pharmacologically similar but structurally distinct Na_V activator sea anemone toxins—called calitoxin I and II—are comprised of 79 amino acids and are as yet not allocated to a separate group (Cariello et al., 1989).

Like the α-scorpion toxins, sea anemone toxins act at site 3 and cause pronounced effects on channel inactivation through similar effects on the movement of the domain IV voltage-sensing domain (Rogers et al., 1996). Accordingly, similar phylar and Na_V subtype selectivity has been reported, with some sea anemone toxins displaying selectivity for crustacean or insect Na_V channels, while others also act at mammalian isoforms (Schweitz et al., 1981). In recent years, more-detailed subtype selectivity studies at heterologously expressed mammalian Na_V isoforms have been conducted. Interestingly, ATX-II (Av2) was most selective for human $Na_V1.1$ and $Na_V1.2$ isoforms, while the related AFT-II was not only significantly less potent but also most selective for $Na_V1.4$ (Table 8) (Oliveira et al., 2004). In contrast, cangitoxin-II is most potent at $Na_V1.5$ and $Na_V1.6$, with little activity at $Na_V1.1$, 1.2, 1.3, 1.4, and 1.7 at 50 nM (Zaharenko et al., 2012). Similar preferential activity at $Na_V1.5$ was also observed for δ-Actitoxin-Bcg1a, although the subtype selectivity was relatively modest at higher concentrations (Zaharenko et al., 2012). The largely unexplored potential for subtype-selective modulation of insect and mammalian Na_V isoforms is also illustrated by CgNa, which affects the insect channel $DmNa_V1$/tipE, $Na_V1.3$, and $Na_V1.6$ with high affinity in the absence of effects at other TTX-S mammalian isoforms (Billen, Debaveye, et al., 2010). In contrast, the type III toxin Av3 preferentially

Table 8 Potency of Selected Sea Anemone Toxins at $Na_V1.1–1.8$

Toxin	Mechanism of Action	$Na_V1.1$	$Na_V1.2$	$Na_V1.3$	$Na_V1.4$	$Na_V1.5$	$Na_V1.6$	$Na_V1.7$	$Na_V1.8$	References
Bc-III	Inhibits inactivation	300 nM	1449 nM	1458 nM	821 nM	307 nM	900 nM	n.d.	n.d.	Oliveira et al. (2004)
AFT-II	Inhibits inactivation	391 nM	1998 nM	460 nM	31 nM	62.5 nM	300 nM	n.d.	n.d.	Oliveira et al. (2004)
ATX-II (Av2)	Inhibits inactivation	6 nM	8 nM	759 nM	109 nM	49 nM	180 nM	n.d.	n.d.	Oliveira et al. (2004)
CGTX-II	Inhibits inactivation	Inactive (50 nM)	Inactive (50 nM)	Inactive (50 nM)	Inactive (50 nM)	Active (50 nM)	Active (50 nM)	Inactive (50 nM)	n.d.	Zaharenko et al. (2012)
CgNa	Inhibits inactivation	Inactive	Inactive	662 nM	Inactive	3060 nM	249 nM	Inactive	n.d.	Billen, Debaveye, Beress, Garateix, and Tytgat (2010)

The Na_V subtype that each toxin is most potent at and any subtype with less than 10-fold selectivity is highlighted in gray.

affects insect channels, with only minor effects on $Na_V1.5$ (Moran et al., 2007). As for the α-scorpion toxins, the channel domains and residues contributing to these subtype-selective pharmacological effects remain to be determined, and may provide additional insight into the structural basis for activity at insect Na_V channels, which are unlikely to be a relevant prey target in the case of sea anemones.

1.5.2.4 μ/β-Spider Toxins

Spider venoms are a rich source of peptides as the venom from individual species can contain up to 1000 disulfide-bonded peptides. Given that an estimated 0.01% of peptides have been characterized, spider venom-derived toxins represent a particularly rich source of Na_V modulators (Klint et al., 2012). The nomenclature of spider toxins is homologous to that of the conotoxins, with μ-spider toxins inhibiting Na_V channels, β-spider toxins shifting the voltage dependence of activation to either more depolarized or hyperpolarized potentials (Fig. 2D and E), and δ-spider toxins delaying fast inactivation of Na_V channels (discussed later) (King, Gentz, Escoubas, & Nicholson, 2008). However, in contrast to the conotoxins, while μ-spider toxins inhibit Na_V channels, they typically act as gating modifiers rather than pore blockers by binding to sites 3 and/or site 4 (Klint et al., 2012). Recently, spider toxins that act on Na_V channels have been classed into 12 families based on sequence homology and manually curated for grouping based on residues of particular importance, with spider peptides belonging to families 1, 2, and 3 among the best-characterized Na_V inhibitors (Table 9) (Klint et al., 2012). In particular, subtype selectivity for $Na_V1.7$ has made spider peptides particularly valuable not only as pharmacological tools but also as potential drug leads. The most selective $Na_V1.7$ spider peptide described to date is β/ω-TRTX-Tp2a (ProTx-II), which inhibits $Na_V1.7$ with 87–500-fold selectivity over the other $Na_V1.2$–1.8 (Schmalhofer et al., 2008). Another notable example is ω-TRTX-Gr2a (also known as GTx1–15, GpTx-1—originally described as a $Ca_V3.1$ inhibitor), which inhibits $Na_V1.7$ with 30–500-fold selectivity over the major off-targets $Na_V1.4$, $Na_V1.5$, and $Na_V1.6$ (Deuis, Wingerd, et al., 2016; Ono et al., 2011). Unfortunately, many peptides from spider venom are promiscuous ion channel modulators, with several also affecting function of various subtypes of the voltage-gated potassium and calcium channels. This caveat can make use of these toxins as pharmacological tools, and interpretation of in vivo or in vitro effects on neuronal activity, difficult.

Table 9 Potency of Selected Spider Toxins at $Na_V1.1–1.8$

Family	Toxin	Mechanism of Action	$Na_V1.1$	$Na_V1.2$	$Na_V1.3$	$Na_V1.4$	$Na_V1.5$	$Na_V1.6$	$Na_V1.7$	$Na_V1.8$	Known Off-Targets	References
1	ω-TRTX-Gr2a (GpTx-1/ GTx1–15)	Traps channel in closed state	6 μM	5 μM	22 μM	326 μM	140 μM	17 μM	0.58 μM	68 μM	$Ca_V3.1$	Deuis, Wingerd, et al. (2016) and Ono, Kimura, and Kubo (2011)
1	μ-TRTX-Hh2a (Huwentoxin-IV)	Traps channel in closed state	n.d	150 nM	338 nM	400 nM	>10 μM	n.d	26 nM	n.d		Xiao et al. (2008)
1	β-TRTX-Ps1a (phrixotoxin 3)	Causes a depolarizing shift in the voltage dependence of activation	610 nM	0.6 nM	42 nM	288 nM	72 nM	n.d	n.d	≈2 μM		Bosmans et al. (2006)
1	μ-TRTX-Tp1a (ProTx-III)	Traps channel in closed state	0.5 μM	0.3 μM	0.9 μM	>5 μM	>5 μM	0.29 μM	0.22 μM	>5 μM		Cardoso et al. (2015)
1	μ-TRTX-Hhn2a (hainantoxin-III)	Traps channel in closed state	n.d	n.d	0.89 μM	>10 μM	>10 μM	n.d	0.15 μM	>10 μM		Liu et al. (2013) and Zhang et al. (2015)
1	μ-TRTX-Hhn1b (hainantoxin-IV)	Traps channel in closed state	n.d	36 nM	375 nM	>1 μM	>1 μM	n.d	21 nM	>10 μM		Cai et al. (2015) and Liu et al. (2003)

Continued

Table 9 Potency of Selected Spider Toxins at $Na_V1.1–1.8$—cont'd

Family	Toxin	Mechanism of Action	$Na_V1.1$	$Na_V1.2$	$Na_V1.3$	$Na_V1.4$	$Na_V1.5$	$Na_V1.6$	$Na_V1.7$	$Na_V1.8$	Known Off-Targets	References
2	β/ω-TRTX-Tp1a (ProTx-I)	Causes a depolarizing shift in the voltage dependence of activation	n.d	<730 nM	n.d	n.d	<730 nM	n.d	51 nM	27 nM	$K_V1.3$, $K_V2.1$, $Ca_V3.1$, $Ca_V3.3$	Bladen, Hamid, Souza, and Zamponi (2014) and Middleton et al. (2002)
2	μ-TRTX-Pn3a	Causes a depolarizing shift in the voltage dependence of activation	37 nM	124 nM	210 nM	144 nM	800 nM	129 nM	0.9 nM	50 μM	2 μM	Deuis et al. (2017)
3	β-TRTX-Gr1a (GrTx1)	Causes a depolarizing shift in the voltage dependence of activation	0.63 μM	0.23 μM	0.77 μM	1.3 μM	22 μM	0.63 μM	0.37 μM	n.d	$K_V11.1$	Clement et al. (2007) and Redaelli et al. (2010)
3	β/ω-TRTX-Tp2a (ProTx-II)	Causes a depolarizing shift in the voltage dependence of activation	16 nM	41 nM	102 nM	39 nM	79 nM	26 nM	0.3 nM	146 nM	$Ca_V3.1$, $Ca_V3.2$	Bladen et al. (2014), Flinspach et al. (2017), and Schmalhofer et al. (2008)

The Na_V subtype that each toxin is most potent at and any subtype with less than 10-fold selectivity is highlighted in gray.

1.5.2.5 μO-Conotoxins

The μO-conotoxins are a small family of hydrophobic peptides stabilized by an inhibitory cysteine knot motif that also cause *net* Na_V channel inhibition. However, they belong to the O- rather than M-superfamily of conotoxins and are structurally and functionally quite dissimilar from the μ-conotoxins, as exemplified by the pharmacology of MrVIA, MrVIB, and more recently, MfVIA (Deuis, Dekan, et al., 2016; Vetter et al., 2012; Wilson, Zhang, et al., 2011). Specifically, the μO-conotoxins act as gating modifiers at a poorly defined binding site that overlaps at least partially with the binding sites of the δ-conotoxins and β-scorpion toxins, as depolarization-induced relief of inhibition was mapped to the β-scorpion toxin binding site on the domain II voltage-sensor, while in binding experiments, MrVIA was able to displace δ-conotoxin TxVIA (Ekberg et al., 2006; Leipold et al., 2007). Apart from their extraordinarily high hydrophobicity, making them difficult to synthesize or express recombinantly, they are remarkable for a number of reasons. The μO-conotoxins most potently affect $Na_V1.8$, a TTX-R isoform that is affected by very few venom peptides (Table 10) (Deuis, Dekan, et al., 2016; Vetter et al., 2012). Intriguingly, despite small but significant hyperpolarizing shifts in the voltage dependence of activation, typically associated with Na_V activators, they decrease peak Na^+ current and act as analgesics in vivo (Fig. 2E) (Deuis, Dekan, et al., 2016; Ekberg et al., 2006; Vetter et al., 2012). In addition, their pharmacology is heavily influenced by the presence of auxiliary β subunits, which affects the on-rate of block in particular (Wilson, Zhang, et al., 2011). Like several μ-theraphotoxins, the μO-conotoxins also interact with lipid membranes, with mutation of two glutamic acid residues (E5/E8) in MfVIA to positively charged arginines improving lipid interactions and potency at $Na_V1.8$ (Deuis, Dekan, et al., 2016).

1.5.2.6 μO§ GVIIJ

The sole member of the newly defined μO§ conotoxins, GVIIJ (Table 11), is defined by a unique structure, binding site, and mechanism of action. The 35 amino acid peptide is, like many other Na_V modulators, stabilized by three disulfide bonds; however, a seventh S-cysteinylated cysteine residue is available for covalent modification of the Na_V channel in a novel binding site. This site, designated site 8, is located in the domain II pore region, specifically the S5 transmembrane segment (Gajewiak et al., 2014). Intriguingly, coexpression of the β2 or β4 but not β1 or β3 subunit abolished block, and mutation of a single residue, L869C, in $Na_V1.5$, improved activity more than 1000-fold (Gajewiak et al., 2014). This

Table 10 Potency of Selected μO-Conotoxins Toxins at $Na_V1.1–1.8$

Toxin	Mechanism of Action	$Na_V1.1$	$Na_V1.2$	$Na_V1.3$	$Na_V1.4$	$Na_V1.5$	$Na_V1.6$	$Na_V1.7$	$Na_V1.8$	References
MrVIB	Traps channel in closed state	n.d	≈1 μM	≈1 μM	222 nM	≈1 μM	n.d	≈1 μM	102 nM	Ekberg et al. (2006) and Zorn et al. (2006)
MfVIA	Traps channel in closed state	3 μM	6 μM	2 μM	81 nM	4 μM	5 μM	6 μM	529 nM	Vetter et al. (2012)

The Na_V subtype that each toxin is most potent at and any subtype with less than 10-fold selectivity is highlighted in gray.

Table 11 Potency of $GVIIJ_{SSG}$ at $Na_V1.1–1.8$

Toxin	Mechanism of Action	$Na_V1.1$	$Na_V1.2$	$Na_V1.3$	$Na_V1.4$	$Na_V1.5$	$Na_V1.6$	$Na_V1.7$	$Na_V1.8$	Reference
$GVIIJ_{SSG}$	Inhibits channel—mechanism unknown	11 nM	11 nM	15 nM	47 nM	207 μM	360 nM	41 nM	inactive	Gajewiak et al. (2014)

The Na_V subtype that each toxin is most potent at and any subtype with less than 10-fold selectivity is highlighted in gray.

remarkable pharmacological activity was used to determine that action potentials in A-fibers are likely mediated by $Na_V1.6$ coexpressed with the β2 or β4 subunit (Wilson et al., 2015).

1.5.2.7 ι-Conotoxins

The ι-conotoxins are also a small, poorly defined class of peptides that likely affect Na_V gating and comprise two members currently, ι-RXIA and ι-LtIIIA (Lewis et al., 2012). These peptides are structurally diverse, with the 46-residue ι-RXIA belonging to the I superfamily, while the 17-residue ι-LtIIIA belongs to the M-superfamily (Buczek et al., 2007; Jimenez et al., 2003; Wang et al., 2009). It is currently unclear whether RXIA and LtIIIA share a binding site, or even similar pharmacological activity, as LtIIIA enhances peak whole cell Na^+ current in sensory neurons (Wang et al., 2009), while RXIA affects the voltage dependence of activation at $Na_V1.6$, 1.2, and 1.7 (Fiedler et al., 2008). However, given that these peptides have no effect on channel inactivation, they are likely distinct from the δ-conotoxins discussed later.

1.5.2.8 δ-Conotoxins and δ-Toxins From Spider Venom

The δ-conotoxins are another class of conotoxins that act on sodium channels, but unlike the μ and μO-conotoxins previously described, they cause slowing of Na_V channel inactivation, similar to toxins that bind to receptor site 3 (Leipold, Hansel, Olivera, Terlau, & Heinemann, 2005). Despite similar activity to site 3 toxins, δ-conotoxins bind to an alternate neurotoxin site, designated site 6, which is made up of amino acid residues in DIV S4 (Fainzilber et al., 1994). Limited data are available on subtype selectivity of δ-conotoxins as they are highly hydrophobic and difficult to synthesize or express (Lewis et al., 2012); however, studies on δ-EVIA, which affects inactivation of $Na_V1.2$, 1.3, and 1.6 but not 1.4 or $Na_V1.5$, suggest that subtype-selective Na_V modulation by the δ-conotoxins is possible (Barbier et al., 2004).

In addition, a recently described excitatory peptide from the vermivirous *Conus suturatus*, SuVIA, affects voltage dependence of activation at $Na_V1.7$ with little effect on inactivation (Jin et al., 2015). This activity suggests a divergent binding site to other δ-conotoxins, and perhaps more appropriate classification of this peptide as an ιO-conotoxin based on its pharmacological effect and structural superfamily. Indeed, like ι-RXIA, SuVIA was most potent at $Na_V1.6$, albeit full subtype selectivity remains to be determined.

Analogous to the δ-conotoxins are the δ-theraphotoxins, δ-actinopoditoxins, δ-ctenitoxins, and δ-hexatoxins from spider venoms. These peptides also act as gating modifier toxins that inhibit inactivation of mammalian voltage-gated sodium channels. Consistent with this activity, δ-toxins from spider venom are generally considered to act at site 3, interacting with amino acid residues located on the S1–2 and/or S3–4 linker of DIV, although experimental evidence for this has been obtained for only a few peptides (Corzo et al., 2003; de Lima et al., 2002; Gilles et al., 2002; Osteen et al., 2016). For example, Magi 4 (δ-hexatoxin-Mg1a) from *Macrothele gigas* displaced the radiolabeled site 3 toxin LqhαIT but not the site 6 toxin δ-conotoxin TxVIA (Corzo et al., 2003), as did δ-hexatoxin-Hv1a, albeit this toxin—in contrast to the α-scorpion toxins—does not distinguish between mammalian and cockroach channels but instead binds poorly to the locust Na_V channel (Gilles et al., 2002). Interestingly, δ-hexatoxin-Hv1a and -Ar1a appear to stabilize distinct subconductance states as differential allosteric effects with the site 2 toxins batrachotoxin and veratridine were observed (Little, Wilson, et al., 1998; Little, Zappia, et al., 1998; Nicholson, Walsh, Little, & Tyler, 1998). At the organism level, δ-toxins from spider venom cause spastic paralysis of insects (Little, Wilson, et al., 1998; Nicholson, 2007), pain, as well as autonomic and somatic symptoms such as sweating, salivation, lacrimation, and muscle fasciculations that can be attributed to the prolongation of action potentials induced by these toxins (Nicholson, Little, & Birinyi-Strachan, 2004). Despite these profound effects on neuronal function, as well as interesting phyla-specific effects, detailed subtype selectivity studies have not been carried out systematically at the full Na_V isoform panel. One notable exception is δ-theraphotoxin-Hm1a, which is a selective modulator of $Na_V1.1$ channels (EC_{50} 38 ± 6 nM) with at least fivefold selectivity over $Na_V1.2$–$Na_V1.8$ (Osteen et al., 2016).

1.5.2.9 Snake Toxins

δ-Calliotoxin is the first three-finger toxin (3FTx) recently identified from snake venom to act on Na_V channels. δ-Calliotoxin activates Na_V channels by causing a small hyperpolarizing shift in the voltage dependence of activation and delaying fast inactivation, an effect similar to toxins acting at site 3 and site 4, although the exact binding site of δ-calliotoxin is not yet known (Yang et al., 2016). The full selectivity of δ-calliotoxin at human $Na_V1.1$–1.9 and other species orthologs remains to be determined.

2. CONCLUSION

2.1 Toxins as Tool Compounds: Insights and Future Directions

The activity and selectivity of toxins provide us with a unique opportunity to study the role of individual Na_V subtypes in clinically relevant conditions, including pain, epilepsy, and cardiac arrhythmias. Indeed, detailed structure–activity studies have been carried out by the pharmaceutical industry on the $Na_V1.7$ selective peptides GpTx-1 (Amgen Inc.), HwTxIV (MedImmune/Astra Zeneca), and CcoTx1 (Pfizer Inc.), highlighting intense industry interest in the field of developing toxin-based therapeutics (Murray et al., 2015; Revell et al., 2013; Shcherbatko et al., 2016). However, while several Na_V subtype-selective toxins are available, selective activators and inhibitors for *all* individual Na_V subtypes have not been described, and full Na_V selectivity data are not available for the majority of toxins. This is due in part, to the historical approach of characterizing Na_V channel activity of toxins using manual patch-clamp electrophysiology, a technique that remains the standard for measuring Na_V channel function, despite being laborious and requiring significant technical expertise to perform. In the last decade, higher-throughput methods to screen and profile the activity of Na_V channel modulators in heterologous expression systems have been developed, including fluorescence-based assays and more recently automated patch-clamp electrophysiology, which allow full characterization of Na_V subtype selectivity of toxins in a number of days, as opposed to weeks. Therefore, venom-derived toxins remain a promising and relatively uncharacterized source of novel and selective Na_V channel modulators, with the potential for use as research tools and/or clinical drug leads.

CONFLICT OF INTEREST

The authors declare no conflicts of interest.

ACKNOWLEDGMENTS

This work was supported by NHMRC project grant APP1102267, APP1125766, and an ARC Future Fellowship to I.V.

REFERENCES

Ahern, C. A. (2013). What activates inactivation? *The Journal of General Physiology*, *142*(2), 97–100.

Akopian, A. N., Sivilotti, L., & Wood, J. N. (1996). A tetrodotoxin-resistant voltage-gated sodium channel expressed by sensory neurons. *Nature*, *379*(6562), 257–262.

Amaya, F., Decosterd, I., Samad, T. A., Plumpton, C., Tate, S., Mannion, R. J., et al. (2000). Diversity of expression of the sensory neuron-specific TTX-resistant voltage-gated-sodium ion channels SNS and SNS2. *Molecular and Cellular Neurosciences*, *15*(4), 331–342.

Armstrong, C. M. (2006). Na channel inactivation from open and closed states. *Proceedings of the National Academy of Sciences of the United States of America*, *103*(47), 17991–17996.

Armstrong, C. M., & Bezanilla, F. (1977). Inactivation of the sodium channel II. Gating current experiments. *The Journal of General Physiology*, *70*(5), 567–590.

Armstrong, C. M., Bezanilla, F., & Rojas, E. (1973). Destruction of sodium conductance inactivation in squid axons perfused with pronase. *The Journal of General Physiology*, *62*(4), 375–391.

Bähring, R., & Covarrubias, M. (2011). Mechanisms of closed-state inactivation in voltage-gated ion channels. *The Journal of Physiology*, *589*(Pt. 3), 461–479.

Barbier, J., Lamthanh, H., Le Gall, F., Favreau, P., Benoit, E., Chen, H., et al. (2004). A delta-conotoxin from Conus ermineus venom inhibits inactivation in vertebrate neuronal Na+ channels but not in skeletal and cardiac muscles. *Journal of Biological Chemistry*, *279*(6), 4680–4685.

Barnett, D. W., Pressel, D. M., & Misler, S. (1995). Voltage-dependent Na+ and Ca2+ currents in human pancreatic islet β-cells: Evidence for roles in the generation of action potentials and insulin secretion. *Pflügers Archiv—European Journal of Physiology*, *431*(2), 272–282.

Barres, B. A., Chun, L. L. Y., & Corey, D. P. (1988). Ion channel expression by white matter glia: I. Type 2 astrocytes and oligodendrocytes. *GLIA*, *1*(1), 10–30.

Barres, B. A., Chun, L. L., & Corey, D. P. (1989). Glial and neuronal forms of the voltage-dependent sodium channel: Characteristics and cell-type distribution. *Neuron*, *2*(4), 1375–1388.

Beneski, D. A., & Catterall, W. A. (1980). Covalent labeling of protein components of the sodium channel with a photoactivable derivative of scorpion toxin. *Proceedings of the National Academy of Sciences of the United States of America*, 77(1), 639–643.

Berta, T., Poirot, O., Pertin, M., Ji, R. R., Kellenberger, S., & Decosterd, I. (2008). Transcriptional and functional profiles of voltage-gated Na(+) channels in injured and non-injured DRG neurons in the SNI model of neuropathic pain. *Molecular and Cellular Neurosciences*, *37*(2), 196–208.

Billen, B., Debaveye, S., Beress, L., Garateix, A., & Tytgat, J. (2010). Phyla- and subtype-selectivity of CgNa, a Na channel toxin from the venom of the giant Caribbean Sea anemone Condylactis gigantea. *Frontiers in Pharmacology*, *1*, 133.

Billen, B., Vassilevski, A., Nikolsky, A., Debaveye, S., Tytgat, J., & Grishin, E. (2010). Unique bell-shaped voltage-dependent modulation of Na+ channel gating by novel insect-selective toxins from the spider Agelena orientalis. *Journal of Biological Chemistry*, *285*(24), 18545–18554.

Black, J. A., Liu, S., & Waxman, S. G. (2009). Sodium channel activity modulates multiple functions in microglia. *GLIA*, *57*(10), 1072–1081.

Black, J. A., Renganathan, M., & Waxman, S. G. (2002). Sodium channel Na(v)1.6 is expressed along nonmyelinated axons and it contributes to conduction. *Brain Research. Molecular Brain Research*, *105*(1–2), 19–28.

Black, J. A., Westenbroek, R. E., Catterall, W. A., & Waxman, S. G. (1995). Type II brain sodium channel expression in non-neuronal cells: Embryonic rat osteoblasts. *Brain Research. Molecular Brain Research*, *34*(1), 89–98.

Bladen, C., Hamid, J., Souza, I. A., & Zamponi, G. W. (2014). Block of T-type calcium channels by protoxins I and II. *Molecular Brain*, 7, 36.

Boiko, T., Rasband, M. N., Levinson, S. R., Caldwell, J. H., Mandel, G., Trimmer, J. S., et al. (2001). Compact myelin dictates the differential targeting of two sodium channel isoforms in the same axon. *Neuron*, *30*(1), 91–104.

Bosmans, F., Rash, L., Zhu, S., Diochot, S., Lazdunski, M., Escoubas, P., et al. (2006). Four novel tarantula toxins as selective modulators of voltage-gated sodium channel subtypes. *Molecular Pharmacology*, *69*(2), 419–429.

Bosmans, F., & Swartz, K. J. (2010). Targeting voltage sensors in sodium channels with spider toxins. *Trends in Pharmacological Sciences*, *31*(4), 175–182.

Bosmans, F., & Tytgat, J. (2007a). Sea anemone venom as a source of insecticidal peptides acting on voltage-gated Na+ channels. *Toxicon*, *49*(4), 550–560.

Bosmans, F., & Tytgat, J. (2007b). Voltage-gated sodium channel modulation by scorpion alpha-toxins. *Toxicon*, *49*(2), 142–158.

Brackenbury, W. J., & Djamgoz, M. B. (2006). Activity-dependent regulation of voltage-gated Na+ channel expression in Mat-LyLu rat prostate cancer cell line. *The Journal of Physiology*, *573*(Pt. 2), 343–356.

Buczek, O., Wei, D., Babon, J. J., Yang, X., Fiedler, B., Chen, P., et al. (2007). Structure and sodium channel activity of an excitatory I1-superfamily conotoxin. *Biochemistry*, *46*(35), 9929–9940.

Burgess, D. L., Kohrman, D. C., Galt, J., Plummer, N. W., Jones, J. M., Spear, B., et al. (1995). Mutation of a new sodium channel gene, Scn8a, in the mouse mutant 'motor endplate disease'. *Nature Genetics*, *10*(4), 461–465.

Cai, T., Luo, J., Meng, E., Ding, J., Liang, S., Wang, S., et al. (2015). Mapping the interaction site for the tarantula toxin hainantoxin-IV (beta-TRTX-Hn2a) in the voltage sensor module of domain II of voltage-gated sodium channels. *Peptides*, *68*, 148–156.

Camargos, T. S., Bosmans, F., Rego, S. C., Mourao, C. B., & Schwartz, E. F. (2015). The scorpion toxin Tf2 from Tityus fasciolatus promotes Nav1.3 opening. *PloS One*, *10*(6), e0128578.

Campos, F. V., Chanda, B., Beirao, P. S., & Bezanilla, F. (2007). Beta-scorpion toxin modifies gating transitions in all four voltage sensors of the sodium channel. *Journal of General Physiology*, *130*(3), 257–268.

Campos, F. V., Chanda, B., Beirao, P. S., & Bezanilla, F. (2008). Alpha-scorpion toxin impairs a conformational change that leads to fast inactivation of muscle sodium channels. *Journal of General Physiology*, *132*(2), 251–263.

Cardoso, F. C., Dekan, Z., Rosengren, K. J., Erickson, A., Vetter, I., Deuis, J. R., et al. (2015). Identification and characterization of ProTx-III [mu-TRTX-Tp1a], a new voltage-gated sodium channel inhibitor from venom of the Tarantula Thrixopelma pruriens. *Molecular Pharmacology*, *88*(2), 291–303.

Cariello, L., de Santis, A., Fiore, F., Piccoli, R., Spagnuolo, A., Zanetti, L., et al. (1989). Calitoxin, a neurotoxic peptide from the sea anemone Calliactis parasitica: Amino acid sequence and electrophysiological properties. *Biochemistry*, *28*(6), 2484–2489.

Carrithers, M. D., Chatterjee, G., Carrithers, L. M., Offoha, R., Iheagwara, U., Rahner, C., et al. (2009). Regulation of podosome formation in macrophages by a splice variant of the sodium channel SCN8A. *Journal of Biological Chemistry*, *284*(12), 8114–8126.

Carrithers, M. D., Dib-Hajj, S., Carrithers, L. M., Tokmoulina, G., Pypaert, M., Jonas, E. A., et al. (2007). Expression of the voltage-gated sodium channel NaV1.5 in the macrophage late endosome regulates endosomal acidification. *Journal of Immunology*, *178*(12), 7822–7832.

Catterall, W. A. (1977). Membrane potential-dependent binding of scorpion toxin to the action potential Na+ ionophore. Studies with a toxin derivative prepared by lactoperoxidase-catalyzed iodination. *Journal of Biological Chemistry*, *252*(23), 8660–8668.

Catterall, W. A. (1979). Binding of scorpion toxin to receptor sites associated with sodium channels in frog muscle. Correlation of voltage-dependent binding with activation. *The Journal of General Physiology*, *74*(3), 375–391.
Catterall, W. A. (1980). Neurotoxins that act on voltage-sensitive sodium channels in excitable membranes. *Annual Review of Pharmacology and Toxicology*, *20*, 15–43.
Catterall, W. A. (1986). Molecular properties of voltage-sensitive sodium channels. *Annual Review of Biochemistry*, *55*, 953–985.
Catterall, W. A., & Beress, L. (1978). Sea anemone toxin and scorpion toxin share a common receptor site associated with the action potential sodium ionophore. *The Journal of Biological Chemistry*, *253*(20), 7393–7396.
Cestele, S., & Catterall, W. A. (2000). Molecular mechanisms of neurotoxin action on voltage-gated sodium channels. *Biochimie*, *82*(9–10), 883–892.
Cestele, S., Qu, Y., Rogers, J. C., Rochat, H., Scheuer, T., & Catterall, W. A. (1998). Voltage sensor-trapping: Enhanced activation of sodium channels by beta-scorpion toxin bound to the S3-S4 loop in domain II. *Neuron*, *21*(4), 919–931.
Cestele, S., Yarov-Yarovoy, V., Qu, Y., Sampieri, F., Scheuer, T., & Catterall, W. A. (2006). Structure and function of the voltage sensor of sodium channels probed by a beta-scorpion toxin. *Journal of Biological Chemistry*, *281*(30), 21332–21344.
Chahine, M., Bennett, P. B., George, A. L., Jr., & Horn, R. (1994). Functional expression and properties of the human skeletal muscle sodium channel. *Pflügers Archiv—European Journal of Physiology*, *427*(1–2), 136–142.
Chahine, M., & O'Leary, M. E. (2011). Regulatory role of voltage-gated Na channel beta subunits in sensory neurons. *Frontiers in Pharmacology*, *2*, 70.
Chanda, B., & Bezanilla, F. (2002). Tracking voltage-dependent conformational changes in skeletal muscle sodium channel during activation. *Journal of General Physiology*, *120*(5), 629–645.
Chang, N. S., French, R. J., Lipkind, G. M., Fozzard, H. A., & Dudley, S., Jr. (1998). Predominant interactions between mu-conotoxin Arg-13 and the skeletal muscle Na+ channel localized by mutant cycle analysis. *Biochemistry*, *37*(13), 4407–4419.
Chau, R., Kalaitzis, J. A., & Neilan, B. A. (2011). On the origins and biosynthesis of tetrodotoxin. *Aquatic Toxicology*, *104*(1–2), 61–72.
Cheah, C. S., Yu, F. H., Westenbroek, R. E., Kalume, F. K., Oakley, J. C., Potter, G. B., et al. (2012). Specific deletion of NaV1.1 sodium channels in inhibitory interneurons causes seizures and premature death in a mouse model of Dravet syndrome. *Proceedings of the National Academy of Sciences of the United States of America*, *109*(36), 14646–14651.
Chiu, S. Y., Schrager, P., & Ritchie, J. M. (1984). Neuronal-type Na+ and K+ channels in rabbit cultured Schwann cells. *Nature*, *311*(5982), 156–157.
Claes, L., Del-Favero, J., Ceulemans, B., Lagae, L., Van Broeckhoven, C., & De Jonghe, P. (2001). De novo mutations in the sodium-channel gene SCN1A cause severe myoclonic epilepsy of infancy. *American Journal of Human Genetics*, *68*(6), 1327–1332.
Clare, J. J., Tate, S. N., Nobbs, M., & Romanos, M. A. (2000). Voltage-gated sodium channels as therapeutic targets. *Drug Discovery Today*, *5*(11), 506–520.
Clement, H., Odell, G., Zamudio, F. Z., Redaelli, E., Wanke, E., Alagon, A., et al. (2007). Isolation and characterization of a novel toxin from the venom of the spider Grammostola rosea that blocks sodium channels. *Toxicon*, *50*(1), 65–74.
Cohen, L., Ilan, N., Gur, M., Stuhmer, W., Gordon, D., & Gurevitz, M. (2007). Design of a specific activator for skeletal muscle sodium channels uncovers channel architecture. *Journal of Biological Chemistry*, *282*(40), 29424–29430.
Cologna, C. T., Peigneur, S., Rustiguel, J. K., Nonato, M. C., Tytgat, J., & Arantes, E. C. (2012). Investigation of the relationship between the structure and function of Ts2, a neurotoxin from Tityus serrulatus venom. *The FEBS Journal*, *279*(8), 1495–1504.

Corzo, G., Gilles, N., Satake, H., Villegas, E., Dai, L., Nakajima, T., et al. (2003). Distinct primary structures of the major peptide toxins from the venom of the spider Macrothele gigas that bind to sites 3 and 4 in the sodium channel. *FEBS Letters*, *547*(1–3), 43–50.

Cox, J. J., Reimann, F., Nicholas, A. K., Thornton, G., Roberts, E., Springell, K., et al. (2006). An SCN9A channelopathy causes congenital inability to experience pain. *Nature*, *444*(7121), 894–898.

Cummins, T. R., Aglieco, F., & Dib-Hajj, S. D. (2002). Critical molecular determinants of voltage-gated sodium channel sensitivity to mu-conotoxins GIIIA/B. *Molecular Pharmacology*, *61*(5), 1192–1201.

Dabby, R., Sadeh, M., Broitman, Y., Yosovich, K., Dickman, R., & Leshinsky-Silver, E. (2016). Painful small fiber neuropathy with gastroparesis: A new phenotype with a novel mutation in the SCN10A gene. *Journal of Clinical Neuroscience*, *26*, 84–88.

de la Vega, R. C., & Possani, L. D. (2007). Novel paradigms on scorpion toxins that affects the activating mechanism of sodium channels. *Toxicon*, *49*(2), 171–180.

de Lima, M. E., Stankiewicz, M., Hamon, A., de Figueiredo, S. G., Cordeiro, M. N., Diniz, C. R., et al. (2002). The toxin Tx4(6–1) from the spider Phoneutria nigriventer slows down Na(+) current inactivation in insect CNS via binding to receptor site 3. *Journal of Insect Physiology*, *48*(1), 53–61.

DeCaen, P. G., Yarov-Yarovoy, V., Sharp, E. M., Scheuer, T., & Catterall, W. A. (2009). Sequential formation of ion pairs during activation of a sodium channel voltage sensor. *Proceedings of the National Academy of Sciences of the United States of America*, *106*(52), 22498–22503.

DeCaen, P. G., Yarov-Yarovoy, V., Zhao, Y., Scheuer, T., & Catterall, W. A. (2008). Disulfide locking a sodium channel voltage sensor reveals ion pair formation during activation. *Proceedings of the National Academy of Sciences of the United States of America*, *105*(39), 15142–15147.

Deuis, J. R., Dekan, Z., Inserra, M. C., Lee, T. H., Aguilar, M. I., Craik, D. J., et al. (2016). Development of a muO-conotoxin analogue with improved lipid membrane interactions and potency for the analgesic sodium channel NaV1.8. *Journal of Biological Chemistry*, *291*(22), 11829–11842.

Deuis, J. R., Dekan, Z., Wingerd, J. S., Smith, J. J., Munasinghe, N. R., Bhola, R. F., et al. (2017). Pharmacological characterisation of the highly NaV1.7 selective spider venom peptide Pn3a. *Scientific Reports*, 7, 40883.

Deuis, J. R., Wingerd, J. S., Winter, Z., Durek, T., Dekan, Z., Sousa, S. R., et al. (2016). Analgesic effects of GpTx-1, PF-04856264 and CNV1014802 in a mouse model of NaV1.7-mediated pain. *Toxins*, *8*(3).

Deuis, J. R., Zimmermann, K., Romanovsky, A. A., Possani, L. D., Cabot, P. J., Lewis, R. J., et al. (2013). An animal model of oxaliplatin-induced cold allodynia reveals a crucial role for Nav1.6 in peripheral pain pathways. *Pain*, *154*(9), 1749–1757.

Dib-Hajj, S. D., Fjell, J., Cummins, T. R., Zheng, Z., Fried, K., LaMotte, R., et al. (1999). Plasticity of sodium channel expression in DRG neurons in the chronic constriction injury model of neuropathic pain. *Pain*, *83*(3), 591–600.

Dib-Hajj, S. D., Yang, Y., Black, J. A., & Waxman, S. G. (2013). The Na(V)1.7 sodium channel: From molecule to man. *Nature Reviews. Neuroscience*, *14*(1), 49–62.

Diss, J. K., Archer, S. N., Hirano, J., Fraser, S. P., & Djamgoz, M. B. (2001). Expression profiles of voltage-gated Na(+) channel alpha-subunit genes in rat and human prostate cancer cell lines. *Prostate*, *48*(3), 165–178.

Djouhri, L., Fang, X., Okuse, K., Wood, J. N., Berry, C. M., & Lawson, S. N. (2003). The TTX-resistant sodium channel Nav1.8 (SNS/PN3): Expression and correlation with membrane properties in rat nociceptive primary afferent neurons. *Journal of Physiology*, *550*(Pt. 3), 739–752.

Donatsch, P., Lowe, D. A., Richardson, B. P., & Taylor, P. (1977). The functional significance of sodium channels in pancreatic beta cell membranes. *Journal of Physiology*, *267*(2), 357–376.

Drenth, J. P., Finley, W. H., Breedveld, G. J., Testers, L., Michiels, J. J., Guillet, G., et al. (2001). The primary erythermalgia-susceptibility gene is located on chromosome 2q31-32. *American Journal of Human Genetics*, *68*(5), 1277–1282.

Durek, T., Vetter, I., Wang, C. I., Motin, L., Knapp, O., Adams, D. J., et al. (2013). Chemical engineering and structural and pharmacological characterization of the alpha-scorpion toxin OD1. *ACS Chemical Biology*, *8*(6), 1215–1222.

Eberhardson, M., & Grapengiesser, E. (1999). Role of voltage-dependent Na + channels for rhythmic Ca2 + signalling in glucose-stimulated mouse pancreatic beta-cells. *Cellular Signalling*, *11*(5), 343–348.

Ekberg, J., Jayamanne, A., Vaughan, C. W., Aslan, S., Thomas, L., Mould, J., et al. (2006). muO-conotoxin MrVIB selectively blocks Nav1.8 sensory neuron specific sodium channels and chronic pain behavior without motor deficits. *Proceedings of the National Academy of Sciences of the United States of America*, *103*(45), 17030–17035.

Escayg, A., MacDonald, B. T., Meisler, M. H., Baulac, S., Huberfeld, G., An-Gourfinkel, I., et al. (2000). Mutations of SCN1A, encoding a neuronal sodium channel, in two families with GEFS+2. *Nature Genetics*, *24*(4), 343–345.

Faber, C. G., Lauria, G., Merkies, I. S., Cheng, X., Han, C., Ahn, H. S., et al. (2012). Gain-of-function Nav1.8 mutations in painful neuropathy. *Proceedings of the National Academy of Sciences of the United States of America*, *109*(47), 19444–19449.

Fainzilber, M., Kofman, O., Zlotkin, E., & Gordon, D. (1994). A new neurotoxin receptor site on sodium channels is identified by a conotoxin that affects sodium channel inactivation in molluscs and acts as an antagonist in rat brain. *Journal of Biological Chemistry*, *269*(4), 2574–2580.

Fertleman, C. R., Baker, M. D., Parker, K. A., Moffatt, S., Elmslie, F. V., Abrahamsen, B., et al. (2006). SCN9A mutations in paroxysmal extreme pain disorder: Allelic variants underlie distinct channel defects and phenotypes. *Neuron*, *52*(5), 767–774.

Fiedler, B., Zhang, M. M., Buczek, O., Azam, L., Bulaj, G., Norton, R. S., et al. (2008). Specificity, affinity and efficacy of iota-conotoxin RXIA, an agonist of voltage-gated sodium channels Na(V)1.2, 1.6 and 1.7. *Biochemical Pharmacology*, *75*(12), 2334–2344.

Flinspach, M., Xu, Q., Piekarz, A. D., Fellows, R., Hagan, R., Gibbs, A., et al. (2017). Insensitivity to pain induced by a potent selective closed-state Nav1.7 inhibitor. *Scientific Reports*, 7, 39662.

Fraser, S. P., Diss, J. K. J., Chioni, A. M., Mycielska, M. E., Pan, H., Yamaci, R. F., et al. (2005). Voltage-gated sodium channel expression and potentiation of human breast cancer metastasis. *Clinical Cancer Research*, *11*(15), 5381–5389.

Frazao, B., Vasconcelos, V., & Antunes, A. (2012). Sea anemone (Cnidaria, Anthozoa, Actiniaria) toxins: An overview. *Marine Drugs*, *10*(8), 1812–1851.

Fukuoka, T., Kobayashi, K., Yamanaka, H., Obata, K., Dai, Y., & Noguchi, K. (2008). Comparative study of the distribution of the alpha-subunits of voltage-gated sodium channels in normal and axotomized rat dorsal root ganglion neurons. *Journal of Comparative Neurology*, *510*(2), 188–206.

Fung, L. W., Kwok, S. L., & Tsui, K. W. (2015). SCN8A mutations in Chinese children with early onset epilepsy and intellectual disability. *Epilepsia*, *56*(8), 1319–1320.

Gajewiak, J., Azam, L., Imperial, J., Walewska, A., Green, B. R., Bandyopadhyay, P. K., et al. (2014). A disulfide tether stabilizes the block of sodium channels by the conotoxin muO section sign-GVIIJ. *Proceedings of the National Academy of Sciences of the United States of America*, *111*(7), 2758–2763.

Gardella, E., Becker, F., Moller, R. S., Schubert, J., Lemke, J. R., Larsen, L. H., et al. (2016). Benign infantile seizures and paroxysmal dyskinesia caused by an SCN8A mutation. *Annals of Neurology*, *79*(3), 428–436.

Garrison, S. R., Weyer, A. D., Barabas, M. E., Beutler, B. A., & Stucky, C. L. (2014). A gain-of-function voltage-gated sodium channel 1.8 mutation drives intense hyperexcitability of A- and C-fiber neurons. *Pain*, *155*(5), 896–905.

Gilles, N., Harrison, G., Karbat, I., Gurevitz, M., Nicholson, G. M., & Gordon, D. (2002). Variations in receptor site-3 on rat brain and insect sodium channels highlighted by binding of a funnel-web spider delta-atracotoxin. *European Journal of Biochemistry*, *269*(5), 1500–1510.

Gilles, N., Krimm, I., Bouet, F., Froy, O., Gurevitz, M., Lancelin, J. M., et al. (2000). Structural implications on the interaction of scorpion alpha-like toxins with the sodium channel receptor site inferred from toxin iodination and pH-dependent binding. *Journal of Neurochemistry*, *75*(4), 1735–1745.

Goldberg, Y. P., MacFarlane, J., MacDonald, M. L., Thompson, J., Dube, M. P., Mattice, M., et al. (2007). Loss-of-function mutations in the Nav1.7 gene underlie congenital indifference to pain in multiple human populations. *Clinical Genetics*, *71*(4), 311–319.

Goldin, A. L. (2003). Mechanisms of sodium channel inactivation. *Current Opinion in Neurobiology*, *13*(3), 284–290.

Goldin, A. L., Barchi, R. L., Caldwell, J. H., Hofmann, F., Howe, J. R., Hunter, J. C., et al. (2000). Nomenclature of voltage-gated sodium channels. *Neuron*, *28*(2), 365–368.

Goral, R. O., Leipold, E., Nematian-Ardestani, E., & Heinemann, S. H. (2015). Heterologous expression of Na1.9 chimeras in various cell systems. *Pflügers Archiv—European Journal of Physiology*, *467*, 2423–2435.

Guy, H. R., & Seetharamulu, P. (1986). Molecular model of the action potential sodium channel. *Proceedings of the National Academy of Sciences*, *83*(2), 508–512.

Hackett, J. D., Wisecaver, J. H., Brosnahan, M. L., Kulis, D. M., Anderson, D. M., Bhattacharya, D., et al. (2013). Evolution of saxitoxin synthesis in cyanobacteria and dinoflagellates. *Molecular Biology and Evolution*, *30*(1), 70–78.

Hains, B. C., Saab, C. Y., Klein, J. P., Craner, M. J., & Waxman, S. G. (2004). Altered sodium channel expression in second-order spinal sensory neurons contributes to pain after peripheral nerve injury. *Journal of Neuroscience*, *24*(20), 4832–4839.

Hamon, A., Gilles, N., Sautiere, P., Martinage, A., Kopeyan, C., Ulens, C., et al. (2002). Characterization of scorpion alpha-like toxin group using two new toxins from the scorpion Leiurus quinquestriatus hebraeus. *European Journal of Biochemistry*, *269*(16), 3920–3933.

Han, C., Vasylyev, D., Macala, L. J., Gerrits, M. M., Hoeijmakers, J. G., Bekelaar, K. J., et al. (2014). The G1662S NaV1.8 mutation in small fibre neuropathy: Impaired inactivation underlying DRG neuron hyperexcitability. *Journal of Neurology, Neurosurgery, and Psychiatry*, *85*(5), 499–505.

Hartshorne, R. P., & Catterall, W. A. (1984). The sodium channel from rat brain. Purification and subunit composition. *The Journal of Biological Chemistry*, *259*(3), 1667–1675.

Heinemann, S. H., Terlau, H., Stuhmer, W., Imoto, K., & Numa, S. (1992). Calcium channel characteristics conferred on the sodium channel by single mutations. *Nature*, *356*(6368), 441–443.

Heron, S. E., Crossland, K. M., Andermann, E., Phillips, H. A., Hall, A. J., Bleasel, A., et al. (2002). Sodium-channel defects in benign familial neonatal-infantile seizures. *Lancet*, *360*(9336), 851–852.

Hille, B. (2001). *Ion channels of excitable membranes*. Sunderland, MA: Sinauer Associates.

Hodgkin, A. L., & Huxley, A. F. (1952a). The components of membrane conductance in the giant axon of Loligo. *The Journal of Physiology, 116*(4), 473–496.
Hodgkin, A. L., & Huxley, A. F. (1952b). Currents carried by sodium and potassium ions through the membrane of the giant axon of Loligo. *The Journal of Physiology, 116*(4), 449–472.
Hodgkin, A. L., & Huxley, A. F. (1952c). The dual effect of membrane potential on sodium conductance in the giant axon of Loligo. *The Journal of Physiology, 116*(4), 497–506.
Hodgkin, A. L., & Huxley, A. F. (1952d). A quantitative description of membrane current and its application to conduction and excitation in nerve. *The Journal of Physiology, 117*(4), 500–544.
Holford, M., Zhang, M. M., Gowd, K. H., Azam, L., Green, B. R., Watkins, M., et al. (2009). Pruning nature: Biodiversity-derived discovery of novel sodium channel blocking conotoxins from Conus bullatus. *Toxicon, 53*(1), 90–98.
Horn, R., Patlak, J., & Stevens, C. F. (1981). Sodium channels need not open before they inactivate. *Nature, 291*(5814), 426–427.
Huang, J., Han, C., Estacion, M., Vasylyev, D., Hoeijmakers, J. G., Gerrits, M. M., et al. (2014). Gain-of-function mutations in sodium channel Na(v)1.9 in painful neuropathy. *Brain, 137*(Pt. 6), 1627–1642.
Hui, K., Lipkind, G., Fozzard, H. A., & French, R. J. (2002). Electrostatic and steric contributions to block of the skeletal muscle sodium channel by mu-conotoxin. *Journal of General Physiology, 119*(1), 45–54.
Jimenez, E. C., Shetty, R. P., Lirazan, M., Rivier, J., Walker, C., Abogadie, F. C., et al. (2003). Novel excitatory Conus peptides define a new conotoxin superfamily. *Journal of Neurochemistry, 85*(3), 610–621.
Jin, A. H., Israel, M. R., Inserra, M. C., Smith, J. J., Lewis, R. J., Alewood, P. F., et al. (2015). delta-Conotoxin SuVIA suggests an evolutionary link between ancestral predator defence and the origin of fish-hunting behaviour in carnivorous cone snails. *Proceedings of the Royal Society of London B: Biological Sciences, 282*(1811).
Jurkat-Rott, K., Holzherr, B., Fauler, M., & Lehmann-Horn, F. (2010). Sodium channelopathies of skeletal muscle result from gain or loss of function. *Pflügers Archiv—European Journal of Physiology, 460*(2), 239–248.
Kaplan, M. R., Cho, M. H., Ullian, E. M., Isom, L. L., Levinson, S. R., & Barres, B. A. (2001). Differential control of clustering of the sodium channels Na(v)1.2 and Na(v) 1.6 at developing CNS nodes of Ranvier. *Neuron, 30*(1), 105–119.
King, G. F., Gentz, M. C., Escoubas, P., & Nicholson, G. M. (2008). A rational nomenclature for naming peptide toxins from spiders and other venomous animals. *Toxicon, 52*(2), 264–276.
Klint, J. K., Senff, S., Rupasinghe, D. B., Er, S. Y., Herzig, V., Nicholson, G. M., et al. (2012). Spider-venom peptides that target voltage-gated sodium channels: Pharmacological tools and potential therapeutic leads. *Toxicon, 60*(4), 478–491.
Kohrman, D. C., Plummer, N. W., Schuster, T., Jones, J. M., Jang, W., Burgess, D. L., et al. (1995). Insertional mutation of the motor endplate disease (med) locus on mouse chromosome 15. *Genomics, 26*(2), 171–177.
Korkosh, V. S., Zhorov, B. S., & Tikhonov, D. B. (2014). Folding similarity of the outer pore region in prokaryotic and eukaryotic sodium channels revealed by docking of conotoxins GIIIA, PIIIA, and KIIIA in a NavAb-based model of Nav1.4. *Journal of General Physiology, 144*(3), 231–244.
Korotzer, A. R., & Cotman, C. W. (1992). Voltage-gated currents expressed by rat microglia in culture. *GLIA, 6*(2), 81–88.
Kostyuk, P. G., Veselovsky, N. S., & Tsyndrenko, A. Y. (1981). Ionic currents in the somatic membrane of rat dorsal root ganglion neurons-I. Sodium currents. *Neuroscience, 6*(12), 2423–2430.

Kuo, C. C., Chen, W. Y., & Yang, Y. C. (2004). Block of tetrodotoxin-resistant Na+ channel pore by multivalent cations: Gating modification and Na+ flow dependence. *Journal of General Physiology*, *124*(1), 27–42.

Leffler, A., Herzog, R. I., Dib-Hajj, S. D., Waxman, S. G., & Cummins, T. R. (2005). Pharmacological properties of neuronal TTX-resistant sodium channels and the role of a critical serine pore residue. *Pflügers Archiv—European Journal of Physiology*, *451*(3), 454–463.

Leipold, E., DeBie, H., Zorn, S., Borges, A., Olivera, B. M., Terlau, H., et al. (2007). muO conotoxins inhibit NaV channels by interfering with their voltage sensors in domain-2. *Channels (Austin, Tex.)*, *1*(4), 253–262.

Leipold, E., Hansel, A., Borges, A., & Heinemann, S. H. (2006). Subtype specificity of scorpion beta-toxin Tz1 interaction with voltage-gated sodium channels is determined by the pore loop of domain 3. *Molecular Pharmacology*, *70*(1), 340–347.

Leipold, E., Hansel, A., Olivera, B. M., Terlau, H., & Heinemann, S. H. (2005). Molecular interaction of delta-conotoxins with voltage-gated sodium channels. *FEBS Letters*, *579*(18), 3881–3884.

Leo, S., D'Hooge, R., & Meert, T. (2010). Exploring the role of nociceptor-specific sodium channels in pain transmission using Nav1.8 and Nav1.9 knockout mice. *Behavioural Brain Research*, *208*(1), 149–157.

Lewis, R. J., Dutertre, S., Vetter, I., & Christie, M. J. (2012). Conus venom peptide pharmacology. *Pharmacological Reviews*, *64*(2), 259–298.

Li, R. A., Ennis, I. L., French, R. J., Dudley, S. C., Jr., Tomaselli, G. F., & Marban, E. (2001). Clockwise domain arrangement of the sodium channel revealed by (mu)-conotoxin (GIIIA) docking orientation. *Journal of Biological Chemistry*, *276*(14), 11072–11077.

Li, R. A., Ennis, I. L., Xue, T., Nguyen, H. M., Tomaselli, G. F., Goldin, A. L., et al. (2003). Molecular basis of isoform-specific micro-conotoxin block of cardiac, skeletal muscle, and brain Na+ channels. *Journal of Biological Chemistry*, *278*(10), 8717–8724.

Lindia, J. A., Kohler, M. G., Martin, W. J., & Abbadie, C. (2005). Relationship between sodium channel NaV1.3 expression and neuropathic pain behavior in rats. *Pain*, *117*(1–2), 145–153.

Linford, N. J., Cantrell, A. R., Qu, Y., Scheuer, T., & Catterall, W. A. (1998). Interaction of batrachotoxin with the local anesthetic receptor site in transmembrane segment IVS6 of the voltage-gated sodium channel. *Proceedings of the National Academy of Sciences of the United States of America*, *95*(23), 13947–13952.

Linnertz, R., Wurm, A., Pannicke, T., Krugel, K., Hollborn, M., Hartig, W., et al. (2011). Activation of voltage-gated Na(+) and Ca(2)(+) channels is required for glutamate release from retinal glial cells implicated in cell volume regulation. *Neuroscience*, *188*, 23–34.

Little, M. J., Wilson, H., Zappia, C., Cestele, S., Tyler, M. I., Martin-Eauclaire, M. F., et al. (1998). Delta-atracotoxins from Australian funnel-web spiders compete with scorpion alpha-toxin binding on both rat brain and insect sodium channels. *FEBS Letters*, *439*(3), 246–252.

Little, M. J., Zappia, C., Gilles, N., Connor, M., Tyler, M. I., Martin-Eauclaire, M. F., et al. (1998). delta-Atracotoxins from Australian funnel-web spiders compete with scorpion alpha-toxin binding but differentially modulate alkaloid toxin activation of voltage-gated sodium channels. *Journal of Biological Chemistry*, *273*(42), 27076–27083.

Liu, Z., Cai, T., Zhu, Q., Deng, M., Li, J., Zhou, X., et al. (2013). Structure and function of hainantoxin-III, a selective antagonist of neuronal tetrodotoxin-sensitive voltage-gated sodium channels isolated from the Chinese bird spider Ornithoctonus hainana. *Journal of Biological Chemistry*, *288*(28), 20392–20403.

Liu, Z., Dai, J., Chen, Z., Hu, W., Xiao, Y., & Liang, S. (2003). Isolation and characterization of hainantoxin-IV, a novel antagonist of tetrodotoxin-sensitive sodium channels from the Chinese bird spider Selenocosmia hainana. *Cellular and Molecular Life Sciences, 60*(5), 972–978.

Liu, M., Yang, K. C., & Dudley, S. C., Jr. (2016). Cardiac sodium channel mutations: Why so many phenotypes? *Current Topics in Membranes, 78*, 513–559.

Logan, M. M., Toma, T., Thomas-Tran, R., & Du Bois, J. (2016). Asymmetric synthesis of batrachotoxin: Enantiomeric toxins show functional divergence against NaV. *Science, 354*(6314), 865–869.

Maertens, C., Cuypers, E., Amininasab, M., Jalali, A., Vatanpour, H., & Tytgat, J. (2006). Potent modulation of the voltage-gated sodium channel Nav1.7 by OD1, a toxin from the scorpion Odonthobuthus doriae. *Molecular Pharmacology, 70*(1), 405–414.

Mantegazza, M., Gambardella, A., Rusconi, R., Schiavon, E., Annesi, F., Cassulini, R. R., et al. (2005). Identification of an Nav1.1 sodium channel (SCN1A) loss-of-function mutation associated with familial simple febrile seizures. *Proceedings of the National Academy of Sciences of the United States of America, 102*(50), 18177–18182.

Martin, F., Ufodiama, C., Watt, I., Bland, M., & Brackenbury, W. J. (2015). Therapeutic value of voltage-gated sodium channel inhibitors in breast, colorectal, and prostate cancer: A systematic review. *Frontiers in Pharmacology, 6*, 273.

Middleton, R. E., Warren, V. A., Kraus, R. L., Hwang, J. C., Liu, C. J., Dai, G., et al. (2002). Two tarantula peptides inhibit activation of multiple sodium channels. *Biochemistry, 41*(50), 14734–14747.

Minett, M. S., Falk, S., Santana-Varela, S., Bogdanov, Y. D., Nassar, M. A., Heegaard, A. M., et al. (2014). Pain without nociceptors? Nav1.7-independent pain mechanisms. *Cell Reports, 6*(2), 301–312.

Misra, S. N., Kahlig, K. M., & George, A. L., Jr. (2008). Impaired NaV1.2 function and reduced cell surface expression in benign familial neonatal-infantile seizures. *Epilepsia, 49*(9), 1535–1545.

Mitrovic, N., George, A. L., Jr., Horn, R., & Horn, D. (2000). Role of domain 4 in sodium channel slow inactivation. *Journal of General Physiology, 115*(6), 707–717.

Moran, Y., Gordon, D., & Gurevitz, M. (2009). Sea anemone toxins affecting voltage-gated sodium channels—Molecular and evolutionary features. *Toxicon, 54*(8), 1089–1101.

Moran, Y., Kahn, R., Cohen, L., Gur, M., Karbat, I., Gordon, D., et al. (2007). Molecular analysis of the sea anemone toxin Av3 reveals selectivity to insects and demonstrates the heterogeneity of receptor site-3 on voltage-gated Na+ channels. *Biochemical Journal, 406*(1), 41–48.

Murray, J. K., Ligutti, J., Liu, D., Zou, A., Poppe, L., Li, H., et al. (2015). Engineering potent and selective analogs of GpTx-1, a tarantula venom peptide antagonist of the NaV1.7 sodium channel. *Journal of Medicinal Chemistry, 58*, 2299–2314.

Narahashi, T. (1972). Mechanism of action of tetrodotoxin and saxitoxin on excitable membranes. *Federation Proceedings, 31*(3), 1124–1132.

Narahashi, T. (1977). Toxic chemicals as probes of nerve membrane function. *Advances in Experimental Medicine and Biology, 84*, 407–445.

Nassar, M. A., Baker, M. D., Levato, A., Ingram, R., Mallucci, G., McMahon, S. B., et al. (2006). Nerve injury induces robust allodynia and ectopic discharges in Nav1.3 null mutant mice. *Molecular Pain, 2*, 33.

Nicholson, G. M. (2007). Insect-selective spider toxins targeting voltage-gated sodium channels. *Toxicon, 49*(4), 490–512.

Nicholson, G. M., Little, M. J., & Birinyi-Strachan, L. C. (2004). Structure and function of delta-atracotoxins: Lethal neurotoxins targeting the voltage-gated sodium channel. *Toxicon, 43*(5), 587–599.

Nicholson, E., & Randall, A. D. (2009). Na(v)1.5 sodium channels in a human microglial cell line. *Journal of Neuroimmunology, 215*(1–2), 25–30.

Nicholson, G. M., Walsh, R., Little, M. J., & Tyler, M. I. (1998). Characterisation of the effects of robustoxin, the lethal neurotoxin from the Sydney funnel-web spider Atrax robustus, on sodium channel activation and inactivation. *Pflügers Archiv—European Journal of Physiology*, *436*(1), 117–126.

Noda, M., Shimizu, S., Tanabe, T., Takai, T., Kayano, T., Ikeda, T., et al. (1984). Primary structure of Electrophorus electricus sodium channel deduced from cDNA sequence. *Nature*, *312*(5990), 121–127.

Noda, M., Suzuki, H., Numa, S., & Stuhmer, W. (1989). A single point mutation confers tetrodotoxin and saxitoxin insensitivity on the sodium channel II. *FEBS Letters*, *259*(1), 213–216.

O'Brien, B. J., Caldwell, J. H., Ehring, G. R., Bumsted O'Brien, K. M., Luo, S., & Levinson, S. R. (2008). Tetrodotoxin-resistant voltage-gated sodium channels Nav1.8 and Nav1.9 are expressed in the retina. *Journal of Comparative Neurology*, *508*(6), 940–951.

Oliveira, J. S., Redaelli, E., Zaharenko, A. J., Cassulini, R. R., Konno, K., Pimenta, D. C., et al. (2004). Binding specificity of sea anemone toxins to Nav 1.1-1.6 sodium channels: Unexpected contributions from differences in the IV/S3-S4 outer loop. *Journal of Biological Chemistry*, *279*(32), 33323–33335.

Ong, B.-H., Tomaselli, G. F., & Balser, J. R. (2000). A structural rearrangement in the sodium channel pore linked to slow inactivation and use dependence. *The Journal of General Physiology*, *116*(5), 653–662.

Ono, S., Kimura, T., & Kubo, T. (2011). Characterization of voltage-dependent calcium channel blocking peptides from the venom of the tarantula Grammostola rosea. *Toxicon*, *58*(3), 265–276.

Osteen, J. D., Herzig, V., Gilchrist, J., Emrick, J. J., Zhang, C., Wang, X., et al. (2016). Selective spider toxins reveal a role for the Nav1.1 channel in mechanical pain. *Nature*, *534*(7608), 494–499.

Papadatos, G. A., Wallerstein, P. M., Head, C. E., Ratcliff, R., Brady, P. A., Benndorf, K., et al. (2002). Slowed conduction and ventricular tachycardia after targeted disruption of the cardiac sodium channel gene Scn5a. *Proceedings of the National Academy of Sciences of the United States of America*, *99*(9), 6210–6215.

Payandeh, J., Gamal El-Din, T. M., Scheuer, T., Zheng, N., & Catterall, W. A. (2012). Crystal structure of a voltage-gated sodium channel in two potentially inactivated states. *Nature*, *486*(7401), 135–139.

Payandeh, J., Scheuer, T., Zheng, N., & Catterall, W. A. (2011). The crystal structure of a voltage-gated sodium channel. *Nature*, *475*(7356), 353–358.

Pedraza Escalona, M., & Possani, L. D. (2013). Scorpion beta-toxins and voltage-gated sodium channels: Interactions and effects. *Frontiers in Bioscience (Landmark edition)*, *18*, 572–587.

Penzotti, J. L., Fozzard, H. A., Lipkind, G. M., & Dudley, S. C., Jr. (1998). Differences in saxitoxin and tetrodotoxin binding revealed by mutagenesis of the Na+ channel outer vestibule. *Biophysical Journal*, *75*(6), 2647–2657.

Piccolino, M. (2006). Luigi Galvani's path to animal electricity. *Comptes Rendus Biologies*, *329*(5–6), 303–318.

Pintar, A., Possani, L. D., & Delepierre, M. (1999). Solution structure of toxin 2 from Centruroides noxius Hoffmann, a β-scorpion neurotoxin acting on sodium channels1. *Journal of Molecular Biology*, *287*(2), 359–367.

Planells-Cases, R., Caprini, M., Zhang, J., Rockenstein, E. M., Rivera, R. R., Murre, C., et al. (2000). Neuronal death and perinatal lethality in voltage-gated sodium channel alpha(II)-deficient mice. *Biophysical Journal*, *78*(6), 2878–2891.

Quintero-Hernandez, V., Jimenez-Vargas, J. M., Gurrola, G. B., Valdivia, H. H., & Possani, L. D. (2013). Scorpion venom components that affect ion-channels function. *Toxicon*, *76*, 328–342.

Ragsdale, D. S., McPhee, J. C., Scheuer, T., & Catterall, W. A. (1994). Molecular determinants of state-dependent block of Na+ channels by local anesthetics. *Science*, *265*(5179), 1724–1728.

Raman, I. M., Sprunger, L. K., Meisler, M. H., & Bean, B. P. (1997). Altered subthreshold sodium currents and disrupted firing patterns in Purkinje neurons of Scn8a mutant mice. *Neuron*, *19*(4), 881–891.

Redaelli, E., Cassulini, R. R., Silva, D. F., Clement, H., Schiavon, E., Zamudio, F. Z., et al. (2010). Target promiscuity and heterogeneous effects of tarantula venom peptides affecting Na+ and K+ ion channels. *Journal of Biological Chemistry*, *285*(6), 4130–4142.

Revell, J. D., Lund, P. E., Linley, J. E., Metcalfe, J., Burmeister, N., Sridharan, S., et al. (2013). Potency optimization of Huwentoxin-IV on hNav1.7: A neurotoxin TTX-S sodium-channel antagonist from the venom of the Chinese bird-eating spider Selenocosmia huwena. *Peptides*, *44*, 40–46.

Rogers, J. C., Qu, Y., Tanada, T. N., Scheuer, T., & Catterall, W. A. (1996). Molecular determinants of high affinity binding of alpha-scorpion toxin and sea anemone toxin in the S3-S4 extracellular loop in domain IV of the Na+ channel alpha subunit. *Journal of Biological Chemistry*, *271*(27), 15950–15962.

Rosker, C., Lohberger, B., Hofer, D., Steinecker, B., Quasthoff, S., & Schreibmayer, W. (2007). The TTX metabolite 4,9-anhydro-TTX is a highly specific blocker of the Na(v1.6) voltage-dependent sodium channel. *American Journal of Physiology. Cell Physiology*, *293*(2), C783–C789.

Rowe, A. H., Xiao, Y., Scales, J., Linse, K. D., Rowe, M. P., Cummins, T. R., et al. (2011). Isolation and characterization of CvIV4: A pain inducing alpha-scorpion toxin. *PloS One*, *6*(8). e23520

Roy, M. L., & Narahashi, T. (1992). Differential properties of tetrodotoxin-sensitive and tetrodotoxin-resistant sodium channels in rat dorsal root ganglion neurons. *Journal of Neuroscience*, *12*(6), 2104–2111.

Sangameswaran, L., Fish, L. M., Koch, B. D., Rabert, D. K., Delgado, S. G., Ilnicka, M., et al. (1997). A novel tetrodotoxin-sensitive, voltage-gated sodium channel expressed in rat and human dorsal root ganglia. *Journal of Biological Chemistry*, *272*(23), 14805–14809.

Schaller, K. L., Krzemien, D. M., Yarowsky, P. J., Krueger, B. K., & Caldwell, J. H. (1995). A novel, abundant sodium channel expressed in neurons and glia. *The Journal of Neuroscience*, *15*(5 Pt. 1), 3231–3242.

Schiavon, E., Sacco, T., Cassulini, R. R., Gurrola, G., Tempia, F., Possani, L. D., et al. (2006). Resurgent current and voltage sensor trapping enhanced activation by a beta-scorpion toxin solely in Nav1.6 channel. Significance in mice Purkinje neurons. *Journal of Biological Chemistry*, *281*(29), 20326–20337.

Schmalhofer, W. A., Calhoun, J., Burrows, R., Bailey, T., Kohler, M. G., Weinglass, A. B., et al. (2008). ProTx-II, a selective inhibitor of NaV1.7 sodium channels, blocks action potential propagation in nociceptors. *Molecular Pharmacology*, *74*(5), 1476–1484.

Schweitz, H., Vincent, J. P., Barhanin, J., Frelin, C., Linden, G., Hugues, M., et al. (1981). Purification and pharmacological properties of eight sea anemone toxins from Anemonia sulcata, Anthopleura xanthogrammica, Stoichactis giganteus, and Actinodendron plumosum. *Biochemistry*, *20*(18), 5245–5252.

Shcherbatko, A., Rossi, A., Foletti, D., Zhu, G., Bogin, O., Galindo Casas, M., et al. (2016). Engineering highly potent and selective microproteins against Nav1.7 sodium channel for treatment of pain. *Journal of Biological Chemistry*, *291*(27), 13974–13986.

Simidu, U., Noguchi, T., Hwang, D. F., Shida, Y., & Hashimoto, K. (1987). Marine bacteria which produce tetrodotoxin. *Applied and Environmental Microbiology*, *53*(7), 1714–1715.

Simkin, D., & Bendahhou, S. (2011). Skeletal muscle Na channel disorders. *Frontiers in Pharmacology*, *2*, 63.

Sontheimer, H., Black, J. A., Ransom, B. R., & Waxman, S. G. (1992). Ion channels in spinal cord astrocytes in vitro. I. Transient expression of high levels of Na+ and K+ channels. *Journal of Neurophysiology*, *68*(4), 985–1000.

Sontheimer, H., & Waxman, S. G. (1992). Ion channels in spinal cord astrocytes in vitro. II. Biophysical and pharmacological analysis of two Na+ current types. *Journal of Neurophysiology*, *68*(4), 1001–1011.

Stephan, M. M., Potts, J. F., & Agnew, W. S. (1994). The micro skeletal muscle sodium channel: Mutation E403Q eliminates sensitivity to tetrodotoxin but not to mu-conotoxins GIIIA and GIIIB. *Journal of Membrane Biology*, *137*(1), 1–8.

Strachan, L. C., Lewis, R. J., & Nicholson, G. M. (1999). Differential actions of pacific ciguatoxin-1 on sodium channel subtypes in mammalian sensory neurons. *Journal of Pharmacology and Experimental Therapeutics*, *288*(1), 379–388.

Stuhmer, W., Conti, F., Suzuki, H., Wang, X., Noda, M., Yahagi, N., et al. (1989). Structural parts involved in activation and inactivation of the sodium channel. *Nature*, *339*(6226), 597–603.

Sugawara, T., Tsurubuchi, Y., Agarwala, K. L., Ito, M., Fukuma, G., Mazaki-Miyazaki, E., et al. (2001). A missense mutation of the Na+ channel alpha II subunit gene Na(v)1.2 in a patient with febrile and a febrile seizures causes channel dysfunction. *Proceedings of the National Academy of Sciences of the United States of America*, *98*(11), 6384–6389.

Tan, J., Liu, Z., Wang, R., Huang, Z. Y., Chen, A. C., Gurevitz, M., et al. (2005). Identification of amino acid residues in the insect sodium channel critical for pyrethroid binding. *Molecular Pharmacology*, *67*(2), 513–522.

Tanaka, B. S., Zhao, P., Dib-Hajj, F. B., Morisset, V., Tate, S., Waxman, S. G., et al. (2016). A gain-of-function mutation in Nav1.6 in a case of trigeminal neuralgia. *Molecular Medicine*, *22*, 338–348.

Terlau, H., Heinemann, S. H., Stuhmer, W., Pusch, M., Conti, F., Imoto, K., et al. (1991). Mapping the site of block by tetrodotoxin and saxitoxin of sodium channel II. *FEBS Letters*, *293*(1–2), 93–96.

Thomas-Tran, R., & Du Bois, J. (2016). Mutant cycle analysis with modified saxitoxins reveals specific interactions critical to attaining high-affinity inhibition of hNaV1.7. *Proceedings of the National Academy of Sciences of the United States of America*, *113*(21), 5856–5861.

Toledo-Aral, J. J., Moss, B. L., He, Z. J., Koszowski, A. G., Whisenand, T., Levinson, S. R., et al. (1997). Identification of PN1, a predominant voltage-dependent sodium channel expressed principally in peripheral neurons. *Proceedings of the National Academy of Sciences of the United States of America*, *94*(4), 1527–1532.

Trainer, V. L., Baden, D. G., & Catterall, W. A. (1994). Identification of peptide components of the brevetoxin receptor site of rat brain sodium channels. *Journal of Biological Chemistry*, *269*(31), 19904–19909.

Trudeau, M. M., Dalton, J. C., Day, J. W., Ranum, L. P., & Meisler, M. H. (2006). Heterozygosity for a protein truncation mutation of sodium channel SCN8A in a patient with cerebellar atrophy, ataxia, and mental retardation. *Journal of Medical Genetics*, *43*(6), 527–530.

Van Wart, A., Trimmer, J. S., & Matthews, G. (2007). Polarized distribution of ion channels within microdomains of the axon initial segment. *Journal of Comparative Neurology*, *500*(2), 339–352.

Veeramah, K. R., O'Brien, J. E., Meisler, M. H., Cheng, X., Dib-Hajj, S. D., Waxman, S. G., et al. (2012). De novo pathogenic SCN8A mutation identified by whole-genome sequencing of a family quartet affected by infantile epileptic encephalopathy and SUDEP. *American Journal of Human Genetics*, *90*(3), 502–510.

Vetter, I., Dekan, Z., Knapp, O., Adams, D. J., Alewood, P. F., & Lewis, R. J. (2012). Isolation, characterization and total regioselective synthesis of the novel muO-conotoxin

MfVIA from Conus magnificus that targets voltage-gated sodium channels. *Biochemical Pharmacology, 84*(4), 540–548.
Walker, J. R., Novick, P. A., Parsons, W. H., McGregor, M., Zablocki, J., Pande, V. S., et al. (2012). Marked difference in saxitoxin and tetrodotoxin affinity for the human nociceptive voltage-gated sodium channel (Nav1.7) [corrected]. *Proceedings of the National Academy of Sciences of the United States of America, 109*(44), 18102–18107.
Wang, L., Liu, J., Pi, C., Zeng, X., Zhou, M., Jiang, X., et al. (2009). Identification of a novel M-superfamily conotoxin with the ability to enhance tetrodotoxin sensitive sodium currents. *Archives of Toxicology, 83*(10), 925–932.
Wang, S. Y., & Wang, G. K. (2003). Voltage-gated sodium channels as primary targets of diverse lipid-soluble neurotoxins. *Cellular Signalling, 15*(2), 151–159.
Wang, J., Yarov-Yarovoy, V., Kahn, R., Gordon, D., Gurevitz, M., Scheuer, T., et al. (2011). Mapping the receptor site for alpha-scorpion toxins on a Na+ channel voltage sensor. *Proceedings of the National Academy of Sciences of the United States of America, 108*(37), 15426–15431.
Wanke, E., Zaharenko, A. J., Redaelli, E., & Schiavon, E. (2009). Actions of sea anemone type 1 neurotoxins on voltage-gated sodium channel isoforms. *Toxicon, 54*(8), 1102–1111.
Waxman, S. G., Kocsis, J. D., & Black, J. A. (1994). Type III sodium channel mRNA is expressed in embryonic but not adult spinal sensory neurons, and is reexpressed following axotomy. *Journal of Neurophysiology, 72*(1), 466–470.
Westenbroek, R. E., Bischoff, S., Fu, Y., Maier, S. K., Catterall, W. A., & Scheuer, T. (2013). Localization of sodium channel subtypes in mouse ventricular myocytes using quantitative immunocytochemistry. *Journal of Molecular and Cellular Cardiology, 64*, 69–78.
Westenbroek, R. E., Merrick, D. K., & Catterall, W. A. (1989). Differential subcellular localization of the RI and RII Na+ channel subtypes in central neurons. *Neuron, 3*(6), 695–704.
Wilson, M. J., Yoshikami, D., Azam, L., Gajewiak, J., Olivera, B. M., Bulaj, G., et al. (2011). mu-Conotoxins that differentially block sodium channels NaV1.1 through 1.8 identify those responsible for action potentials in sciatic nerve. *Proceedings of the National Academy of Sciences of the United States of America, 108*(25), 10302–10307.
Wilson, M. J., Zhang, M. M., Azam, L., Olivera, B. M., Bulaj, G., & Yoshikami, D. (2011). Navbeta subunits modulate the inhibition of Nav1.8 by the analgesic gating modifier muO-conotoxin MrVIB. *Journal of Pharmacology and Experimental Therapeutics, 338*(2), 687–693.
Wilson, M. J., Zhang, M. M., Gajewiak, J., Azam, L., Rivier, J. E., Olivera, B. M., et al. (2015). Alpha- and beta-subunit composition of voltage-gated sodium channels investigated with mu-conotoxins and the recently discovered muO section sign-conotoxin GVIIJ. *Journal of Neurophysiology, 113*(7), 2289–2301.
Xiao, Y., Bingham, J. P., Zhu, W., Moczydlowski, E., Liang, S., & Cummins, T. R. (2008). Tarantula huwentoxin-IV inhibits neuronal sodium channels by binding to receptor site 4 and trapping the domain II voltage sensor in the closed configuration. *Journal of Biological Chemistry, 283*(40), 27300–27313.
Yanagawa, Y., Abe, T., & Satake, M. (1986). Blockade of [3H]lysine-tetrodotoxin binding to sodium channel proteins by conotoxin GIII. *Neuroscience Letters, 64*(1), 7–12.
Yang, D. C., Deuis, J. R., Dashevsky, D., Dobson, J., Jackson, T. N., Brust, A., et al. (2016). The snake with the scorpion's sting: Novel three-finger toxin sodium channel activators from the venom of the long-glanded blue coral snake (Calliophis bivirgatus). *Toxins, 8*(10).
Yang, M., Kozminski, D. J., Wold, L. A., Modak, R., Calhoun, J. D., Isom, L. L., et al. (2012). Therapeutic potential for phenytoin: Targeting Na(v)1.5 sodium channels to

reduce migration and invasion in metastatic breast cancer. *Breast Cancer Research and Treatment*, *134*(2), 603–615.
Yang, Y., Wang, Y., Li, S., Xu, Z., Li, H., Ma, L., et al. (2004). Mutations in SCN9A, encoding a sodium channel alpha subunit, in patients with primary erythermalgia. *Journal of Medical Genetics*, *41*(3), 171–174.
Yao, S., Zhang, M. M., Yoshikami, D., Azam, L., Olivera, B. M., Bulaj, G., et al. (2008). Structure, dynamics, and selectivity of the sodium channel blocker mu-conotoxin SIIIA. *Biochemistry*, *47*(41), 10940–10949.
Zaharenko, A. J., Schiavon, E., Ferreira, W. A., Jr., Lecchi, M., de Freitas, J. C., Richardson, M., et al. (2012). Characterization of selectivity and pharmacophores of type 1 sea anemone toxins by screening seven Na(v) sodium channel isoforms. *Peptides*, *34*(1), 158–167.
Zhang, M. M., Green, B. R., Catlin, P., Fiedler, B., Azam, L., Chadwick, A., et al. (2007). Structure/function characterization of micro-conotoxin KIIIA, an analgesic, nearly irreversible blocker of mammalian neuronal sodium channels. *Journal of Biological Chemistry*, *282*(42), 30699–30706.
Zhang, M. M., Gruszczynski, P., Walewska, A., Bulaj, G., Olivera, B. M., & Yoshikami, D. (2010). Cooccupancy of the outer vestibule of voltage-gated sodium channels by micro-conotoxin KIIIA and saxitoxin or tetrodotoxin. *Journal of Neurophysiology*, *104*(1), 88–97.
Zhang, F., Liu, Y., Zhang, C., Li, J., Yang, Z., Gong, X., et al. (2015). Natural mutations change the affinity of mu-theraphotoxin-Hhn2a to voltage-gated sodium channels. *Toxicon*, *93*, 24–30.
Zhang, M. M., McArthur, J. R., Azam, L., Bulaj, G., Olivera, B. M., French, R. J., et al. (2009). Synergistic and antagonistic interactions between tetrodotoxin and mu-conotoxin in blocking voltage-gated sodium channels. *Channels (Austin, Tex.)*, *3*(1), 32–38.
Zhang, M. M., Wilson, M. J., Azam, L., Gajewiak, J., Rivier, J. E., Bulaj, G., et al. (2013). Co-expression of Na(V)beta subunits alters the kinetics of inhibition of voltage-gated sodium channels by pore-blocking mu-conotoxins. *British Journal of Pharmacology*, *168*(7), 1597–1610.
Zhang, J. Z., Yarov-Yarovoy, V., Scheuer, T., Karbat, I., Cohen, L., Gordon, D., et al. (2011). Structure-function map of the receptor site for beta-scorpion toxins in domain II of voltage-gated sodium channels. *Journal of Biological Chemistry*, *286*(38), 33641–33651.
Zhao, P., Barr, T. P., Hou, Q., Dib-Hajj, S. D., Black, J. A., Albrecht, P. J., et al. (2008). Voltage-gated sodium channel expression in rat and human epidermal keratinocytes: Evidence for a role in pain. *Pain*, *139*(1), 90–105.
Zhu, S., Peigneur, S., Gao, B., Lu, X., Cao, C., & Tytgat, J. (2012). Evolutionary diversification of Mesobuthus alpha-scorpion toxins affecting sodium channels. *Molecular & Cellular Proteomics*, *11*(1)M111 012054.
Zhu, L., Peigneur, S., Gao, B., Tytgat, J., & Zhu, S. (2013). Two recombinant alpha-like scorpion toxins from Mesobuthus eupeus with differential affinity toward insect and mammalian Na(+) channels. *Biochimie*, *95*(9), 1732–1740.
Zorn, S., Leipold, E., Hansel, A., Bulaj, G., Olivera, B. M., Terlau, H., et al. (2006). The muO-conotoxin MrVIA inhibits voltage-gated sodium channels by associating with domain-3. *FEBS Letters*, *580*(5), 1360–1364.
Zsiros, E., Kis-Toth, K., Hajdu, P., Gaspar, R., Bielanska, J., Felipe, A., et al. (2009). Developmental switch of the expression of ion channels in human dendritic cells. *Journal of Immunology*, *183*(7), 4483–4492.

CHAPTER FOUR

Role of Nonneuronal TRPV4 Signaling in Inflammatory Processes

Pradeep Rajasekhar*,†, Daniel P. Poole*,†,‡, Nicholas A. Veldhuis*,†,‡,1

*Monash Institute of Pharmaceutical Sciences, Monash University, Melbourne, VIC, Australia
†Australian Research Council Centre of Excellence in Convergent Bio-Nano Science and Technology, Parkville, VIC, Australia
‡The University of Melbourne, Parkville, VIC, Australia
[1]Corresponding author: e-mail address: nicholas.veldhuis@monash.edu

Contents

Abstract

Transient receptor potential (TRP) ion channels are important signaling components in nociceptive and inflammatory pathways. This is attributed to their ability to function as polymodal sensors of environmental stimuli (chemical and mechanical) and as effector molecules in receptor signaling pathways. TRP vanilloid 4 (TRPV4) is a non-selective cation channel that is activated by multiple endogenous stimuli including

Advances in Pharmacology, Volume 79
ISSN 1054-3589
http://dx.doi.org/10.1016/bs.apha.2017.03.002

shear stress, membrane stretch, and arachidonic acid metabolites. TRPV4 contributes to many important physiological processes and dysregulation of its activity is associated with chronic conditions of metabolism, inflammation, peripheral neuropathies, musculoskeletal development, and cardiovascular regulation. Mechanosensory and receptor- or lipid-mediated signaling functions of TRPV4 have historically been attributed to central and peripheral neurons. However, with the development of potent and selective pharmacological tools, transgenic mice and improved molecular and imaging techniques, many new roles for TRPV4 have been revealed in nonneuronal cells. In this chapter, we discuss these recent findings and highlight the need for greater characterization of TRPV4-mediated signaling in nonneuronal cell types that are either directly associated with neurons or indirectly control their excitability through release of sensitizing cellular factors. We address the integral role of these cells in sensory and inflammatory processes as well as their importance when considering undesirable on-target effects that may be caused by systemic delivery of TRPV4-selective pharmaceutical agents for treatment of chronic diseases. In future, this will drive a need for targeted drug delivery strategies to regulate such a diverse and promiscuous protein.

NONSTANDARD ABBREVIATIONS

CNS central nervous system
EDHF endothelium-derived hyperpolarizing factor
GI gastrointestinal
GPCR G protein-coupled receptor
NO nitric oxide
PNS peripheral nervous system
SGC satellite glial cell
TNF tumor necrosis factor
TRP transient receptor potential
TRPV4 transient receptor potential vanilloid 4

1. INTRODUCTION

Transient receptor potential (TRP) ion channels are a super family of homologous tetrameric nonselective cation channels that perform sensory and signaling functions throughout the body. TRP channels can increase intracellular levels of cations including Ca^{2+} to trigger cellular secretory events. Although their nociceptive and neurogenic inflammatory roles are well established, there are many other cell types in which TRP channels play a role in the secretion of cellular or metabolic factors that influence neuronal activity.

The TRP vanilloid 4 (TRPV4) ion channel has the unique ability to enable many different cell types to "respond" to their cellular environment. TRPV4 functions both as a sensor at the surface of load-bearing and pressure-sensing cells, and as an effector molecule for a number of distinct cell types that are integral to immune, inflammatory, and metabolic pathways. These cells have many overlapping functions, including barrier formation (gastrointestinal (GI), blood–brain barrier, skin), inflammatory signaling, wound healing and sensing of mechanical pressure. They all participate in complex networks of interconnecting cells that are essential for survival. Yet intriguingly, mice with a functional deletion of TRPV4 thrive and do not exhibit any obvious associated sensory or inflammatory phenotypes. Despite any redundancies in TRPV4 function, these knockout mice have proven invaluable to our understanding of the different cell types and physiological processes to which TRPV4 contributes. Furthermore, multiple human TRPV4 mutations associated with inflammatory, metabolic, and musculoskeletal disorders have been identified (Nilius & Voets, 2013). While loss of TRPV4 activity may not be detrimental, mutations that change trafficking or activity (e.g., gain of function) suggests that altered TRPV4 Ca^{2+} signaling may have deleterious consequences (Lamande et al., 2011).

The initial characterization of TRPV4 function and expression was predominantly targeted toward neurons of the peripheral nervous system (PNS) and central nervous system (CNS). It is now established that TRPV4 is functionally expressed by neurons in the hippocampus, sensory ganglia, myenteric plexus of the colon as well as by sympathetic and parasympathetic nerve fibers (Alessandri-Haber et al., 2003; Fichna et al., 2015; Li et al., 2013). In addition, TRPV4 promotes diverse systemic functions, including vasodilation, bladder voiding, wound healing, and ciliary beating frequency. In preclinical studies, it has also been demonstrated to play a role in chronic inflammatory conditions including arthritis and inflammatory bowel disease, and to mediate thermal and mechanical hyperalgesia (White et al., 2016).

The availability of robust pharmacological tools (agonists and antagonists) as well as different TRPV4 knockout mice have made it possible to explore the functional roles of TRPV4. TRPV4 can be activated by warm temperatures (>27°C), cell swelling, mechanical stress, and arachidonic acid or its metabolites (eicosanoic acids) that are generated by inflammatory processes or receptor-mediated signaling (reviewed by White et al., 2016). TRP channels also function as G protein-coupled receptor (GPCR) signaling effectors, where activation of GPCRs such as the bradykinin B2 receptor, protease-activated receptor 2 (PAR2), histamine H1 receptor, and P2Y1 purinoceptor can increase kinase activity and production of lipid signaling mediators to enhance TRP channel activity and cell surface expression (Veldhuis, Poole, Grace, McIntyre, & Bunnett, 2015). Together, these examples illustrate that there are numerous primary and secondary mechanisms in place to modulate TRP channel signaling.

In this chapter, we review some of the new physiological roles for TRPV4 in nonneuronal cells. It is an inherently promiscuous channel that interacts with many proteins and initiates unique functions, many of which can regulate neuronal activity. A trend is emerging, where the functional effects of TRPV4 activation are not necessarily directly mediated by neurogenic mechanisms, but through actions at glial cells, immune cells, epithelia, and vasculature closely associated with these neurons. To assess the potential for future therapeutic intervention of TRPV4 activity, a deeper exploration of the roles of TRPV4 in different cells is required, so that we may distinguish the cellular source of TRPV4-mediated pronociceptive or proinflammatory signals. TRPV4-mediated signaling and secretion are addressed as key mechanisms for cell–cell communication, and knowledge gaps in these mechanisms are discussed.

2. EPITHELIAL AND ENDOTHELIAL CELLS

Epithelial and endothelial cells form important biological barriers within organs and vascular systems. An important feature of these cell types is tight intercellular junctions that separate different compartments within the body and provide protection from external environmental factors, including noxious chemical irritants in food or air, foreign cells, and exposure to UV radiation. Afferent terminals innervate these barriers to provide sensory feedback to the CNS and conversely, to enable efferent processes to regulate barrier secretion and absorption, immune responses, and contraction of adjacent muscle cells.

2.1 Colonic Epithelial Cells

TRP channels expressed throughout the digestive tract mediate sensory processing of taste and visceral sensation and contribute to neurogenic regulation of GI motility, absorption, and secretion. In addition, TRP channels have emerged as therapeutic targets due to their contribution to the onset and exacerbation of chronic conditions of the GI tract, including inflammatory bowel disease, gastroesophageal reflux disease, pancreatitis, and functional bowel disorders such as irritable bowel syndrome (reviewed by Holzer, 2011; Poole, Lieu, Veldhuis, Rajasekhar, & Bunnett, 2015). Although TRPV4 expressed by visceral afferents contribute to these disorders, less is known about the role of TRPV4 in colonic epithelia or other GI-localized cells. A comprehensive study by Vergnolle and colleagues has confirmed functional expression of TRPV4 in both human and mouse colonocytes (D'Aldebert et al., 2011). Although no difference could be detected in human tissue isolated from IBD and non-IBD patients, upregulation of TRPV4 mRNA, and immunoreactivity in colonic epithelia was demonstrated in the dextran sulfate sodium model of ulcerative colitis. Furthermore, intracolonic administration of the weak TRPV4 agonist 4α-phorbol-12,13-didecanoate (4αPDD, 3–24 h) increased colonic tissue inflammation scores in mice and the production of proinflammatory chemokines, including interleukin-6 (IL-6) and monocyte chemotactic protein 1 (MCP-1) (D'Aldebert et al., 2011). This demonstrates an important secretory function in colonic epithelia that were supported by 4αPDD-mediated cytokine secretion in colonocyte cultures. Indeed, TRPV4 is associated with the secretion of chemokines and other factors by nonneuronal cells to enhance neuronal excitability and activate proinflammatory pathways. Examples of these interactions are illustrated in Table 1.

The clinical use of nonsteroidal antiinflammatory drugs (NSAIDs) is associated with the development of inflammatory damage to the GI tract. The involvement of TRPV4 in NSAID-induced colonic inflammation has also been demonstrated experimentally through pharmacological and genetic downregulation of TRPV4 activity (Yamawaki et al., 2014).

2.2 Keratinocytes

Keratinocytes in the skin, esophagus, and cornea are important barrier-forming cells that provide the first line of defense to the external environment. Since the discovery of warmth-induced TRPV4-mediated currents in keratinocytes (Chung, Lee, Mizuno, Suzuki, & Caterina, 2004), new roles for TRPV4 in these cells are emerging. TRPV4 expression by skin keratinocytes has been confirmed through comparison of immunolabeling in tissues from wild-type and $TRPV4^{-/-}$ mice. TRPV4 interacts with cytoskeletal components including β-actin and β-catenin, and consequently regulates Ca^{2+}-dependent formation of adherens junctions (Sokabe, Fukumi-Tominaga, Yonemura, Mizuno, & Tominaga, 2010). In the same study, the thickness and dye permeability of the cornified epidermal layer were assessed

Table 1 TRPV4-Dependent Mechanisms and Mediators in Nonneuronal Cells

Cell Type	Mediator/Mechanism	References
Stretch/Hypoosmolarity-Mediated Secretion and Direct Neuronal Activation		
Esophageal keratinocytes	ATP	Mihara, Boudaka, Sugiyama, Moriyama, and Tominaga (2011)
Urothelial cells	ATP	Beckel et al. (2015) and Mochizuki et al. (2009)
Astrocytes	Glutamate	Takano et al. (2005)
Agonist-Induced Inflammatory Cytokine Secretion		
Mouse colon; Colonic epithelial cells (Caco-2, T84 cell lines)	IL-8, MIG, IP-10, MCP-1, RANTES	D'Aldebert et al. (2011)
Macrophage	IL-1β, IL-10	Scheraga et al. (2016)
T-cells	IFN-ɣ, IL-2	Majhi et al. (2015)
Microglia	TNF	Konno et al. (2012)
Synoviocyte	IL-8	Itoh et al. (2009)
Esophageal epithelial cells	IL-8 (IL-1β induced)	Ueda, Shikano, Kamiya, Joh, and Ugawa (2011)
Stretch or Ligand-Mediated Endothelial Relaxation and Edema		
Endothelial cells	Ca^{2+}-mediated regulation of junctions Nitric oxide Endothelium-derived hyperpolarizing factor	Mendoza et al. (2010) and Sukumaran et al. (2013)

IFN-ɣ, interferon gamma; IL, interleukin; IP-10, interferon gamma-induced protein 10, also known as CXCL10; MCP-1, monocyte chemotactic protein 1 also known as CCL2; MIG, monokine induced by gamma interferon also known as CXCL9; PNS, peripheral nervous system; RANTES, regulated on activation, normal T cell expressed and secreted also known as CCL5; TNF, tumor necrosis factor.

as a measure of barrier formation, and differences between wild-type and TRPV4$^{-/-}$ mice could only be observed following chemical disruption of the dermal layer. UVB (short wavelength ultraviolet radiation) increases expression and Ca^{2+} permeability of TRPV4 on epidermal keratinocytes, causing skin tissue damage, increased expression of endothelin-1, and subsequent sunburn-mediated nociceptive signaling (Moore et al., 2013). Recently, keratinocyte-selective inducible TRPV4 knockout mice have also defined a new role for TRPV4 activity in histaminergic itch via a mitogen-activated protein kinase (ERK1/2) signaling cascade (Chen et al., 2016). Together, these findings support a model in which keratinocytes act as both itch- and pain-generating cells. TRPV4-dependent ERK signaling may promote secretion of cellular factors that transmit these signals to primary afferents, but this is yet to be characterized in detail.

TRPV4 is expressed by epithelial cells of the esophagus. This has been demonstrated in human and mouse esophageal tissue and the human esophageal epithelial cell line, HET-1A (Ueda et al., 2011). TRPV4 activation by heat, mechanical stimuli (stretch), or endogenous agonists can induce TRPV4-mediated currents and ATP release, and these are absent in TRPV4$^{-/-}$ mice. It has been proposed that TRPV4-mediated ATP release may stimulate purinergic receptors on esophageal vagal mechanosensitive afferent terminals, thus implicating keratinocyte-TRPV4 in esophageal mechanotransduction and heat hypersensitivity (Mihara et al., 2011; Ueda et al., 2011).

2.3 Urothelial Cells

The close cellular association and communication between urothelial cells of the urinary bladder wall and extrinsic afferent terminals are an important sensory pathway for timely urine expulsion. While TRPV4 may perform a mechanosensory function in primary afferents that innervate the bladder, high levels of TRPV4 expression have also been detected in the urothelium of mouse, rat, and human tissue suggesting a urothelial component to TRPV4-mediated bladder regulation (Birder et al., 2007; Janssen et al., 2011; Yamada et al., 2009). A mouse model of cyclophosphamide-induced cystitis, known to cause dysregulation of bladder voiding, is associated with enhanced TRPV4 activity and poor bladder storage. Although the cellular mechanisms through which TRPV4 influences bladder function were not determined, this study provided the first demonstration of the small molecule HC-067047 as a highly potent compound with TRPV4-selective antagonist activity (Everaerts et al., 2010).

Similar to keratinocytes, studies in human urothelium demonstrated TRPV4 association with α-catenin and localization to adherens junctions, are consistent with bladder stretch (distention) induced TRPV4 activity (Janssen et al., 2011). Furthermore, activation of urothelial TRPV4 is hypothesized to promote pannexin channel-mediated ATP release (Beckel et al., 2015; Mochizuki et al., 2009). This phenomenon has also been observed in airway epithelia and is consistent with the concept of non-neuronal TRPV4 regulation of afferents via an ATP-purinergic signaling pathway (Seminario-Vidal et al., 2011).

2.4 Vascular Endothelial Cells

Endothelial cells form the inner lining of blood vessels and control vascular contractility via intercellular regulation of the outer smooth muscle cell layer. Since early observations of heat-induced TRPV4 activity in mouse aortic endothelial cells (Watanabe et al., 2002), studies have shown that TRPV4 is exquisitely regulated by multiple mechanisms to maintain smooth muscle vascular tone. Furthermore, while TRPV4 activity on sensory neurons promotes neurogenic edema and plasma extravasation at the site of injury, direct activation of endothelial TRPV4 increases endothelial cell permeability and edema, most likely by coupling to the calcium-activated potassium channel $K_{Ca}3.1$ and calcium-activated chloride channels (CaCC) (Simonsen, Wandall-Frostholm, Olivan-Viguera, & Kohler, 2016), or by regulation of cytoskeletal and junction proteins, as described earlier. All of these cellular processes have recently been reviewed in detail (Filosa, Yao, & Rath, 2013; White et al., 2016).

When assessing the validity of TRPV4 as a therapeutic target, it is important to discuss how dysregulation of TRPV4 can impact vasodilation and edema. At its most extreme, exogenous activation by systemic administration of a potent, selective TRPV4 agonist (GSK1016790A) caused significant vessel relaxation and reduced cardiac output, which was interpreted as circulatory collapse (Willette et al., 2008). In contrast, TRPV4 antagonists have been explored for treatment of pulmonary edema (endothelial cell permeability and acute lung injury) caused by congestive heart failure and endothelial stretch (Jian, King, Al-Mehdi, Liedtke, & Townsley, 2008). Inhibition of TRPV4 using GSK2193874 prevents pulmonary edema in a mouse model of heart failure (Thorneloe et al., 2012) and another TRPV4 antagonist GSK2798745 is currently in phase II clinical trials for treating symptoms of congestive heart failure (NTC02497937). Together, while systemic activation of TRPV4 is detrimental, antagonism of TRPV4 is reported to be well tolerated and a potential therapeutic strategy (Balakrishna et al., 2014; Thorneloe et al., 2012; Ye et al., 2012).

A more detailed understanding of the cellular processes associated with TRPV4 function in endothelia and smooth muscle cells is required, if these pathways are to be therapeutically exploited. The vascular endothelium communicates with smooth muscle cells through Ca^{2+}-dependent release of cellular factors to influence contractility. Evidence suggests that TRPV4 on endothelial and smooth muscle cells participates in transduction of all Ca^{2+}-dependent vasodilatory factors: potassium, endothelial nitric oxide synthase (eNOS)-generated nitric oxide, arachidonic acid metabolites such prostaglandins and eicosanoids (generated by epoxygenase and cytochrome P450 enzymes, respectively), and endothelium-derived hyperpolarizing factor (EDHF) (Dahan et al., 2012; Earley, Heppner, Nelson, & Brayden, 2005; Sonkusare et al., 2012; Watanabe et al., 2002).

In endothelia, TRPV4 is activated by receptor signaling or shear stress associated with luminal blood flow and can participate in distinct signaling processes that are dependent upon the extent of activation. A detailed Ca^{2+}-imaging study using expression of an endothelial-restricted GFP-based Ca^{2+} sensor, GCaMP, has demonstrated how low-level agonist or acetylcholine/muscarinic receptor activation of few TRPV4 channels can generate intermittent, localized Ca^{2+} influx events known as "Ca^{2+} sparklets." These sparklets mediate NO or EDHF production and release (Sonkusare et al., 2012) and can stimulate Ca^{2+}-sensitive small-conductance and intermediate- potassium channels (e.g., $K_{Ca}3.1$) to enhance processes leading to vascular relaxation, but can also increase the potential for edema and circulatory collapse to occur (Sukumaran et al., 2013; Wandall-Frostholm et al., 2015).

Modulation of vascular tone can also be achieved through TRPV4 activity on smooth muscle cells. As illustrated in Fig. 1, endothelial release of arachidonic metabolites can directly activate smooth muscle cell TRPV4. This results in much larger increases in intracellular Ca^{2+} through coordinated ryanodine receptor store-operated (endoplasmic reticulum) Ca^{2+} release, and activation of Ca^{2+}-sensitive large conductance (BK_{Ca}) potassium channels (Dahan et al., 2012; Earley et al., 2005; Watanabe et al., 2002).

3. GLIAL CELLS

Glial cells are no longer considered structural cells that merely support neuronal health, development, and function. More recently, they have been established as multifaceted cells that perform immunoprotective roles, control neuronal excitability, and mediate signaling between neurons and blood vessels. In instances where nerve injury or inflammatory neuropathies lead to neuropathic pain, glial cells can be activated, and work synergistically with immune cells to lower activation thresholds in dorsal root ganglion (DRG)

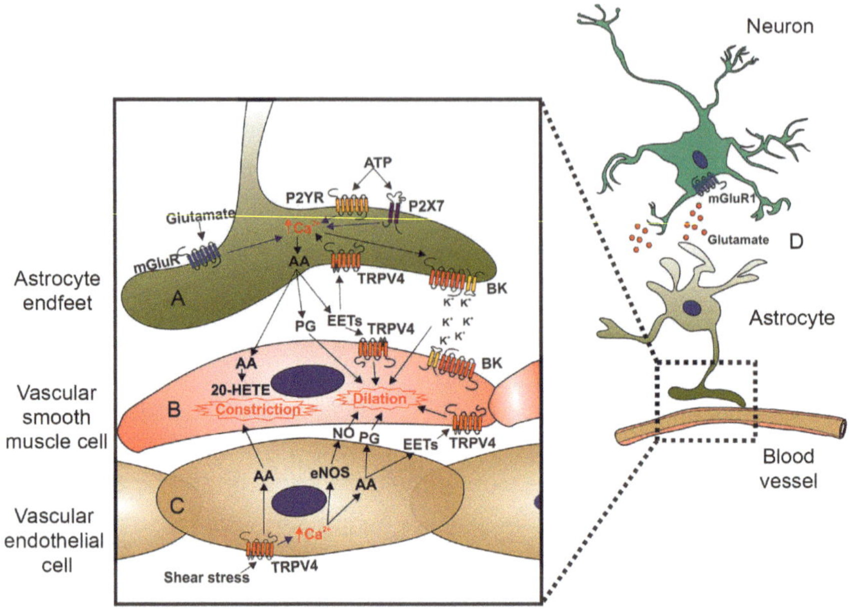

Fig. 1 TRPV4 and regulation of blood vessels in the brain: (A) Glutamate or ATP released by neurons in the brain can activate the mGluR glutamate receptor or P2Y and P2X7 purinoceptors on astrocytes, respectively. This increases intracellular calcium ($[Ca^{2+}]_i$) and generation of arachidonic acid (AA) and its metabolites: prostaglandins (PG) and epoxyeicosatrienoic acid (EET). (B) PG and EET can dilate blood vessels and the related 20-hydroxyeicosatetraenoic acid (20-HETE) can constrict vessels. Calcium-dependent K^+ channels (BK) on astrocytes or smooth muscle cells are activated by increased $[Ca^{2+}]_i$. This releases K^+ ions and causes dilation of blood vessels. (C) Shear stress from blood flow can increase $[Ca^{2+}]_i$ in endothelial cells via TRPV4, increasing eNOS activity and release of the vasodilator nitric oxide (NO). (D) Astrocytic glutamate release activates neuronal mGluR1, resulting in increased hippocampal neuron excitatory postsynaptic currents.

and second-order spinal neurons that mediate pain transmission (Scholz & Woolf, 2007). Glial cells of the PNS (satellite glia and Müller glia) and CNS (astrocytes and microglia) share similarities in the coexpression of TRPV4 and the aquaporin 4 (AQP4) water channel. While this suggests a role for glia in cell swelling and water retention, many other glial signaling functions are emerging and may involve TRPV4 activity.

3.1 Astrocytes

Astrocytes are glial cells of the CNS that perform multiple roles in the regulation of neuronal activity. Their projections make contact with adjacent synapses, other astrocytes and also extend branched projections that terminate with endfeet enveloping capillaries and arterioles. Thus, they are in the perfect position to mediate communication between neurons and cerebral microcirculation (Fig. 1). They can respond to synaptic activity and dampen neuronal responses to decrease pain perception and can also stimulate neuronal activity by increased Ca^{2+} signaling and secretion of "gliotransmitters" such as glutamate and ATP, or Ca^{2+}-activated potassium release through BK_{Ca} channels (Kang, Xu, Xu, Nedergaard, & Kang, 2005; Kim et al., 2016; Pannasch & Rouach, 2013; Takano et al., 2005). TRPV4 is expressed in only a subset of astrocytes, but can stimulate an interconnecting glial network through gap junctions to increase Ca^{2+} levels and glutamate release. This initiates neuronal excitatory postsynaptic currents (Fig. 1). Importantly, astrocyte-derived TRPV4-mediated glutamate signaling was confirmed by stimulation with a TRPV4 agonist and by measuring excitability of $TRPV4^{-/-}$ hippocampal neurons that were cocultured with wild-type astrocytes (Shibasaki, Ikenaka, Tamalu, Tominaga, & Ishizaki, 2014).

TRPV4 expression is confined to a discrete subpopulation of astrocytes localized at the interface of the brain and extracerebral liquid spaces, where coexpression with AQP4 is necessary for volume homeostasis (Benfenati et al., 2007, 2011). This is consistent with TRPV4 activity regulating neurovascular coupling (Dunn, Hill-Eubanks, Liedtke, & Nelson, 2013) and in pathogenesis following cerebral hypoxia (Butenko et al., 2012). Although the underlying mechanisms are not entirely clear, it is proposed to involve TRPV4-mediated increases in Ca^{2+} levels, leading to production of arachidonic acid-derived endogenous lipids such as prostaglandins and eicosanoids, which initiate smooth muscle relaxation and vessel dilation (Earley & Brayden, 2015; Filosa et al., 2013). Nitric oxide synthase activity and NO production can also be increased by endothelial TRPV4 activity to mediate relaxation. This is consistent with TRPV4-mediated NO production in other cell types including the myenteric plexus (Fichna et al., 2015).

3.2 Microglia

Microglia are the resident immune cells of the CNS that maintain neuronal health through protection against proinflammatory or ischemic insult. Like astrocytes, microglia are in close association with neurons and express functional TRPV4. Intriguingly, concurrent stimulation of microglia with a TRPV4 agonist (4αPDD) and the proinflammatory lipopolysaccharide (LPS) can diminish microglial release of tumor necrosis factor (TNF) and an ischemia-related β-galactoside-binding lectin, known as galectin-3 (Konno et al., 2012). This is proposed to be caused by TRPV4-mediated membrane depolarization, leading to Ca^{2+}-dependent suppression of microglial activity. In contrast, TRPV4 activity in other immune cells, as described in detail below, promotes increased production of proinflammatory cytokines, and elevated expression of cell surface markers associated with inflammation and increased phagocytic activity.

3.3 Satellite Glia

Satellite glial cells (SGCs) ensheath the somata of sensory neurons located in dorsal root and trigeminal ganglia. With neural-crest embryonic origins, these SGCs are distinct from glia of the CNS, yet appear to share many functional similarities with astrocytes. Although relatively little is known about how these cells contribute to the development of pain, SGCs express inwardly rectifying Kir4.1 potassium channels to reduce extracellular availability of potassium and dampen activity of DRG neurons (Takeda, Takahashi, Nasu, & Matsumoto, 2011; Tang, Schmidt, Perez-Leighton, & Kofuji, 2010; Vit, Ohara, Bhargava, Kelley, & Jasmin, 2008). In addition, our own studies have revealed that, like astrocytes, a subset of SGCs express functional TRPV4 and these channels can be acutely sensitized by the metabotropic purinoceptor, P2Y1. These experiments were performed exclusively on SGCs in association with neurons and suggest that ATP release from neurons can increase SGC Ca^{2+} signaling via a P2Y1 and protein kinase C (PKC)-dependent mechanism (Rajasekhar, Poole, Liedtke, Bunnett, & Veldhuis, 2015). Other complementary studies demonstrate that SGCs release ATP and glutamate upon increases in intracellular Ca^{2+} (Suadicani et al., 2010; Wagner et al., 2014). Further studies are required to confirm if signaling from this P2Y1–TRPV4 axis provides a positive feedback loop to enhance neuronal excitability.

3.4 Müller Glia

Since the first observations of retinal glial cells by Heinrich Müller in 1851, Müller glia have been established as important supporting cells for retinal development and health by contributing to maintenance of retinal structure and function (Bhattacharjee & Sanyal, 1975). In the retina, Müller glia express TRPV4, whereas retinal astrocytes and microglia do not (Ryskamp et al., 2011). Similar to the cerebral astrocytes, Müller glia also coexpress AQP4 and TRPV4, and these proteins may function synergistically for sensing and responding to osmotic stresses. Further studies are required to determine if TRPV4 activity or expression is altered in chronic pathological states associated with retinal damage, such as diabetes, traumatic ocular injury, or glaucoma (Jo et al., 2015; Ryskamp et al., 2014, 2011).

4. IMMUNE AND SECRETORY CELLS

In the innate immune system, macrophages, dendritic cells, and epithelia perform critical roles in the acute phase of detection and defense against pathogen exposure. These cells express pattern-recognition receptors such as Toll-like receptors (TLRs) that can bind and identify foreign particulates (e.g., proteins, lipids, sugars) and initiate signaling processes that lead to phagocytosis and cytokine production, to eliminate microorganisms and amplify the immune response (Akira, Uematsu, & Takeuchi, 2006).

As discussed below, a number of immune cell-related studies have demonstrated that pharmacological inhibition or genetic deletion of TRPV4 reduces the severity of inflammation in mouse models of age-related osteoarthritis, histaminergic itch, ventilator-induced lung injury, and systemic inflammation observed in models of sepsis. Immune cell-mediated cytokine release is a major component of these inflammatory conditions and can lead to neuronal sensitization and pain. Further characterization of TRPV4 secretory functions in immune cells may be valuable for addressing inflammatory conditions that pose significant clinical and economic burden worldwide.

4.1 Macrophages

Macrophages are highly mobile, responsive, shape-shifting innate immune cells that can bind and recognize foreign material for pathogen elimination. A genomic characterization of macrophages has confirmed the transcriptional presence of TRPV4 and many other ion channels (Groot-Kormelink, Fawcett, Wright, Gosling, & Kent, 2012) and these channels are proposed to regulate signaling processes including phagocytosis, an internalization mechanism for isolating and digesting foreign particulate material for subsequent antigen presentation. Indeed, LPS-stimulation of cultured bone marrow-derived macrophages requires TRPV4 for Ca^{2+}-dependent actin remodeling, phagocytosis of *Escherichia coli*, and cytokine production (decreased IL-1β and increased IL-10 production). This suggests that TRPV4 activity and LPS-induced TLR-mediated signaling pathways may be codependent. TRPV4 is also proposed to contribute to upregulation of phagocytosis in affected tissue in a mechanosensitive manner, potentially caused by elevated inflammation and edema increasing osmotic stress or extracellular matrix (ECM) stiffness (Scheraga et al., 2016). TRPV4 promotes the Ca^{2+}-dependent production of superoxide and nitric oxide, as confirmed through adoptive transfer of wild-type and TRPV4$^{-/-}$ alveolar macrophages to TRPV4$^{-/-}$ and wild-type mice, respectively. These are key signaling intermediates that enhance inflammation and lung damage by increasing vascular permeability (edema) and hypoxic or metabolic stress (Groot-Kormelink et al., 2012; Hamanaka et al., 2010; Scheraga et al., 2016).

4.2 T Cells

Flow cytometry and functional screening of TRP channels in the Jurkat human T cell line and mouse splenic T cells have demonstrated that TRPV4 and the capsaicin-sensitive TRPV1 ion channel contribute to Ca^{2+}-dependent T cell activation (Majhi et al., 2015). Within the acquired immune system, T cells eliminate pathogens by releasing specific cytokines to promote macrophage and B cell chemotaxis and activation. Naïve T cells express an array of store-operated and signaling-regulated ion channels. These channels are stimulated when T cells encounter antigen presenting cells, leading to elevated Ca^{2+} signaling and upregulation of transcriptional activity (Vig & Kinet, 2009). Once activated, they increase production and presentation of T cell activation markers (e.g., CD25 and CD69) and cytokine production. Thus, while TRPV4 can be pharmacologically controlled in T cells to regulate receptor expression and acquired inflammatory responses, this may be challenging in pathophysiological settings due to potential redundancies in the T cell channelome (Majhi et al., 2015).

4.3 Chondrocytes

As a mechanosensitive and proinflammatory channel, TRPV4 was readily identified as a mediator of mechanotransduction and arthritic conditions in load-bearing joints. Some inconsistencies in the precise role of TRPV4 in these pathophysiological states have been observed, where osteoarthritis (OA) and skeletal dysplasia are associated with global TRPV4 knockout mice studied in age-related and obesity models and also with gain-of-function TRPV4 mutations identified in humans (Clark & Malcangio, 2012; Lamande et al., 2011; O'Conor, Griffin, Liedtke, & Guilak, 2013;

O'Conor et al., 2016). Although contradictory, these findings highlight the complexity of TRPV4 Ca^{2+} flux in multiple cell types and indicate that a global knockout for a functionally diverse gene such as TRPV4 may lead to masked or misleading phenotypes in some cases. Sources of TRPV4-dependent inflammation and nociception in joints may arise from one or more cell types including chondrocytes, osteoclasts, synoviocytes, macrophages, or adipocytes and collectively these cells can modulate bone growth and density, and release of inflammatory factors into the synovial space (Itoh et al., 2009; Ye et al., 2012). A role for chondrocyte-mediated TRPV4 activity has been determined, and chondrocyte-selective knockout mice have recently been used to demonstrate that a loss of TRPV4 expression and activity in the cells reduces progression of physiological (age-related) but not pathophysiological (injury-induced) OA (O'Conor et al., 2016).

Chondrocytes are cartilage-secreting cells that perform essential roles within joints. They respond to mechanical pressure by mediating mechanotransduction, which involves changes in $[Ca^{2+}]_i$ and kinase signaling (e.g., ERK1/2 activity), and subsequent transcriptional changes that promote expression and secretion of proteins that change extracellular joint composition. A comprehensive review of these pathways indicates the TRPV4-mediated Ca^{2+} signaling regulates the transcriptional control of many processes through cAMP-CREB (cyclic AMP response element-binding protein) pathways (McNulty, Leddy, Liedtke, & Guilak, 2015).

Therapeutic intervention may be achieved with administration of TRPV4 antagonists or siRNA gene silencing, inhibition of upstream receptor signaling partners (e.g., protease-activated PAR2) or inhibition of micro-RNAs that upregulate TRPV4 activity and NO production (Hu, Zhu, & Wang, 2013; McNulty et al., 2015).

4.4 Myofibroblasts

Fibroblasts are present in almost every organ of the body and are quiescent under normal conditions. However, in acute inflammatory states, dysregulation of immune responses and the wound healing process can upregulate the activation and differentiation of fibroblasts into myofibroblasts, leading to excessive production of ECM components and fibrosis (Wynn, 2011; Wynn & Ramalingam, 2012). Primary human and murine fibroblasts express functional TRPV4, and its activity potentiates TGF-β1-mediated differentiation into myofibroblasts (Rahaman et al., 2014). $TRPV4^{-/-}$ mice were protected from profibrotic effects in a bleomycin-induced lung fibrosis model. Although the expression levels of TRPV4 were not different between fibroblasts isolated from healthy control and idiopathic pulmonary fibrosis patients, fibroblasts from the latter showed increased TRPV4 activity quantified by increases in Ca^{2+} influx. This study proposes a model wherein matrix stiffness in the lung sensitizes TRPV4 to mediate myofibroblast differentiation. However, it should be noted that increased expression and activity of proteases such as cathepsins and elastase in pulmonary disorders (Koslowski, Knoch, Kuhlisch, Seidel, & Kasper, 2003; Obayashi et al., 1997; Withana et al., 2016; Yamanouchi et al., 1998) can sensitize TRPV4 via actions on protease-activated receptor 2-mediated signaling in other cell types (Zhao et al., 2014, 2015). Indeed, many studies have described the role of PAR1 and PAR2 in fibroblasts and in the development of pulmonary fibrosis (Borensztajn et al., 2010; Scotton et al., 2009). Thus, proteases may perform a central role in the increased activity of TRPV4 in fibroblasts under pathophysiological conditions for potentiation of TGF-β1-induced myofibroblast differentiation and pulmonary fibrosis.

5. CONCLUSION

Many cell types express TRPV4 and this is often overlooked and underappreciated, especially in the context of neurogenic inflammation and pain. Nonneuronal cells closely associated with neurons (e.g., "gliotransmitter" release by glial cells) and indirect mechanisms typically associated with TRPV4-mediated edema or immune cell infiltration can contribute to both inflammation and nociception. The majority of the current literature focuses on TRPV4 expression by afferent neurons and how activation of these neurons by endogenous TRPV4 agonists can exacerbate inflammation and pain.

By addressing many similarities and differences in TRPV4 function throughout the body, this review has more specifically discussed TRPV4 activity in immune, epithelial, and secretory cells. A common emerging theme is the TRPV4-mediated increase in $[Ca^{2+}]_i$ inducing the release of cytokines, ATP, and glutamate in multiple cell types. In addition, there are several observations indicating that TRPV4 activity increases inflammatory cytokine production and secretion. While these findings suggest an important role for TRPV4 in chronic inflammatory conditions and neuropathic pain, it is very difficult to differentiate these proinflammatory roles from other physiological outcomes such as wound healing, long-term dampening of neuronal responses, and immune cell clearance. TRPV4 is widely expressed throughout the body and is implicated in a variety of physiological processes. The availability of pharmacological tools (specific agonists and antagonists) as well as genetic tools (global and tissue specific TRPV4 knockout mice) has been instrumental in probing functional expression of TRPV4 in different tissues.

Compared to other TRP channel superfamily members, TRPV4 has the greatest number of disease causing mutations in humans, which are collectively referred to as channelopathies. Mutations lead to dysfunctional signaling that underlies arthropathies, skeletal dysplasias, and peripheral neuropathies. There has been much discussion about why TRPV4 knockout mice have very mild phenotypes, considering the widespread expression of this channel (Nilius & Voets, 2013; White et al., 2016). This is consistent with studies in the clinic, where the successful phase I clinical trial of GSK2798745 demonstrated minimal adverse effects of TRPV4 antagonists in humans. Perhaps only in phase II clinical trials will the benefits of blocking TRPV4 in pathophysiological conditions be revealed. Mild TRPV4 knockout phenotypes may be caused by redundancy mechanisms via upregulation of other ion channels with similar distribution patterns or functions, or other inherent compensatory mechanisms. To account for this, it would be useful to perform a comparison of normal function and disease in tissue-specific conditional (inducible) TRPV4 knockouts (especially in tissues with high TRPV4 expression) and global knockouts. Potential examples include examination of vascular function and pulmonary edema in endothelial-specific TRPV4 knockout mice, and characterization of the development, severity, and resolution of inflammatory diseases in mice that selectively lack functional TRPV4 in macrophages or other immune cells.

It is tempting to speculate that future studies with these genetic tools may alternatively reveal roles for TRPV4 *both* in the onset and clearance of chronic inflammation. This would further complicate the discussion surrounding the use of TRPV4 agonists or antagonists for the treatment of chronic diseases. Furthermore, the multitude of varied roles for TRPV4 is both fascinating and frightening, when considering potential on-target effects that would be observed without careful control of tissue-selective drug delivery.

CONFLICT OF INTEREST

The authors have no conflicts of interest to declare.

ACKNOWLEDGMENTS

Research by the authors is supported by the ARC Centre of Excellence in Convergent Bio-Nano Science and Technology (N.A.V.), NHMRC Australia grant APP1083480 (D.P.P.), and an Australian Government Research Training Program Scholarship (P.R.).

REFERENCES

Akira, S., Uematsu, S., & Takeuchi, O. (2006). Pathogen recognition and innate immunity. *Cell, 124*(4), 783–801. http://dx.doi.org/10.1016/j.cell.2006.02.015.

Alessandri-Haber, N., Yeh, J. J., Boyd, A. E., Parada, C. a., Chen, X., Reichling, D. B., et al. (2003). Hypotonicity induces TRPV4-mediated nociception in rat. *Neuron, 39*, 497–511.

Balakrishna, S., Song, W., Achanta, S., Doran, S. F., Liu, B., Kaelberer, M. M., et al. (2014). TRPV4 inhibition counteracts edema and inflammation and improves pulmonary function and oxygen saturation in chemically induced acute lung injury. *American Journal of Physiology. Lung Cellular and Molecular Physiology, 307*(2), L158–L172. http://dx.doi.org/10.1152/ajplung.00065.2014.

Beckel, J. M., Daugherty, S. L., Tyagi, P., Wolf-Johnston, A. S., Birder, L. A., Mitchell, C. H., et al. (2015). Pannexin 1 channels mediate the release of ATP into the lumen of the rat urinary bladder. *The Journal of Physiology, 593*(8), 1857–1871. http://dx.doi.org/10.1113/jphysiol.2014.283119.

Benfenati, V., Amiry-Moghaddam, M., Caprini, M., Mylonakou, M. N., Rapisarda, C., Ottersen, O. P., et al. (2007). Expression and functional characterization of transient receptor potential vanilloid-related channel 4 (TRPV4) in rat cortical astrocytes. *Neuroscience, 148*, 876–892. http://dx.doi.org/10.1016/j.neuroscience.2007.06.039.

Benfenati, V., Caprini, M., Dovizio, M., Mylonakou, M. N., Ferroni, S., Ottersen, O. P., et al. (2011). An aquaporin-4/transient receptor potential vanilloid 4 (AQP4/TRPV4) complex is essential for cell-volume control in astrocytes. *Proceedings of the National Academy of Sciences of the United States of America, 108*(6), 2563–2568. http://dx.doi.org/10.1073/pnas.1012867108.

Bhattacharjee, J., & Sanyal, S. (1975). Developmental origin and early differentiation of retinal Muller cells in mice. *Journal of Anatomy, 120*(Pt. 2), 367–372.

Birder, L., Kullmann, F. A., Lee, H., Barrick, S., de Groat, W., Kanai, A., et al. (2007). Activation of urothelial transient receptor potential vanilloid 4 by 4alpha-phorbol 12,13-didecanoate contributes to altered bladder reflexes in the rat. *The Journal of Pharmacology and Experimental Therapeutics, 323*(1), 227–235. http://dx.doi.org/10.1124/jpet.107.125435.

Borensztajn, K., Bresser, P., van der Loos, C., Bot, I., van den Blink, B., den Bakker, M. A., et al. (2010). Protease-activated receptor-2 induces myofibroblast differentiation and tissue factor up-regulation during bleomycin-induced lung injury: Potential role in pulmonary fibrosis. *The American Journal of Pathology, 177*(6), 2753–2764. http://dx.doi.org/10.2353/ajpath.2010.091107.

Butenko, O., Dzamba, D., Benesova, J., Honsa, P., Benfenati, V., Rusnakova, V., et al. (2012). The increased activity of TRPV4 channel in the astrocytes of the adult rat hippocampus after cerebral hypoxia/ischemia. *PloS One*, 7(6), e39959. http://dx.doi.org/10.1371/journal.pone.0039959.

Chen, Y., Fang, Q., Wang, Z., Zhang, J. Y., MacLeod, A. S., Hall, R. P., et al. (2016). Transient receptor potential vanilloid 4 ion channel functions as a pruriceptor in epidermal keratinocytes to evoke histaminergic itch. *The Journal of Biological Chemistry, 291*(19), 10252–10262. http://dx.doi.org/10.1074/jbc.M116.716464.

Chung, M. K., Lee, H., Mizuno, A., Suzuki, M., & Caterina, M. J. (2004). TRPV3 and TRPV4 mediate warmth-evoked currents in primary mouse keratinocytes. *The Journal of Biological Chemistry, 279*(20), 21569–21575. http://dx.doi.org/10.1074/jbc.M401872200.

Clark, A. K., & Malcangio, M. (2012). Microglial signalling mechanisms: Cathepsin S and fractalkine. *Experimental Neurology, 234*(2), 283–292. http://dx.doi.org/10.1016/j.expneurol.2011.09.012.

Dahan, D., Ducret, T., Quignard, J. F., Marthan, R., Savineau, J. P., & Esteve, E. (2012). Implication of the ryanodine receptor in TRPV4-induced calcium response in pulmonary arterial smooth muscle cells from normoxic and chronically hypoxic rats. *American Journal of Physiology. Lung Cellular and Molecular Physiology, 303*(9), L824–L833. http://dx.doi.org/10.1152/ajplung.00244.2011.

D'Aldebert, E., Cenac, N., Rousset, P., Martin, L., Rolland, C., Chapman, K., et al. (2011). Transient receptor potential vanilloid 4 activated inflammatory signals by intestinal epithelial cells and colitis in mice. *Gastroenterology, 140*, 275–285. http://dx.doi.org/10.1053/j.gastro.2010.09.045.

Dunn, K. M., Hill-Eubanks, D. C., Liedtke, W. B., & Nelson, M. T. (2013). TRPV4 channels stimulate Ca2+-induced Ca2+ release in astrocytic endfeet and amplify neurovascular coupling responses. *Proceedings of the National Academy of Sciences of the United States of America, 110*(15), 6157–6162. http://dx.doi.org/10.1073/pnas.1216514110.

Earley, S., & Brayden, J. E. (2015). Transient receptor potential channels in the vasculature. *Physiological Reviews, 95*(2), 645–690. http://dx.doi.org/10.1152/physrev.00026.2014.

Earley, S., Heppner, T. J., Nelson, M. T., & Brayden, J. E. (2005). TRPV4 forms a novel Ca2+ signaling complex with ryanodine receptors and BKCa channels. *Circulation Research, 97*(12), 1270–1279. http://dx.doi.org/10.1161/01.RES.0000194321.60300.d6.

Everaerts, W., Zhen, X., Ghosh, D., Vriens, J., Gevaert, T., Gilbert, J. P., et al. (2010). Inhibition of the cation channel TRPV4 improves bladder function in mice and rats with cyclophosphamide-induced cystitis. *Proceedings of the National Academy of Sciences of the United States of America, 107*(44), 19084–19089. http://dx.doi.org/10.1073/pnas.1005333107.

Fichna, J., Poole, D. P., Veldhuis, N., MacEachern, S. J., Saur, D., Zakrzewski, P. K., et al. (2015). Transient receptor potential vanilloid 4 inhibits mouse colonic motility by activating NO-dependent enteric neurotransmission. *Journal of Molecular Medicine (Berlin, Germany), 93*(12), 1297–1309. http://dx.doi.org/10.1007/s00109-015-1336-5.

Filosa, J. A., Yao, X., & Rath, G. (2013). TRPV4 and the regulation of vascular tone. *Journal of Cardiovascular Pharmacology, 61*(2), 113–119. http://dx.doi.org/10.1097/FJC.0b013e318279ba42.

Groot-Kormelink, P. J., Fawcett, L., Wright, P. D., Gosling, M., & Kent, T. C. (2012). Quantitative GPCR and ion channel transcriptomics in primary alveolar macrophages and macrophage surrogates. *BMC Immunology, 13*, 57. http://dx.doi.org/10.1186/1471-2172-13-57.

Hamanaka, K., Jian, M. Y., Townsley, M. I., King, J. A., Liedtke, W., Weber, D. S., et al. (2010). TRPV4 channels augment macrophage activation and ventilator-induced lung injury. *American Journal of Physiology. Lung Cellular and Molecular Physiology, 299*(3), L353–L362. http://dx.doi.org/10.1152/ajplung.00315.2009.

Holzer, P. (2011). TRP channels in the digestive system. *Current Pharmaceutical Biotechnology, 12*(1), 24–34. http://dx.doi.org/10.2174/138920111793937862.

Hu, F., Zhu, W., & Wang, L. (2013). MicroRNA-203 up-regulates nitric oxide expression in temporomandibular joint chondrocytes via targeting TRPV4. *Archives of Oral Biology, 58*(2), 192–199. http://dx.doi.org/10.1016/j.archoralbio.2012.08.013.

Itoh, Y., Hatano, N., Hayashi, H., Onozaki, K., Miyazawa, K., & Muraki, K. (2009). An environmental sensor, TRPV4 is a novel regulator of intracellular Ca2+ in human synoviocytes. *American Journal of Physiology. Cell Physiology*, *297*(5), C1082–C1090. http://dx.doi.org/10.1152/ajpcell.00204.2009.

Janssen, D. A., Hoenderop, J. G., Jansen, K. C., Kemp, A. W., Heesakkers, J. P., & Schalken, J. A. (2011). The mechanoreceptor TRPV4 is localized in adherence junctions of the human bladder urothelium: A morphological study. *The Journal of Urology*, *186*(3), 1121–1127. http://dx.doi.org/10.1016/j.juro.2011.04.107.

Jian, M. Y., King, J. A., Al-Mehdi, A. B., Liedtke, W., & Townsley, M. I. (2008). High vascular pressure-induced lung injury requires P450 epoxygenase-dependent activation of TRPV4. *American Journal of Respiratory Cell and Molecular Biology*, *38*(4), 386–392. http://dx.doi.org/10.1165/rcmb.2007-0192OC.

Jo, A. O., Ryskamp, D. A., Phuong, T. T., Verkman, A. S., Yarishkin, O., MacAulay, N., et al. (2015). TRPV4 and AQP4 channels synergistically regulate cell volume and calcium homeostasis in retinal Muller glia. *The Journal of Neuroscience*, *35*(39), 13525–13537. http://dx.doi.org/10.1523/JNEUROSCI.1987-15.2015.

Kang, N., Xu, J., Xu, Q., Nedergaard, M., & Kang, J. (2005). Astrocytic glutamate release-induced transient depolarization and epileptiform discharges in hippocampal CA1 pyramidal neurons. *Journal of Neurophysiology*, *94*(6), 4121–4130. http://dx.doi.org/10.1152/jn.00448.2005.

Kim, S. K., Hayashi, H., Ishikawa, T., Shibata, K., Shigetomi, E., Shinozaki, Y., et al. (2016). Cortical astrocytes rewire somatosensory cortical circuits for peripheral neuropathic pain. *The Journal of Clinical Investigation*, *126*(5), 1983–1997. http://dx.doi.org/10.1172/JCI82859.

Konno, M., Shirakawa, H., Iida, S., Sakimoto, S., Matsutani, I., Miyake, T., et al. (2012). Stimulation of transient receptor potential vanilloid 4 channel suppresses abnormal activation of microglia induced by lipopolysaccharide. *Glia*, *60*, 761–770. http://dx.doi.org/10.1002/glia.22306.

Koslowski, R., Knoch, K., Kuhlisch, E., Seidel, D., & Kasper, M. (2003). Cathepsins in bleomycin-induced lung injury in rat. *The European Respiratory Journal*, *22*(3), 427–435.

Lamande, S. R., Yuan, Y., Gresshoff, I. L., Rowley, L., Belluoccio, D., Kaluarachchi, K., et al. (2011). Mutations in TRPV4 cause an inherited arthropathy of hands and feet. *Nature Genetics*, *43*(11), 1142–1146. http://dx.doi.org/10.1038/ng.945.

Li, L., Qu, W., Zhou, L., Lu, Z., Jie, P., Chen, L., et al. (2013). Activation of transient receptor potential vanilloid 4 increases NMDA-activated current in hippocampal pyramidal neurons. *Frontiers in Cellular Neuroscience*, 7, 17. http://dx.doi.org/10.3389/fncel.2013.00017.

Majhi, R. K., Sahoo, S. S., Yadav, M., Pratheek, B. M., Chattopadhyay, S., & Goswami, C. (2015). Functional expression of TRPV channels in T cells and their implications in immune regulation. *The FEBS Journal*, *282*(14), 2661–2681. http://dx.doi.org/10.1111/febs.13306.

McNulty, A. L., Leddy, H. A., Liedtke, W., & Guilak, F. (2015). TRPV4 as a therapeutic target for joint diseases. *Naunyn-Schmiedeberg's Archives of Pharmacology*, *388*(4), 437–450. http://dx.doi.org/10.1007/s00210-014-1078-x.

Mendoza, S. A., Fang, J., Gutterman, D. D., Wilcox, D. A., Bubolz, A. H., Li, R., et al. (2010). TRPV4-mediated endothelial Ca2+ influx and vasodilation in response to shear stress. *American Journal of Physiology. Heart and Circulatory Physiology*, *298*(2), H466–H476. http://dx.doi.org/10.1152/ajpheart.00854.2009.

Mihara, H., Boudaka, A., Sugiyama, T., Moriyama, Y., & Tominaga, M. (2011). Transient receptor potential vanilloid 4 (TRPV4)-dependent calcium influx and ATP release in mouse oesophageal keratinocytes. *The Journal of Physiology*, *589*(Pt. 14), 3471–3482. http://dx.doi.org/10.1113/jphysiol.2011.207829.

Mochizuki, T., Sokabe, T., Araki, I., Fujishita, K., Shibasaki, K., Uchida, K., et al. (2009). The TRPV4 Cation Channel mediates stretch-evoked Ca2+ influx and ATP release in primary urothelial cell cultures. *The Journal of Biological Chemistry*, *284*(32), 21257–21264. http://dx.doi.org/10.1074/jbc.M109.020206.

Moore, C., Cevikbas, F., Pasolli, H. A., Chen, Y., Kong, W., Kempkes, C., et al. (2013). UVB radiation generates sunburn pain and affects skin by activating epidermal TRPV4 ion channels and triggering endothelin-1 signaling. *Proceedings of the National Academy of Sciences of the United States of America*, *110*(34), E3225–E3234. http://dx.doi.org/10.1073/pnas.1312933110.

Nilius, B., & Voets, T. (2013). The puzzle of TRPV4 channelopathies. *EMBO Reports*, *14*(2), 152–163. http://dx.doi.org/10.1038/embor.2012.219.

Obayashi, Y., Yamadori, I., Fujita, J., Yoshinouchi, T., Ueda, N., & Takahara, J. (1997). The role of neutrophils in the pathogenesis of idiopathic pulmonary fibrosis. *Chest*, *112*(5), 1338–1343.

O'Conor, C. J., Griffin, T. M., Liedtke, W., & Guilak, F. (2013). Increased susceptibility of Trpv4-deficient mice to obesity and obesity-induced osteoarthritis with very high-fat diet. *Annals of the Rheumatic Diseases*, *72*(2), 300–304. http://dx.doi.org/10.1136/annrheumdis-2012-202272.

O'Conor, C. J., Ramalingam, S., Zelenski, N. A., Benefield, H. C., Rigo, I., Little, D., et al. (2016). Cartilage-specific knockout of the mechanosensory Ion Channel TRPV4 decreases age-related osteoarthritis. *Scientific Reports*, *6*, 29053. http://dx.doi.org/10.1038/srep29053.

Pannasch, U., & Rouach, N. (2013). Emerging role for astroglial networks in information processing: From synapse to behavior. *Trends in Neurosciences*, *36*(7), 405–417. http://dx.doi.org/10.1016/j.tins.2013.04.004.

Poole, D. P., Lieu, T., Veldhuis, N. A., Rajasekhar, P., & Bunnett, N. W. (2015). Targeting of transient receptor potential channels in digestive disease. In A. Szallasi (Ed.), *TRP channels as therapeutic targets* (pp. 385–403). Elsevier. http://dx.doi.org/10.1016/b978-0-12-420024-1.00021-7.

Rahaman, S. O., Grove, L. M., Paruchuri, S., Southern, B. D., Abraham, S., Niese, K. A., et al. (2014). TRPV4 mediates myofibroblast differentiation and pulmonary fibrosis in mice. *The Journal of Clinical Investigation*, *124*(12), 5225–5238. http://dx.doi.org/10.1172/JCI75331.

Rajasekhar, P., Poole, D. P., Liedtke, W., Bunnett, N. W., & Veldhuis, N. A. (2015). P2Y1 receptor activation of the TRPV4 ion channel enhances purinergic signaling in satellite glial cells. *The Journal of Biological Chemistry*, *290*(48), 29051–29062. http://dx.doi.org/10.1074/jbc.M115.689729.

Ryskamp, D. A., Jo, A. O., Frye, A. M., Vazquez-Chona, F., MacAulay, N., Thoreson, W. B., et al. (2014). Swelling and eicosanoid metabolites differentially gate TRPV4 channels in retinal neurons and glia. *The Journal of Neuroscience*, *34*(47), 15689–15700. http://dx.doi.org/10.1523/jneurosci.2540-14.2014.

Ryskamp, D. A., Witkovsky, P., Barabas, P., Huang, W., Koehler, C., Akimov, N. P., et al. (2011). The polymodal ion channel transient receptor potential vanilloid 4 modulates calcium flux, spiking rate, and apoptosis of mouse retinal ganglion cells. *The Journal of Neuroscience*, *31*(19), 7089–7101. http://dx.doi.org/10.1523/JNEUROSCI.0359-11.2011.

Scheraga, R. G., Abraham, S., Niese, K. A., Southern, B. D., Grove, L. M., Hite, R. D., et al. (2016). TRPV4 mechanosensitive ion channel regulates lipopolysaccharide-stimulated macrophage phagocytosis. *Journal of Immunology*, *196*(1), 428–436. http://dx.doi.org/10.4049/jimmunol.1501688.

Scholz, J., & Woolf, C. J. (2007). The neuropathic pain triad: Neurons, immune cells and glia. *Nature Neuroscience*, *10*(11), 1361–1368. http://dx.doi.org/10.1038/nn1992.

Scotton, C. J., Krupiczojc, M. A., Konigshoff, M., Mercer, P. F., Lee, Y. C., Kaminski, N., et al. (2009). Increased local expression of coagulation factor X contributes to the fibrotic response in human and murine lung injury. *The Journal of Clinical Investigation, 119*(9), 2550–2563. http://dx.doi.org/10.1172/JCI33288.

Seminario-Vidal, L., Okada, S. F., Sesma, J. I., Kreda, S. M., van Heusden, C. A., Zhu, Y., et al. (2011). Rho signaling regulates pannexin 1-mediated ATP release from airway epithelia. *The Journal of Biological Chemistry, 286*(30), 26277–26286. http://dx.doi.org/10.1074/jbc.M111.260562.

Shibasaki, K., Ikenaka, K., Tamalu, F., Tominaga, M., & Ishizaki, Y. (2014). A novel subtype of astrocytes expressing TRPV4 (transient receptor potential vanilloid 4) regulates neuronal excitability via release of gliotransmitters. *The Journal of Biological Chemistry, 289*, 14470–14480. http://dx.doi.org/10.1074/jbc.M114.557132.

Simonsen, U., Wandall-Frostholm, C., Olivan-Viguera, A., & Kohler, R. (2016). Emerging roles of calcium-activated K channels and TRPV4 channels in lung oedema and pulmonary circulatory collapse. *Acta Physiologica (Oxford, England)*. http://dx.doi.org/10.1111/apha.12768.

Sokabe, T., Fukumi-Tominaga, T., Yonemura, S., Mizuno, A., & Tominaga, M. (2010). The TRPV4 channel contributes to intercellular junction formation in keratinocytes. *The Journal of Biological Chemistry, 285*(24), 18749–18758. http://dx.doi.org/10.1074/jbc.M110.103606.

Sonkusare, S. K., Bonev, A. D., Ledoux, J., Liedtke, W., Kotlikoff, M. I., Heppner, T. J., et al. (2012). Elementary Ca2+ signals through endothelial TRPV4 channels regulate vascular function. *Science, 336*(6081), 597–601. http://dx.doi.org/10.1126/science.1216283.

Suadicani, S. O., Cherkas, P. S., Zuckerman, J., Smith, D. N., Spray, D. C., & Hanani, M. (2010). Bidirectional calcium signaling between satellite glial cells and neurons in cultured mouse trigeminal ganglia. *Neuron Glia Biology, 6*(1), 43–51. http://dx.doi.org/10.1017/S1740925X09990408.

Sukumaran, S. V., Singh, T. U., Parida, S., Narasimha Reddy Ch, E., Thangamalai, R., Kandasamy, K., et al. (2013). TRPV4 channel activation leads to endothelium-dependent relaxation mediated by nitric oxide and endothelium-derived hyperpolarizing factor in rat pulmonary artery. *Pharmacological Research, 78*, 18–27. http://dx.doi.org/10.1016/j.phrs.2013.09.005.

Takano, T., Kang, J., Jaiswal, J. K., Simon, S. M., Lin, J. H., Yu, Y., et al. (2005). Receptor-mediated glutamate release from volume sensitive channels in astrocytes. *Proceedings of the National Academy of Sciences of the United States of America, 102*(45), 16466–16471. http://dx.doi.org/10.1073/pnas.0506382102.

Takeda, M., Takahashi, M., Nasu, M., & Matsumoto, S. (2011). Peripheral inflammation suppresses inward rectifying potassium currents of satellite glial cells in the trigeminal ganglia. *Pain, 152*, 2147–2156. http://dx.doi.org/10.1016/j.pain.2011.05.023.

Tang, X., Schmidt, T. M., Perez-Leighton, C. E., & Kofuji, P. (2010). Inwardly rectifying potassium channel Kir4.1 is responsible for the native inward potassium conductance of satellite glial cells in sensory ganglia. *Neuroscience, 166*, 397–407. http://dx.doi.org/10.1016/j.neuroscience.2010.01.005.

Thorneloe, K. S., Cheung, M., Bao, W., Alsaid, H., Lenhard, S., Jian, M. Y., et al. (2012). An orally active TRPV4 channel blocker prevents and resolves pulmonary edema induced by heart failure. *Science Translational Medicine, 4*(159), 159ra148. http://dx.doi.org/10.1126/scitranslmed.3004276.

Ueda, T., Shikano, M., Kamiya, T., Joh, T., & Ugawa, S. (2011). The TRPV4 channel is a novel regulator of intracellular Ca2+ in human esophageal epithelial cells. *American Journal of Physiology. Gastrointestinal and Liver Physiology, 301*(1), G138–G147. http://dx.doi.org/10.1152/ajpgi.00511.2010.

Veldhuis, N. A., Poole, D. P., Grace, M., McIntyre, P., & Bunnett, N. W. (2015). The G protein-coupled receptor-transient receptor potential channel axis: Molecular insights for targeting disorders of sensation and inflammation. *Pharmacological Reviews, 67*(1), 36–73. http://dx.doi.org/10.1124/pr.114.009555.

Vig, M., & Kinet, J. P. (2009). Calcium signaling in immune cells. *Nature Immunology*, *10*(1), 21–27. http://dx.doi.org/10.1038/ni.f.220.

Vit, J.-P., Ohara, P. T., Bhargava, A., Kelley, K., & Jasmin, L. (2008). Silencing the Kir4.1 potassium channel subunit in satellite glial cells of the rat trigeminal ganglion results in pain-like behavior in the absence of nerve injury. *The Journal of Neuroscience*, *28*, 4161–4171. http://dx.doi.org/10.1523/JNEUROSCI.5053-07.2008.

Wagner, L., Warwick, R. a., Pannicke, T., Reichenbach, A., Grosche, A., & Hanani, M. (2014). Glutamate release from satellite glial cells of the murine trigeminal ganglion. *Neuroscience Letters*, *578*, 143–147. http://dx.doi.org/10.1016/j.neulet.2014.06.047.

Wandall-Frostholm, C., Dalsgaard, T., Bajoriūnas, V., Oliván-Viguera, A., Sadda, V., Beck, L., et al. (2015). Genetic deficit of $K_{Ca}3.1$ channels protects against pulmonary circulatory collapse induced by TRPV4 channel activation. *The British Journal of Pharmacology*, *172*(18), 4493–4505. http://dx.doi.org/10.1111/bph.13234.

Watanabe, H., Vriens, J., Suh, S. H., Benham, C. D., Droogmans, G., & Nilius, B. (2002). Heat-evoked activation of TRPV4 channels in a HEK293 cell expression system and in native mouse aorta endothelial cells. *The Journal of Biological Chemistry*, *277*(49), 47044–47051. http://dx.doi.org/10.1074/jbc.M208277200.

White, J. P., Cibelli, M., Urban, L., Nilius, B., McGeown, J. G., & Nagy, I. (2016). TRPV4: Molecular conductor of a diverse orchestra. *Physiological Reviews*, *96*(3), 911–973. http://dx.doi.org/10.1152/physrev.00016.2015.

Willette, R. N., Bao, W., Nerurkar, S., Yue, T. L., Doe, C. P., Stankus, G., et al. (2008). Systemic activation of the transient receptor potential vanilloid subtype 4 channel causes endothelial failure and circulatory collapse: Part 2. *The Journal of Pharmacology and Experimental Therapeutics*, *326*(2), 443–452. http://dx.doi.org/10.1124/jpet.107.134551.

Withana, N. P., Ma, X., McGuire, H. M., Verdoes, M., van der Linden, W. A., Ofori, L. O., et al. (2016). Non-invasive imaging of idiopathic pulmonary fibrosis using cathepsin protease probes. *Scientific Reports*, *6*, 19755. http://dx.doi.org/10.1038/srep19755.

Wynn, T. A. (2011). Integrating mechanisms of pulmonary fibrosis. *The Journal of Experimental Medicine*, *208*(7), 1339–1350. http://dx.doi.org/10.1084/jem.20110551.

Wynn, T. A., & Ramalingam, T. R. (2012). Mechanisms of fibrosis: Therapeutic translation for fibrotic disease. *Nature Medicine*, *18*(7), 1028–1040. http://dx.doi.org/10.1038/nm.2807.

Yamada, T., Ugawa, S., Ueda, T., Ishida, Y., Kajita, K., & Shimada, S. (2009). Differential localizations of the transient receptor potential channels TRPV4 and TRPV1 in the mouse urinary bladder. *The Journal of Histochemistry and Cytochemistry*, *57*(3), 277–287. http://dx.doi.org/10.1369/jhc.2008.951962.

Yamanouchi, H., Fujita, J., Hojo, S., Yoshinouchi, T., Kamei, T., Yamadori, I., et al. (1998). Neutrophil elastase: Alpha-1-proteinase inhibitor complex in serum and bronchoalveolar lavage fluid in patients with pulmonary fibrosis. *The European Respiratory Journal*, *11*(1), 120–125.

Yamawaki, H., Mihara, H., Suzuki, N., Nishizono, H., Uchida, K., Watanabe, S., et al. (2014). Role of transient receptor potential vanilloid 4 activation in indomethacin-induced intestinal damage. *American Journal of Physiology. Gastrointestinal and Liver Physiology*, *307*(1), G33–G40. http://dx.doi.org/10.1152/ajpgi.00105.2013.

Ye, L., Kleiner, S., Wu, J., Sah, R., Gupta, R. K., Banks, A. S., et al. (2012). TRPV4 is a regulator of adipose oxidative metabolism, inflammation, and energy homeostasis. *Cell*, *151*(1), 96–110. http://dx.doi.org/10.1016/j.cell.2012.08.034.

Zhao, P., Lieu, T., Barlow, N., Metcalf, M., Veldhuis, N. A., Jensen, D. D., et al. (2014). Cathepsin S causes inflammatory pain via biased agonism of PAR2 and TRPV4. *The Journal of Biological Chemistry*, *289*(39), 27215–27234. http://dx.doi.org/10.1074/jbc.M114.599712.

Zhao, P., Lieu, T., Barlow, N., Sostegni, S., Haerteis, S., Korbmacher, C., et al. (2015). Neutrophil elastase activates protease-activated receptor-2 (PAR2) and transient receptor potential vanilloid 4 (TRPV4) to cause inflammation and pain. *The Journal of Biological Chemistry*, *290*(22), 13875–13887. http://dx.doi.org/10.1074/jbc.M115.642736.

CHAPTER FIVE

Genetically Encoded Calcium Indicators as Probes to Assess the Role of Calcium Channels in Disease and for High-Throughput Drug Discovery

John J. Bassett*, Gregory R. Monteith*,†,1
*School of Pharmacy, The University of Queensland, Brisbane, QLD, Australia
†Mater Research, The University of Queensland, Brisbane, QLD, Australia
[1]Corresponding author: e-mail address: gregm@uq.edu.au

Contents

Abstract

The calcium ion (Ca^{2+}) is an important signaling molecule implicated in many cellular processes, and the remodeling of Ca^{2+} homeostasis is a feature of a variety of pathologies. Typical methods to assess Ca^{2+} signaling in cells often employ small molecule fluorescent dyes, which are sometimes poorly suited to certain applications such as assessment of cellular processes, which occur over long periods (hours or days) or in vivo experiments. Genetically encoded calcium indicators are a set of tools available for the measurement of Ca^{2+} changes in the cytosol and subcellular compartments, which circumvent some of the inherent limitations of small molecule Ca^{2+} probes. Recent advances in genetically encoded calcium sensors have greatly increased their

Advances in Pharmacology, Volume 79
ISSN 1054-3589
http://dx.doi.org/10.1016/bs.apha.2017.01.001

ability to provide reliable monitoring of Ca^{2+} changes in mammalian cells. New genetically encoded calcium indicators have diverse options in terms of targeting, Ca^{2+} affinity and fluorescence spectra, and this will further enhance their potential use in high-throughput drug discovery and other assays. This review will outline the methods available for Ca^{2+} measurement in cells, with a focus on genetically encoded calcium sensors. How these sensors will improve our understanding of the deregulation of Ca^{2+} handling in disease and their application to high-throughput identification of drug leads will also be discussed.

ABBREVIATIONS

$[Ca^{2+}]_{CYT}$ resting cytosolic free calcium ion concentration
AM acetoxymethyl
ATP adenosine triphosphate
BAPTA 1,2-bis(*o*-aminophenoxy)ethane-*N,N,N',N'*-tetraacetic acid
Ca^{2+} calcium ion
ER endoplasmic reticulum
FLIPR fluorescence imaging plate reader
FRET Förster resonance energy transfer
GECI genetically encoded calcium indicator
GFP green fluorescent protein
IP_3 inositol 1,4,5-trisphosphate
IP_3R 1,4,5-trisphosphate-activated receptor
NFAT nuclear factor of activated T cells
PS1 presenilin-1
RyR ryanodine receptor
SR/ER sarcoplasmic/endoplasmic reticulum
TRP transient receptor potential

1. INTRODUCTION

The calcium ion (Ca^{2+}) is an important intracellular second messenger, the movement of which is responsible for the regulation of a variety of cellular processes. These include proliferation, excitation/contraction coupling, cell death, gene transcription, and cell motility (Berridge, Bootman, & Roderick, 2003; Clapham, 2007). Simultaneous regulation of these and other Ca^{2+}-dependent processes is achieved via a suite of Ca^{2+} channels, pumps, exchangers, and regulators. Together, they function to manipulate the temporal and spatial aspects of the Ca^{2+} signal (Berridge, 2000; Berridge et al., 2003; Prevarskaya, Ouadid-Ahidouch, Skryma, & Shuba, 2014). Plasma membrane Ca^{2+} pumps are responsible for preserving a large plasmalemmal concentration gradient for Ca^{2+}, which consists of a resting cytosolic free Ca^{2+} concentration ($[Ca^{2+}]_{CYT}$) of approximately ~100 nM. This is in stark contrast to the high concentration of free Ca^{2+} in the extracellular space (~1–2 mM) (Berridge, 2000; Clapham, 2007). Fig. 1 outlines the key classes of Ca^{2+} channels located in mammalian cells, with the approximate free Ca^{2+} levels for the cytosol, sarcoplasmic/endoplasmic reticulum (SR/ER), and mitochondria.

Alterations in Ca^{2+} signaling have been linked to the pathophysiology of several diseases including cardiovascular disease, neurological disorders, and cancer (Brini, Cali, Ottolini, & Carafoli, 2014; Fearnley, Roderick, & Bootman, 2011; Monteith, McAndrew, Faddy, & Roberts-Thomson, 2007). Targeting regulators of Ca^{2+} signaling therefore may represent an area of opportunity for the identification of new therapies for such diseases. Modulating Ca^{2+} signaling has already been demonstrated to have clinical relevance. Examples include the L-type voltage-gated Ca^{2+} channel

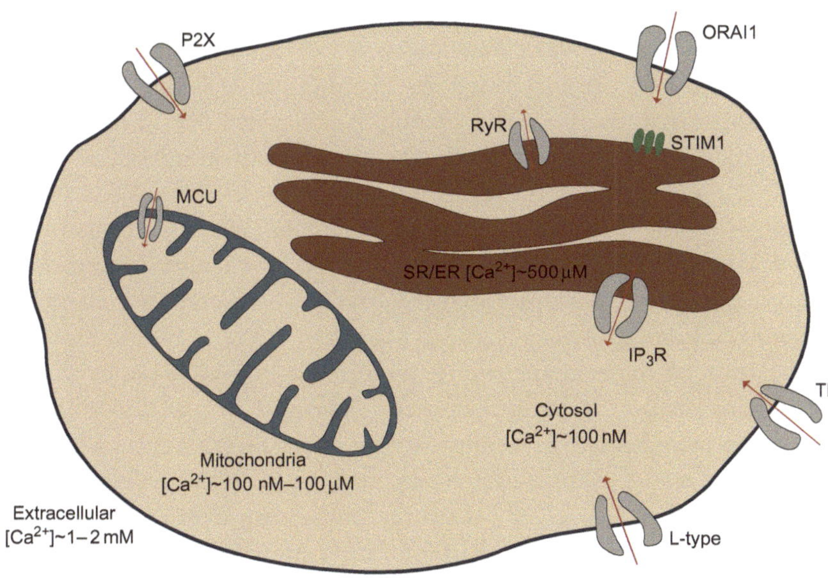

Fig. 1 Schematic representation of a mammalian cell highlighting some of the main Ca^{2+} channel families. Ca^{2+} channels in conjunction with Ca^{2+} pumps, exchangers, and other regulators are responsible for intracellular calcium signaling. Through the action of these proteins, Ca^{2+} concentration gradients are apparent across the plasma membrane and at intracellular organelles such as the endoplasmic reticulum, which can be altered by these channels. *Adapted from Stewart, T. A., Yapa, K. T., & Monteith, G. R. (2015). Altered calcium signaling in cancer cells.* Biochimica et Biophysica Acta, 1848*(10), 2502–2511.*

blockers such as amlodipine and nifedipine, which have been widely used for hypertension (Elliott & Ram, 2011; Godfraind, 2014). Other examples include the N-type Ca^{2+} channel blocker ziconitide which can be used in the treatment of severe chronic pain (Schmidtko, Lotsch, Freynhagen, & Geisslinger, 2010) and the clinical trial of an inhibitor of the Ca^{2+} ion permeable transient receptor potential V4 (TRPV4) channel (GSK2798745) in congestive heart failure patients (GlaxoSmithKline, 2000).

Studies investigating alterations in Ca^{2+} signaling in disease often focus on changes in expression of Ca^{2+} channels, pumps, or their regulators. Some examples include the identification of increased expression of inositol 1,4,5-trisphosphate (IP_3)-activated receptors (IP_3Rs) in cardiomyocytes isolated from spontaneously hypertensives rats, a model of cardiac hypertrophy (Harzheim et al., 2009), and the down regulation of plasma membrane Ca^{2+} ATPase 4 levels in colon cancers (Aung et al., 2009). While studies reporting altered expression of calcium channels and pumps have improved our understanding of many diseases, another important consideration is changes to the Ca^{2+} signal itself. The significance of assessment of Ca^{2+} levels is evident when one considers Ca^{2+} permeable ion channels. Overexpression of a plasmalemmal ion channel per se is unlikely to alter calcium signaling in disease if the channel is not active due to the absence of appropriate stimuli or a lack of appropriate trafficking to the plasma membrane.

Changes in Ca^{2+} signaling in disease is almost always likely to be the result of a symphony of changes, not only due to changes in expression but also due to alterations in protein localization or changes in posttranslational modifications (Stewart, Yapa, & Monteith, 2015). One way to measure the sum of these changes and their impact on disease, is via the measurement of the Ca^{2+} signal directly. Advances in our knowledge of such changes have been catalyzed by improvements in the methods to measure intracellular Ca^{2+}. These improvements have been the development of tools (e.g., small molecule Ca^{2+}-sensitive fluorescent dyes and genetically encoded calcium indicators (GECIs)) and their use with advanced imaging methods. As will be outlined in this review, the recent expansion of GECIs continues to diversify the tools available to measure Ca^{2+} changes in disease. With the range of sensors now available, it is often just a matter of the thoughtful selection of the correct probe for the specific application. This review will focus on GECIs and how these tools can be applied to the study of Ca^{2+} signaling in disease and in high-throughput screening for drug discovery.

2. THE CALCIUM SIGNAL IN DISEASE

Remodeling of intracellular Ca^{2+} signaling is a key component of several diseases (Brini, Ottolini, Cali, & Carafoli, 2013; Missiaen et al., 2000; Roderick & Cook, 2008). Research into pathological changes of Ca^{2+} signaling in neurodegenerative disease, cardiovascular disease, and cancer predominate. In Alzheimer's disease, resting cytosolic free Ca^{2+} has been reported to be elevated (Kuchibhotla, Lattarulo, Hyman, & Bacskai, 2009) and this remodeling of intracellular Ca^{2+} signaling is thought to be the result of several mechanisms (Berridge, 2014). In presenilin (PS1) mutation models of familial Alzheimer's disease, upregulation of ryanodine receptor (RyR) Ca^{2+} channels (Chan, Mayne, Holden, Geiger, & Mattson, 2000) and increased activity of IP_3Rs may enhance Ca^{2+} store release from the SR/ER (Cheung et al., 2008). Given the role of Ca^{2+} signaling in apoptosis and necrosis, this dysregulation of Ca^{2+} present in Alzheimer's disease and other neurodegenerative disorders is speculated to contribute to characteristic neuronal cell death associated with a variety of pathologies (Mattson & Chan, 2003). Changes in the handling of Ca^{2+} have also been identified in cardiac hypertrophy and heart failure. For example, the $Ca_v3.2$ voltage-gated calcium channel has been implicated in cardiac hypertrophy, in mice, $Ca_v3.2$ knockout was found to be protective against induction of cardiac hypertrophy, a process thought to be the consequence of reduced calcineurin/nuclear factor of activated T cells (NFAT) activation (Chiang et al., 2009). The 1,4,5-triphosphate receptor, type 3 (IP_3R3) Ca^{2+} channel, while normally having minimal expression in cardiac tissue, is found to be upregulated in patients with heart failure (Go et al., 1995) and it has been proposed that the result of this upregulation is the sensitization of RyRs to increase Ca^{2+} store release (Harzheim et al., 2009).

As discussed earlier, calcium signaling is integral to normal cell physiology and has an important role in a variety of processes ranging from proliferation and hormone secretion to cell death (Berridge et al., 2003). In cancer, many of these cell functions are altered which can contribute to disease progression (Hanahan & Weinberg, 2011). It is therefore unsurprising that dysregulation of Ca^{2+} signaling is a reported feature of some cancers. Alteration of Ca^{2+} signaling has been identified in cancers of the prostate, breast, colon, and ovaries (Monteith, Davis, & Roberts-Thomson, 2012; Prevarskaya, Zhang, & Barritt, 2007; Roderick & Cook, 2008). As an example, the Ca^{2+} channel TRPV6 can be upregulated in prostate cancer (Peng et al., 2001) and this is thought to function as a mechanism to increase $[Ca^{2+}]_{CYT}$ to promote proliferation (Lehen'kyi, Flourakis, Skryma, & Prevarskaya, 2007). Indeed, levels of TRPV6 have been suggested as a marker of prostate cancer progression (Fixemer, Wissenbach, Flockerzi, & Bonkhoff, 2003). TRPV6 can also be overexpressed in breast cancer (Bolanz, Hediger, & Landowski, 2008; Dhennin-Duthille et al., 2011) and has been associated with the aggressive estrogen receptor-negative subtype (Peters et al., 2012). Several other calcium channels and pumps have been linked to breast cancer, these include other TRP channels such as TRPC1 (Dhennin-Duthille et al., 2011) and TRPM7 (Guilbert et al., 2009), members of the store-operated Ca^{2+} entry family ORAI1 (McAndrew et al., 2011) and ORAI3 (Faouzi et al., 2011), and pumps that are responsible for Ca^{2+} efflux across the plasma membrane such as PMCA2 (Lee, Roberts-Thomson, & Monteith, 2005).

The diversity of disorders associated with altered Ca^{2+} signaling has propelled the need for tools to improve our understanding of the contribution of these changes to disease pathophysiology. With recent advancements, we also now have the capabilities and measurement tools to identify compounds able to disrupt or prevent Ca^{2+} alterations in some diseases that are currently not effectively treated. Therefore, monitoring the Ca^{2+} signal is an increasingly important method for drug discovery.

3. THE CALCIUM SIGNAL AS A TOOL IN BIOMOLECULAR SCREENING

The concept of Ca^{2+} signaling assessment as an endpoint for biomolecular screening in drug discovery is not new; however, recent advances in Ca^{2+} measurement methods including those related to genetically encoded Ca^{2+} indicators will allow further progress in this field. Likewise improvements in high-throughput screening instrumentation are further contributing to the development of this area.

Assays investigating alterations in the Ca^{2+} signal not only provide a platform to better identify the mechanism of Ca^{2+} changes in disease, but they also allow the screening of compounds that are able to alter intracellular Ca^{2+} and the nature of the Ca^{2+} signal. For example, in neuroscience, where Ca^{2+} oscillations can be a surrogate for activity (Smetters, Majewska, & Yuste, 1999), assessment of $[Ca^{2+}]_{CYT}$ may allow the identification of compounds able to alter neuronal activity and synaptic transmission (Woods & Padmanabhan, 2012). Another example is the screening of compounds potentially able to promote cancer cell death induced by chemotherapeutic drugs, through assessment of the high cytosolic or mitochondrial Ca^{2+} levels associated with cell death. Screening for Ca^{2+} changes could allow the identification of lead compounds that are not capable of inducing cell death alone, but able to augment free Ca^{2+} levels to a sufficient extent to promote the effectiveness of existing therapies.

The above examples of assessment of Ca^{2+} levels as a biomolecular screen are easily applied to plate reader devices, such as the fluorescence imaging plate reader (FLIPR^{TETRA}; Molecular Devices, Sunnyvale, CA, USA) for high-throughput assays (Monteith & Bird, 2005). An increasing area of interest is the development of cell-based assays involving high content screening (Mattiazzi Usaj et al., 2016). Instead of a single measurement from a population of cells (such as produced in plate reader assays), high content screening allows dynamic visualization of cells at a single-cell level often with simultaneous assessment of other cellular functions through other fluorescence probes with distinct fluorescence spectra (Zanella, Lorens, & Link, 2010). For example, this has been used in a genome-wide siRNA screen for regulators of Parkin, a gene important in mitochondrial damage in Parkinson's disease (Hasson et al., 2013). Candidate genes were identified by examining Parkin translocation in HeLa cells, determined by loss of nuclear localized green fluorescent protein (GFP)-tagged Parkin (Hasson et al., 2013). This was identified by measuring Parkin-GFP colocalization with spectrally distinct Hoechst 33342 fluorescence, with some hits discarded based on mitochondrial depletion identified by a third fluorescence channel (Hasson et al., 2013). High content screening drastically increases the depth of information uncovered from a bioassay and is well suited to investigation of the nature of Ca^{2+} alterations induced by compounds or extracts from screening libraries. Some examples include the identification of heterogeneity in the response between individual cells and cell populations; changes in subcellular Ca^{2+} levels (e.g., mitochondria), and how these relate to changes in the cytosol; Ca^{2+} oscillation, and Ca^{2+} wave rates; and simultaneous assessment of Ca^{2+} changes with other events (e.g., morphology or transcription factor translocation). When developing such phenotypic measurements of Ca^{2+} signaling success requires streamlined analysis, including features such as automated cell detection and cell tracking. These requirements are common for other high content imaging assays, such as those investigating cellular migration, proliferation, or protein colocalization (Boutros, Heigwer, & Laufer, 2015; Mattiazzi Usaj et al., 2016).

The success of cell-based assays when applied to Ca^{2+} signaling is critically dependent on the method for measuring intracellular calcium. The next focus of this review will be to highlight some of the methods to measure intracellular calcium levels and how these may influence their application to studying disease processes or biomolecular screening. There will be an emphasis on GECIs and how recent developments in this field can be leveraged for these types of assays.

4. METHODS TO MEASURE CYTOSOLIC CALCIUM

The intricacies of intracellular Ca^{2+} signaling are progressively becoming unraveled with advances in the methods to measure intracellular free Ca^{2+}. Development of such methods has highlighted the importance of spatial and temporal aspect of the Ca^{2+} signal for differential regulation of Ca^{2+}-dependent functions (Rudolf, Mongillo, Rizzuto, & Pozzan, 2003). Ca^{2+} indicators are often classified into one of two groups: small molecule fluorescent Ca^{2+} dyes or protein-based GECIs.

4.1 Small Molecule Fluorescent Dyes for the Assessment of Ca^{2+} Signaling

Small molecule fluorescent calcium indicators are organic molecules capable of undergoing a change in fluorescence in response to Ca^{2+} binding. These compounds were developed over 30 years ago (Grynkiewicz, Poenie, & Tsien, 1985; Tsien, Pozzan, & Rink, 1982) and continue to be widely used for Ca^{2+} measurement. Their extensive use is related to their high performance (high fluorescence intensity, large dynamic range, fast kinetics, linear responses) (Lock, Parker, & Smith, 2015; Mank & Griesbeck, 2008), established protocols (Takahashi, Camacho, Lechleiter, & Herman, 1999), and the now vast array of variants available—including a range of Ca^{2+} affinities and emission wavelengths.

Small molecule Ca^{2+} indicators may be intensiometric (or single wavelength) or ratiometric. Intensiometric probes only undergo an increase in fluorescence intensity on binding Ca^{2+}; in contrast, ratiometric probes also exhibit a shift in fluorescence spectra upon Ca^{2+} binding. With appropriate calibration, ratiometric dyes can be used for accurate quantitative assessment of absolute free Ca^{2+} (Bootman, Rietdorf, Collins, Walker, & Sanderson, 2013). Small molecule Ca^{2+} dyes are mostly modeled on the structure of the calcium chelator 1,2-bis(*o*-aminophenoxy)ethane-*N*,*N*,

N',*N'*-tetraacetic acid (BAPTA) coupled to a fluorescent reporter group (Grynkiewicz et al., 1985). This BAPTA structural element has a high affinity for Ca^{2+}, though this structure can be modified to adjust Ca^{2+} affinity to allow detection at a range of Ca^{2+} concentrations (Oheim et al., 2014). Probes are most commonly used in an acetoxymethyl (AM) ester form, allowing free passage of the otherwise highly charged dye across the phospholipid bilayer (Paredes, Etzler, Watts, Zheng, & Lechleiter, 2008). Once the AM ester form has crossed the plasma membrane, intracellular esterases generate the Ca^{2+} sensitive ionized moiety (Thomas et al., 2000).

Some applications for Ca^{2+} measurement are poorly suited to the use of small molecule fluorescent dyes. One example is long-term Ca^{2+} monitoring. Dye leakage is a common occurrence (Palmer & Tsien, 2006; Thomas et al., 2000) and can occur within 30 min of dye loading dependent on cell types and/or experimental conditions (Paredes et al., 2008). This limitation can be particularly evident in some cancer cell lines that express multidrug-resistance proteins that can transport many of these probes (Homolya et al., 1993). Over time, fluorescent dyes also have the tendency to sequester into subcellular Ca^{2+} stores such as the endoplasmic reticulum (ER) (Mank & Griesbeck, 2008) where Ca^{2+} levels may saturate probes appropriate for $[Ca^{2+}]_{CYT}$ measurements. Together, these limitations can reduce the reliability of these indicators for long-term Ca^{2+} measurements.

A further weaknesses of small molecule calcium dyes is their inability to be readily targeted to specific tissues, cell types, or subcellular locations (Demaurex, 2005). Dyes can accumulate in subcellular regions (Oheim et al., 2014), though it is often not without background fluorescence in other areas such as the cytosol (Petrou et al., 2000). One example are members of the rhodamines that can accumulate in the mitochondria that has allowed probes such as Rhod-2 to be used to assess mitochondrial Ca^{2+} changes in mammalian cells (Babcock, Herrington, Goodwin, Park, & Hille, 1997). Fluorescent dyes are also poorly suited to in vivo studies (Helmchen & Waters, 2002; Whitaker, 2010). This is related to challenges in dye loading in vivo, including the inability to load specific cell types, loss of the probe due to efflux mechanisms, and probe sequestration. Although there are some examples where in vivo measurements have been achieved (Helmchen, Svoboda, Denk, & Tank, 1999; Stosiek, Garaschuk, Holthoff, & Konnerth, 2003), such approaches are unsuited to most in vivo applications.

4.2 GECIs for the Assessment of Ca^{2+} Signaling

GECIs can overcome some of the issues associated with small molecule fluorescent dyes. One of the principle advantages of GECIs is that these sensors enable long-term, repeat [Ca^{2+}] measurement. Instead of experiments over minutes or hours, GECIs can allow repeated measurement over an extended period, up to many weeks or months (Aramuni & Griesbeck, 2013). This has led to these sensors being successfully introduced into several organisms for in vivo intracellular Ca^{2+} studies, from *Drosophila* (Tian et al., 2009) to mice (Hasan et al., 2004), to even primates (Santisakultarm et al., 2016).

Arguably, the development and application of GECIs has predominantly been driven by neuroscience research, where the disadvantages of small molecule Ca^{2+} probes are particular evident (Mank & Griesbeck, 2008; Tian, Hires, & Looger, 2012). Unlike small molecule fluorescent Ca^{2+} dyes, GECIs can be readily targeted to specific tissues, cell populations, or subcellular location through the addition of an appropriate promoter or targeting sequence. For example, GECIs allow Ca^{2+} measurement of astrocytes among a population of neurons (Shigetomi, Kracun, Sofroniew, & Khakh, 2010), or can be targeted to presynaptic neurons (Jackson & Burrone, 2016) or even a specific interneuron subtype (Hinckley & Pfaff, 2013). This targeting feature also opens up the investigation of Ca^{2+} handling in particular organelles such as the ER or mitochondria, through the introduction of a targeting sequence (recently reviewed by Suzuki, Kanemaru, & Iino, 2016).

The basic structure of most GECIs consists of a Ca^{2+} sensing element coupled to one or two fluorophores, capable of an alteration in fluorescence with Ca^{2+} binding. Calmodulin is a common binding domain for GECIs. An alternative approach uses troponin C as a binding domain, a protein suggested to have less potential for endogenous interaction (Heim & Griesbeck, 2004).

As outlined later, genetically encoded calcium sensors use either fluorescent or luminescent proteins to report changes in calcium signaling.

4.2.1 Aequorin-Based GECIs

Aequorin is a bioluminescence-based indicator first isolated from the *Aequorea victoria* jellyfish (Shimomura, Johnson, & Saiga, 1962). In the presence of an external cofactor (coelenterazine), aequorin undergoes an irreversible reaction on binding Ca^{2+} to produce a photon of light (Brini, Pinton, Pozzan, & Rizzuto, 1999). Aequorin and its derivatives can be successfully targeted to subcellular locations (Robert, Pinton, Tosello, Rizzuto, & Pozzan, 2000) and represented the first advance in protein-based indicators of Ca^{2+} appropriate for use in the study of Ca^{2+} levels in subcellular organelles. However aequorin-based indicators are dim relative to fluorescent GECIs and for this reason are not ideal for single-cell Ca^{2+} measurements (Ottolini, Cali, & Brini, 2014). Because the probe is consumed during the reaction (Bonora et al., 2013), these indicators are also poorly suited to long-term Ca^{2+} monitoring. This limits the application of aequorin-based indicators, compared with their fluorescent counterparts. A new class of genetically encoded calcium sensors named GAP (GFP-Aequorin Protein) are capable of both Ca^{2+}-dependent luminescence or fluorescence (Rodriguez-Prados, Rojo-Ruiz, Aulestia, Garcia-Sancho, & Alonso, 2015). The ability to perform mean cell population luminescence in conjunction with fluorescence measurements may aid the identification of between-experiment variability (Rodriguez-Prados et al., 2015).

4.2.2 Förster Resonance Energy Transfer-Based GECIs

Fluorescent GECIs were first developed more than 15 years ago (Miyawaki et al., 1997; Romoser, Hinkle, & Persechini, 1997) and exploited the phenomenon of Förster resonance energy transfer (FRET). This occurs when excitation of a donor fluorophore enables nonradiative energy transfer to allow fluorescence of a closely linked second acceptor fluorescent protein (Zhang, Campbell, Ting, & Tsien, 2002). FRET-based Ca^{2+} sensors often link two fluorophores with overlapping excitation/emission spectra via a Ca^{2+}-binding domain. Measurement of Ca^{2+} can be achieved by monitoring the change in FRET signal as a result of a conformational change with Ca^{2+} binding (Romoser et al., 1997). The first major family of FRET-based indicators was termed cameleons, consisting of a blue and green fluorescent protein linked by calmodulin fused to M13, a myosin light chain kinase-binding peptide (Miyawaki et al., 1997). Early versions of cameleons suffered from pH sensitivity, low signal, and photobleaching (Demaurex, 2005; Mank & Griesbeck, 2008), subsequent versions reduced some of these limitations (Palmer, Qin, Park, & McCombs, 2011).

One advantage of FRET-based genetically encoded calcium sensors is the possibility of ratiometric imaging (and thus a superior ability to approximate absolute free Ca^{2+} concentrations) (Rose, Goltstein, Portugues, & Griesbeck, 2014). Ratiometric measurements with FRET sensors can be used to resolve motion artifacts or variations in sensor expression among a tissue population, which can be an advantage for in vivo experiments (Lutcke et al., 2010; Rose et al., 2014). However, these indicators generally have a lower signal-to-noise ratio, decreased brightness and slower kinetics compared to single fluorophore GECIs (Ai, 2015; Tian, Akerboom, Schreiter, & Looger, 2012; Tian, Hires, et al., 2012). FRET-based GECIs have a large spectral bandwidth, limiting capacity to multiplex with fluorescent indicators targeting other parameters (Rose et al., 2014; Tian, Akerboom, et al., 2012).

4.2.3 Single-Wavelength Fluorescent GECIs

Single fluorescent protein calcium indicators were first developed following the observation that GFP can have proteins inserted in its beta-barrel structure and still maintain the ability to fluoresce (Baird, Zacharias, & Tsien, 1999). This led to the development of the Camgaroo family of indicators, consisting of a single fluorophore (circular permutation of yellow fluorescent protein) modified to contain a calmodulin Ca^{2+} -binding domain within its beta-barrel structure (Baird et al., 1999). Although this series formed the basis for future GECI classes, Camgaroos suffered from sensitivity to pH and low brightness (Mank & Griesbeck, 2008; Whitaker, 2010). The Pericams were a subsequent family of single-fluorophore indicators, although these offered some improvements over Camgaroo sensors, pH sensitivity, and low brightness limited use (Mank & Griesbeck, 2008; Pologruto, Yasuda, & Svoboda, 2004; Whitaker, 2010).

First developed at a similar time to the Pericams, another class of single fluorescent protein GECIs are termed GCaMP. These Ca^{2+} sensors consist of a circular permutation of GFP linked to a M13 fragment of myosin light chain kinase at the N-terminus and calmodulin-binding domain at the C-terminus (Nakai, Ohkura, & Imoto, 2001). Like other early GECIs, the first series of GCaMP suffered issues with low brightness, temperature sensitivity, poor expression, and pH sensitivity (Tallini et al., 2006; Whitaker, 2010). An advance came in 2009 with the development of GCaMP3, with several improvements including increased protein stability and dynamic range (Tian et al., 2009). The subsequent GCaMP5 indicators were developed with further improvements in brightness, dynamic range, and affinity for Ca^{2+} (Akerboom et al., 2012). The most recent version of this series, GCaMP6, was developed through screening variants with point mutations from the GCaMP5G structure (Chen et al., 2013). Three of these were selected, named GCaMP6f (fast), GCaMP6m (medium), and GCaMP6s (slow), distinguished by their response kinetics in detecting Ca^{2+} transients (Chen et al., 2013). Though GCaMP6s has slower kinetics than the other GCaMP6 variants, it is the most sensitive of the three sensors

(Chen et al., 2013). In contrast, the fast kinetics of GCaMP6f is likely the preferred variant for the measurement of rapid Ca^{2+} oscillations, like those observed in neurons.

Compared with FRET-based indicators, single fluorescent protein indicators have the advantage of generally more favorable dynamic range, in part due to their typically lower basal fluorescence. This also reduces the potential for photobleaching in long-term assays. However, given measurements of fluorescence intensity is influenced by sensor expression, single fluorescent protein indicators are arguably still best suited to relative measurements of intracellular free Ca^{2+} (Abdul, Ramlal, & Hoosein, 2008; Whitaker, 2010).

5. NEW GECIs

In recent years, there have been considerable gains in performance for genetically encoded Ca^{2+} indicators. A significant improvement came from the development of the GCaMP6 indicators, as for the first time, these indicators had comparable performance (Chen et al., 2013) with regards to sensitivity and kinetics compared with leading small molecular Ca^{2+} -sensitive dyes (e.g., Fluo-4). GCaMP6 indicators have widespread use (Lee, Huang, & Fitzpatrick, 2016; Montijn, Meijer, Lansink, & Pennartz, 2016; Sidik et al., 2016; Theis et al., 2016) and several variants on the original series have since been developed, targeted to various locations. Table 1 outlines the properties of some of these indicators, along with several other GECIs discussed in this review.

Recently, there has also been considerable interest in developing high-performance GECIs capable of fluorescence emission in longer wavelength hues (Zhao et al., 2011), allowing the potential for multicolor Ca^{2+} imaging. This has a major advantage in studies seeking to investigate the Ca^{2+} signaling interactions between two cell populations, or between two cellular compartments (e.g., cytosolic vs mitochondrial; Li et al., 2014). One example includes the GECO series of indicators, which are available with red, blue, or green intensiometric emission (Zhao et al., 2011). Red-shifted indicators have the added advantage of greater tissue penetration, reduced phototoxicity, and less light scattering in vivo (Oheim et al., 2014; Pendin, Greotti, Filadi, & Pozzan, 2015; Rodriguez et al., 2017). Newly developed cytosolic red Ca^{2+} indicators have significantly improved performance relative to previous red indicators (Dana et al., 2016; Inoue et al., 2015). These include R-CaMP2 (Inoue et al., 2015), jRGECO1a (Dana et al., 2016), jRCaMP1a,

Table 1 Properties in vitro of Widely Used Genetically Encoded Calcium Indicators and Those Discussed in This Review

Indicator		Class	Fluorophore (s)	Max Dynamic Range	K_d (nM)	Excitation (nm)	Emission (nm)	References
4mtD3cpv		FRET	ECFP/cpVenus	5.1	760	433	475,528	Palmer et al. (2006)
CEPIA1*er*	G-CEPIA1*er*	Intensiometric	cpEGFP	4.7	672,000	497	511	Suzuki et al. (2014)
	GEM-CEPIA1*er*	Ratiometric	cpEGFP	21.7	558,000	391	462,510	Suzuki et al. (2014)
	R-CEPIA1*er*	Intensiometric	cpmApple	8.8	565,000	562	584	Suzuki et al. (2014)
D1ER		FRET	ECFP,citrine	—	810, 60,000	433	475,529	Palmer, Jin, Reed, and Tsien (2004)
D4ER		FRET	ECFP,citrine	—	195,000	435	475,540	Ravier et al. (2011)
Fast-GCaMPs	Fast-GCaMP3-RS09	Intensiometric	cpEGFP	9.5	690	497	512	Sun et al. (2013)
	Fast-GCaMP6f-RS06	Intensiometric	cpEGFP	18.7	320	488	512	Badura, Sun, Giovannucci, Lynch, and Wang (2014)
	Fast-GCaMP6f-RS09	Intensiometric	cpEGFP	25	520	488	512	Badura et al. (2014)
GAP	goGAP1	Ratiometric/ bioluminescent	GFP variant/ aequorin	—	12,000	403,470	510	Rodriguez-Garcia et al. (2014)
	erGAP3	Ratiometric/ bioluminescent	GFP variant/ aequorin	3	489,000	405,470	535	Navas-Navarro et al. (2016)
GCaMP3		Intensiometric	cpEGFP	12	840	485	510	Tian et al. (2009)
GCaMP5G		Intensiometric	cpEGFP	32.7	460	485	510	Akerboom et al. (2012)
	Lck-GCaMP5G	Intensiometric	cpEGFP	—	—	485	510	Akerboom et al. (2012)

GCaMP6	GCaMP6f	Intensiometric	cpEGFP	51.8	375	497	515	Chen et al. (2013)
	GCaMP6m	Intensiometric	cpEGFP	38.1	167	497	515	Chen et al. (2013)
	GCaMP6s	Intensiometric	cpEGFP	63.2	144	497	515	Chen et al. (2013)
	2mtGCaMP6m	Intensiometric	cpEGFP	—	167	474	515	Hill et al. (2014)
	4mtGCaMP6f	Intensiometric	cpEGFP	—	—	497	515	Tosatto et al. (2016)
	Lck-GCaMP6s	Intensiometric	cpEGFP	—	144	497	515	O'Donnell, Jackson, and Robinson (2016)
	sPA-GCaMP6f	Intensiometric	cpEGFP	—	681	480	513	Berlin et al. (2015)
GCaMP8		Intensiometric	cpEGFP	37.5	200	488	—	Ohkura et al. (2012)
GECO	G-GECO1	Intensiometric	cpEGFP	25	749	496	512	Zhao et al. (2011)
	GEM-GECO1	Ratiometric	cpEGFP	110	340	390	455,511	Zhao et al. (2011)
	R-GECO1	Intensiometric	cpmApple	16	482	561	589	Zhao et al. (2011)
	ER-LAR-GECO1	Intensiometric	cpmApple	10	24,000	561	589	Wu et al. (2014)
	mito-LAR-GECO1.2	Intensiometric	cpmApple	8.7	12,000	557	584	Wu et al. (2014)
	NLS-R-GECO1	Intensiometric	cpmApple	16	482	561	589	Zhao et al. (2011)
	Orai-G-GECO1	Intensiometric	cpEGFP	25	749	496	512	Dynes, Amcheslavsky, and Cahalan (2016)
	Orai-G-GECO1.2	Intensiometric	cpEGFP	23	1150	498	513	Dynes et al. (2016)
go-D1cpv		FRET	ECFP,cpVenus	—	—	425	480,520	Lissandron, Podini, Pizzo, and Pozzan (2010)

Continued

Table 1 Properties in vitro of Widely Used Genetically Encoded Calcium Indicators and Those Discussed in This Review—cont'd

Indicator	Class	Fluorophore (s)	Max Dynamic Range	K_d (nM)	Excitation (nm)	Emission (nm)	References
NLS-GCaMP2	Intensiometric	cpEGFP	—	—	480	508	Bengtson, Freitag, Weislogel, and Bading (2010)
jRCaMP1a	Intensiometric	cpmRuby	3.2	214	570	600	Dana et al. (2016)
jRCaMP1b	Intensiometric	cpmRuby	7.2	712	570	600	Dana et al. (2016)
jRGECO1a	Intensiometric	cpmApple	11.6	148	570	600	Dana et al. (2016)
RCaMP1h	Intensiometric	cpmRuby	10.5	1300	571	594	Akerboom et al. (2013)
R-CaMP2	Intensiometric	cpmApple	4.8	69	565	583	Inoue et al. (2015)
TN-XXL	FRET	ECFP, cp174Citrine	—	800	430	480,535	Mank et al. (2008)
Twitch3	FRET	ECFP, cp174Citrine	7	250	432	475,527	Thestrup et al. (2014)
Twitch4	FRET	ECFP, cp174Citrine	6	2800	432	475,527	Thestrup et al. (2014)
YC3.6	FRET	ECFP, cp173Venus	5.6	250	430	480,530	Nagai, Yamada, Tominaga, Ichikawa, and Miyawaki (2004)
YC-Nano50	FRET	ECFP, cp173Venus	12.5	52.5	430	480,530	Horikawa et al. (2010)

Adapted from Perez Koldenkova, V., & Nagai, T. (2013). Genetically encoded Ca(2+) indicators: Properties and evaluation. *Biochimica et Biophysica Acta, 1833*(7), 1787–1797; Rose, T., Goltstein, P. M., Portugues, R., & Griesbeck, O. (2014). Putting a finishing touch on GECIs. *Frontiers in Molecular Neuroscience,* 7, 88; Suzuki, J., Kanemaru, K., & Iino, M. (2016). Genetically encoded fluorescent indicators for organellar calcium imaging. *Biophysical Journal, 111*(6), 1119–1131.

and jRCaMP1b (Dana et al., 2016). R-CaMP2 and jRGECO1a are derived from the mApple fluorophore, a protein capable of photoswitching (Shaner et al., 2008), which may limit the use of these indicators in certain protocols (Dana et al., 2016). jRCaMP1a and jRCaMP1b have a different fluorophore, mRuby, and were derived by screening mutational variants of RCaMP1h (Dana et al., 2016). These sensors have distinct properties which may make them suitable for different applications; jRCaMP1a has a higher affinity for Ca^{2+} (K_d 214 nM), while jRCaMP1b has a greater dynamic range (Dana et al., 2016).

Other developments in GECIs include the Fast-GCaMPs (Sun et al., 2013), later improved to combine the properties of brightness associated with GCaMP6f (Badura et al., 2014). A GCaMP8 (Ohkura et al., 2012) indicator is also available, though the alternative numbering structure employed by this group should not suggest superiority to GCaMP6 (Broussard, Liang, & Tian, 2014). It has also recently been identified that some GCaMP variants can be photoconverted from green to red, by prolonged exposure with blue-green light at 450–500 nm (Ai et al., 2015). Importantly, these indicators remain Ca^{2+} sensitive (Ai et al., 2015). This can allow the "highlighting" of selective cells among a population in vivo, potentially useful for repeated measurements or distinguishing individual cell morphology (Berlin et al., 2015; Hoi, Matsuda, Nagai, & Campbell, 2013). Differentiating individual cells could also be achieved by the newly developed photoactivatable GCaMP6 series, where cells expressing the Ca^{2+} sensor can be selectively highlighted via excitation at 405 nm (Berlin et al., 2015). Further diversity has come from the targeting of several modern GECIs to various intracellular organelles as described later. In many cases, this has been possible through the development of indicators with lower affinities for Ca^{2+} ions, thus avoiding saturation in organelles with high free Ca^{2+} levels in their lumen (e.g., the ER).

6. TARGETING GECIs

One of the advantages of all GECIs is their ability to be targeted to specific tissues, cell populations, subcellular regions, or organelles. The concept of targeting GECIs has been around for some time; however with recent advances, new efforts have been made to develop sensors that are capable of reliable Ca^{2+} measurement at various cellular sites. GECIs have been targeted to the mitochondria, ER, nucleus, Golgi apparatus, endosomes, peroxisomes, and the subplasmalemmal domain (Demaurex, 2005; Suzuki et al., 2016; Williams, Monif, & Richardson, 2013). Given there is a large variation in the resting-free Ca^{2+} levels between different subcellular organelles (e.g., cytosol ~100 nM vs the ER ~500 μM (Carafoli, 1987; Vandecaetsbeek, Vangheluwe, Raeymaekers, Wuytack, & Vanoevelen, 2011)), care needs to be taken when selecting a GECI to measure Ca^{2+} changes, with an appropriate K_d required for the expected Ca^{2+} level (to avoid indicator saturation). Fig. 2 highlights some examples of targeted GECIs for various intracellular organelles and subcellular locations. Environmental differences such as pH can also vary between organelles and this must also be considered in indicator selection (Perez Koldenkova & Nagai, 2013). The effect of the addition of a targeting sequence likewise needs to be carefully considered, given the possibility of obstruction of normal sensor activity (Suzuki et al., 2016). Low-affinity indicators have been developed for measurement of free Ca^{2+} in the ER lumen. One example is the CEPIA series, which comprises three variants; red (R-CEPIA1*er*), green (G-CEPIA1*er*), or the ratiometric blue/green (GEM-CEPIA1*er*) (Suzuki et al., 2014). The dual emission of GEM-CEPIA1*er* enables the ability to normalize for factors such as variations in sensor expression (Suzuki et al., 2014). GAP Ca^{2+} indicators have also been targeted to the ER and Golgi apparatus (Navas-Navarro et al., 2016; Rodriguez-Garcia et al., 2014) and likewise several FRET-based cameleons have been targeted to various organelles successfully (Demaurex & Frieden, 2003). Aside from organellar targeting, it can be advantageous to monitor Ca^{2+} levels at other locations within the cell, such as the plasma membrane. Indeed localized Ca^{2+} microdomains located near the plasma membrane can have signaling functions independent of global $[Ca^{2+}]_{CYT}$ changes (Rizzuto & Pozzan, 2006). Several GECIs have been targeted to this location (Akerboom et al., 2012; Heim & Griesbeck, 2004; Nagai et al., 2004; Shigetomi et al., 2010). A recent study also described single channel recording of STIM1/ORAI1 interaction in HEK-293A cells with three different GECI-ORAI1 fusions (Dynes et al., 2016).

The increasing array of GECIs available continues to expand the choices available for Ca^{2+} measurement. However, indicators need to be selected based on the specific experimental requirements. Consideration must be given to factors such as the importance of absolute quantitation, impact of phototoxicity, location of Ca^{2+} changes to be measured, and the need for multicolor imaging.

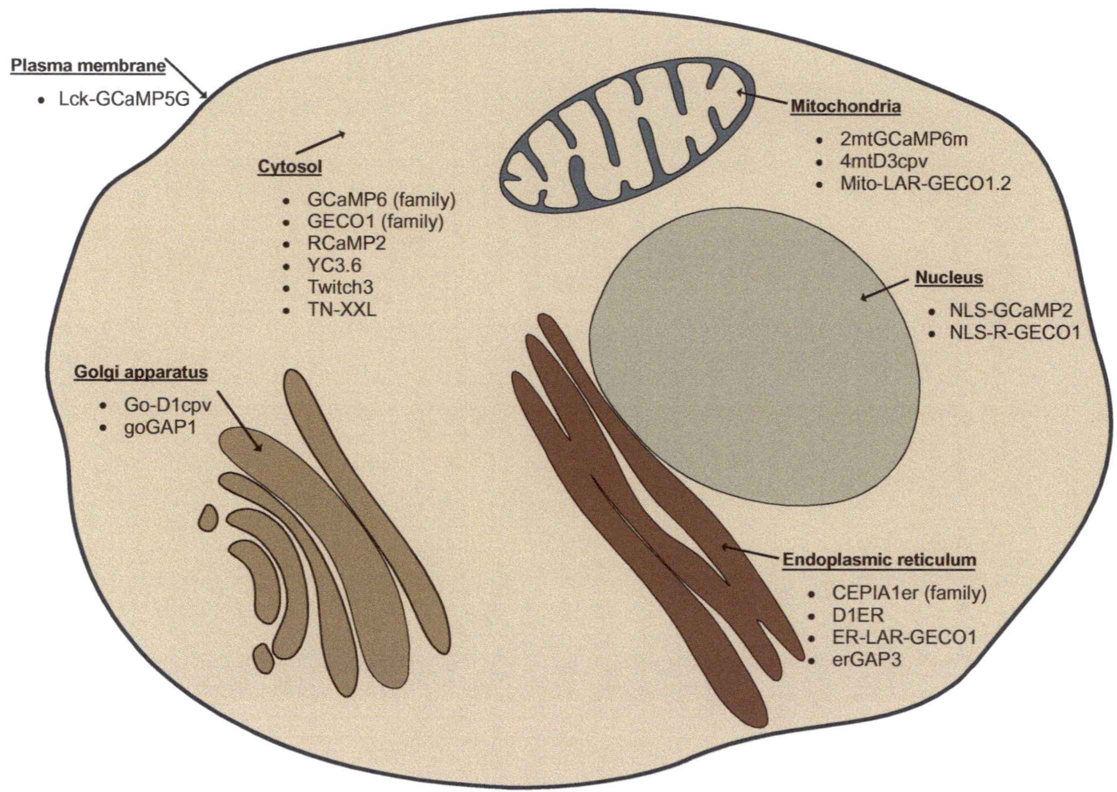

Fig. 2 Examples of genetically encoded calcium indicators targeted to intracellular organelles, subcellular locations, or with cytosolic localization. While not a complete list, this figure highlights some of the commonly applied genetically encoded calcium indicators for Ca^{2+} measurements at various cell locations.

7. APPLICATION OF GECIs IN THE ASSESSMENT OF CALCIUM HOMEOSTASIS IN DISEASE

The application of GECIs has often been focused on studies investigating neuronal physiology. Such work often takes advantage of the ability of GECIs to be targeted to specific cell populations or cell locations, in addition to the suitability of GECIs for chronic imaging (a significant limitation of small molecule fluorescent indicators). There are numerous examples of GECIs being used to better understand the nature of Ca^{2+} signaling changes in disease using both in vitro and in vivo models. Some exemplar studies are outlined later which provide insights into how other areas of biomedical research may utilize GECIs to better understand the role of Ca^{2+} homeostasis remodeling in disease.

In astrocyte neuronal death induced by oxygen deprivation, the plasma membrane targeted Lck-GCaMP6s sensor was able to identify spontaneous Ca^{2+} transients, accompanying mitochondrial disruption (O'Donnell et al., 2016). These were of two distinct phenotypes. The first, a fast transient propagating between mitochondria, while the latter, a newly identified localized Ca^{2+} oscillation at plasma membrane immediately adjacent to mitochondria (O'Donnell et al., 2016). In pluripotent stem cell-derived cardiomyocytes, GCaMP5G was expressed to identify proarrhythmic disruption of Ca^{2+} signaling induced by pharmacological agents (Shinnawi et al., 2015). By coexpressing with a genetically encoded voltage indicator, this model provides the ability to screen compounds that disrupt normal Ca^{2+} dynamics or membrane depolarization (Shinnawi et al., 2015).

GECIs have also been used to characterize Ca^{2+} changes associated with viral infection (Perry, Ramachandran, Utama, & Hyser, 2015). By expressing both R-CEPIA1*er* (targeting the ER) and the cytosolic GCaMP5G (or GCaMP6s) sensor, Perry et al. observed attenuated adenosine triphosphate (ATP)-induced Ca^{2+} transients at the cytosol and ER of both MA-104 and HeLa cells following infection with rotavirus or poliovirus (Perry et al., 2015). The authors also demonstrated the GECIs could be used to monitor Ca^{2+} changes during live cell imaging of viral infection measured over 16 h, identifying increased Ca^{2+} oscillations with rotavirus infection, which could be attenuated with inhibitors of Ca^{2+} influx (Perry et al., 2015). Application of GECIs has extended to other research areas. The expression of GCaMP indicators in somatosensory neurons of live mice enabled the observation of differential neuronal responses dependent on the type of painful stimuli, suggesting future use of this GECI-based model could help elicit the neuronal mechanisms of distinct pain pathways (Emery et al., 2016). Another example used expression of GCaMP indicators in *Toxoplasma gondii* to screen compounds capable of disrupting Ca^{2+} signaling, enabling the authors to identify novel antiparasitic compounds (Sidik et al., 2016).

As already discussed, there is an increasing awareness of the importance of the nature of calcium signaling changes rather than changes in expression of calcium channels in cancer (Stewart et al., 2015); however, GECIs remain relatively underutilized in this research area. Of the few studies that have used GECIs in cancer cells, most have been in breast cancer cells. Indeed over 10 years ago, D1ER (an ER-targeted GECI) was used to monitor ER Ca^{2+} changes because of Bcl-2-mediated ER stress in MCF7 cells (Palmer et al., 2004). The authors identified that Bcl-2 reduced Ca^{2+} levels in the ER by increasing Ca^{2+} leak from internal stores (Palmer et al., 2004) likely via IP_3Rs. A more recent example is the use of a mitochondrial targeted GCaMP6f indicator to identify that mitochondrial calcium uniporter silencing attenuates mitochondrial calcium uptake in MDA-MB-231, MDA-MB-468, and BT-549 breast cancer cells (Tosatto et al., 2016).

Arguably one of the greatest advantages for GECIs is their ability to be used in chronic measurements of Ca^{2+}, a property that favors the use of these sensors in vivo. Repeated Ca^{2+} measurement can be achieved through intravital microscopy (Pittet & Weissleder, 2011). This typically involves the implantation of a window in the model organism allowing the visualization of Ca^{2+} changes (Karreman, Hyenne, Schwab, & Goetz, 2016). For example, implantation of a cranial window was used in an Alzheimer's disease mouse model (APP/PS1 mice) to image neurons expressing the GCaMP6m sensor (Liebscher, Keller, Goltstein, Bonhoeffer, & Hubener, 2016). This enabled the identification of various neuronal Ca^{2+} alterations in this model, including a reduction in the magnitude of neuronal responses in response to visual and motor cues (Liebscher et al., 2016). Expression of the cameleon indicator YC3.6 in neurons of APP mice (another Alzheimer's disease model) also made use of intravital imaging, finding increased Ca^{2+} levels in the dendrites and axons adjacent to amyloid-β plaques with associated morphological changes in part the result of these increases (Kuchibhotla et al., 2008). YC3.6 has also been used in a mouse model of familial hemiplegic migraine type 1 (Eikermann-Haerter et al., 2015). In vivo imaging was achieved via a cranial window allowing the identification of Ca^{2+}

overload associated with changes in $Ca_v2.1$ channels (Eikermann-Haerter et al., 2015). Given the role of calcium signaling in the heart, there is also potential for use of GECIs in vivo in this context (see recent review, Kaestner et al., 2014) and protocols have been published outlining intravital imaging of the heart in live mice (e.g., Vinegoni, Aguirre, Lee, & Weissleder, 2015). One example used the expression of GCaMP3 in human embryonic stem cell-derived cardiomyocytes to confirm functional activity of these cells following transplantation to regenerate myocardium tissue damage in guinea-pigs (Shiba et al., 2012).

Intravital imaging is also a technique to be exploited in in vivo cancer models, where the ability to chronically image cancer cells could further our understanding of tumor progression and metastasis (Ellenbroek & van Rheenen, 2014). An example of this potential is seen by the use of an intravital chamber in p53 knockout mice to measure the disruption of Ca^{2+} dynamics during apoptosis, using the small molecule dye fura-2 (Giorgi et al., 2015). Given the recent progress in both GECIs and intravital imaging, there is likely to be an increase in the use of these sensors to investigate Ca^{2+} signaling changes in cancer in vivo.

8. GECIs AND BIOMOLECULAR SCREENING

Only a few published studies have used GECIs in the context of high-throughput screening in drug discovery; however, there has been wide use of small molecule Ca^{2+} indicators in a variety of G-protein-coupled receptors and ion channel-based biomolecular screens (Behrendt, Germann, Gillen, Hatt, & Jostock, 2004; Herington et al., 2015; Wang et al., 2015). This is a strong indicator of the utility of GECIs in biomolecular screening, given the recent advances in GECIs as discussed throughout this review.

One example, where GECIs have been used in a cell-based screen, was described by Honarnejad et al. (2013). This involved the stable expression of the FRET-based cameleon YC3.6 in HEK-293 cells expressing a PS1 gene mutation associated with Alzheimer's disease. PS1 mutation can augment ER calcium homeostasis, evidenced by a reduction of the magnitude Carbachol-induced ER calcium release (Honarnejad et al., 2013). This group screened 20,000 compounds and was able to identify 53 hits capable of causing recovery of the wild-type ER calcium release, by examining those with the highest FRET signal (Honarnejad et al., 2013). RCaMP1h, a red fluorescent GECI, has recently been used to screen genes capable of altering synaptic vesicles using the model organism *Caenorhabditis elegans* using high content imaging (Wabnig, Liewald, Yu, & Gottschalk, 2015). By incorporating RCaMP1h into postsynaptic body wall muscle, RNA interference allowed identification of genes able to alter synaptic transmission following stimulation of cholinergic neurons. This assay was not without challenges; nematodes were imaged in microwells made from agar and despite identifying five target genes capable of altering Ca^{2+}, this did not translate to a strong phenotype of altered synaptic vesicle trafficking (Wabnig et al., 2015). It is likely that some GECIs are already part of biodiscovery projects within pharmaceutical companies and have not yet been described in journal articles, as has been done with small molecule-based probes (Herington et al., 2015). However, it is clear that further application of GECIs in academia and industry will help accelerate the discovery of a new generation of pharmacological agents capable of modulating calcium signaling in disease.

9. CONCLUSION

The advances in GECIs have been exponential over recent years. Each year incremental improvements are made and new GECIs released. Further development in the properties of fluorescent proteins (including far-red and infrared protein indicators) will enhance this diversity of available Ca^{2+} sensors (Rodriguez et al., 2017). This will assist researchers to avoid spectral overlap, an increasingly important consideration for simultaneous cytosolic/organellar Ca^{2+} measurements (Rose et al., 2014). Advancement will also come from improvements in instrument capabilities and enhancement of software platforms for streamlining analysis.

CONFLICT OF INTEREST

None to declare.

ACKNOWLEDGMENTS

We would like to acknowledge the support of National Health and Medical Research Council (NHMRC; project grants 1079671, 1079672). G.R.M. was supported by the Mater Foundation. The Translational Research Institute is supported by a grant from the Australian Government.

REFERENCES

Abdul, M., Ramlal, S., & Hoosein, N. (2008). Ryanodine receptor expression correlates with tumor grade in breast cancer. *Pathology Oncology Research*, *14*(2), 157–160.

Ai, H. W. (2015). Fluorescent-protein-based probes: General principles and practices. *Analytical and Bioanalytical Chemistry*, *407*(1), 9–15.

Ai, M., Mills, H., Kanai, M., Lai, J., Deng, J., Schreiter, E., et al. (2015). Green-to-red photoconversion of GCaMP. *PloS One*, *10*(9), e0138127.

Akerboom, J., Carreras Calderon, N., Tian, L., Wabnig, S., Prigge, M., Tolo, J., et al. (2013). Genetically encoded calcium indicators for multi-color neural activity imaging and combination with optogenetics. *Frontiers in Molecular Neuroscience*, *6*, 2.

Akerboom, J., Chen, T. W., Wardill, T. J., Tian, L., Marvin, J. S., Mutlu, S., et al. (2012). Optimization of a GCaMP calcium indicator for neural activity imaging. *Journal of Neuroscience*, *32*(40), 13819–13840.

Aramuni, G., & Griesbeck, O. (2013). Chronic calcium imaging in neuronal development and disease. *Experimental Neurology*, *242*, 50–56.

Aung, C. S., Ye, W., Plowman, G., Peters, A. A., Monteith, G. R., & Roberts-Thomson, S. J. (2009). Plasma membrane calcium ATPase 4 and the remodeling of calcium homeostasis in human colon cancer cells. *Carcinogenesis*, *30*(11), 1962–1969.

Babcock, D. F., Herrington, J., Goodwin, P. C., Park, Y. B., & Hille, B. (1997). Mitochondrial participation in the intracellular Ca^{2+} network. *Journal of Cell Biology*, *136*(4), 833–844.

Badura, A., Sun, X. R., Giovannucci, A., Lynch, L. A., & Wang, S. S. (2014). Fast calcium sensor proteins for monitoring neural activity. *Neurophotonics*, *1*(2), 025008.

Baird, G. S., Zacharias, D. A., & Tsien, R. Y. (1999). Circular permutation and receptor insertion within green fluorescent proteins. *Proceedings of the National Academy of Sciences of the United States of America*, *96*(20), 11241–11246.

Behrendt, H. J., Germann, T., Gillen, C., Hatt, H., & Jostock, R. (2004). Characterization of the mouse cold-menthol receptor TRPM8 and vanilloid receptor type-1 VR1 using a fluorometric imaging plate reader (FLIPR) assay. *British Journal of Pharmacology*, *141*(4), 737–745.

Bengtson, C. P., Freitag, H. E., Weislogel, J. M., & Bading, H. (2010). Nuclear calcium sensors reveal that repetition of trains of synaptic stimuli boosts nuclear calcium signaling in CA1 pyramidal neurons. *Biophysical Journal*, *99*(12), 4066–4077.

Berlin, S., Carroll, E. C., Newman, Z. L., Okada, H. O., Quinn, C. M., Kallman, B., et al. (2015). Photoactivatable genetically encoded calcium indicators for targeted neuronal imaging. *Nature Methods*, *12*(9), 852–858.

Berridge, M. J. (2000). The versatility and universality of calcium signalling. *Nature Reviews. Molecular Cell Biology*, *1*(1), 11–21.

Berridge, M. J. (2014). Calcium regulation of neural rhythms, memory and Alzheimer's disease. *Journal of Physiology*, *592*(2), 281–293.

Berridge, M. J., Bootman, M. D., & Roderick, H. L. (2003). Calcium signalling: Dynamics, homeostasis and remodelling. *Nature Reviews. Molecular Cell Biology*, *4*(7), 517–529.

Bolanz, K. A., Hediger, M. A., & Landowski, C. P. (2008). The role of TRPV6 in breast carcinogenesis. *Molecular Cancer Therapeutics*, *7*(2), 271–279.

Bonora, M., Giorgi, C., Bononi, A., Marchi, S., Patergnani, S., Rimessi, A., et al. (2013). Subcellular calcium measurements in mammalian cells using jellyfish photoprotein aequorin-based probes. *Nature Protocols*, *8*(11), 2105–2118.

Bootman, M. D., Rietdorf, K., Collins, T., Walker, S., & Sanderson, M. (2013). Ca^{2+} -sensitive fluorescent dyes and intracellular Ca^{2+} imaging. *Cold Spring Harbor Protocols*, *2013*(2), 83–99.

Boutros, M., Heigwer, F., & Laufer, C. (2015). Microscopy-based high-content screening. *Cell*, *163*(6), 1314–1325.

Brini, M., Cali, T., Ottolini, D., & Carafoli, E. (2014). Neuronal calcium signaling: Function and dysfunction. *Cellular and Molecular Life Sciences*, *71*(15), 2787–2814.

Brini, M., Ottolini, D., Cali, T., & Carafoli, E. (2013). Calcium in health and disease. *Metal Ions in Life Sciences*, *13*, 81–137.

Brini, M., Pinton, P., Pozzan, T., & Rizzuto, R. (1999). Targeted recombinant aequorins: Tools for monitoring [Ca2+] in the various compartments of a living cell. *Microscopy Research and Technique*, *46*(6), 380–389.

Broussard, G. J., Liang, R., & Tian, L. (2014). Monitoring activity in neural circuits with genetically encoded indicators. *Frontiers in Molecular Neuroscience*, 7, 97.

Carafoli, E. (1987). Intracellular calcium homeostasis. *Annual Review of Biochemistry*, *56*, 395–433.

Chan, S. L., Mayne, M., Holden, C. P., Geiger, J. D., & Mattson, M. P. (2000). Presenilin-1 mutations increase levels of ryanodine receptors and calcium release in PC12 cells and cortical neurons. *Journal of Biological Chemistry*, *275*(24), 18195–18200.

Chen, T. W., Wardill, T. J., Sun, Y., Pulver, S. R., Renninger, S. L., Baohan, A., et al. (2013). Ultrasensitive fluorescent proteins for imaging neuronal activity. *Nature*, *499*(7458), 295–300.

Cheung, K. H., Shineman, D., Muller, M., Cardenas, C., Mei, L., Yang, J., et al. (2008). Mechanism of Ca2+ disruption in Alzheimer's disease by presenilin regulation of InsP3 receptor channel gating. *Neuron*, *58*(6), 871–883.

Chiang, C. S., Huang, C. H., Chieng, H., Chang, Y. T., Chang, D., Chen, J. J., et al. (2009). The Ca(v)3.2 T-type Ca(2+) channel is required for pressure overload-induced cardiac hypertrophy in mice. *Circulation Research*, *104*(4), 522–530.

Clapham, D. E. (2007). Calcium signaling. *Cell*, *131*(6), 1047–1058.

Dana, H., Mohar, B., Sun, Y., Narayan, S., Gordus, A., Hasseman, J. P., et al. (2016). Sensitive red protein calcium indicators for imaging neural activity. *eLife*, *5*, e12727.

Demaurex, N. (2005). Calcium measurements in organelles with Ca^{2+}-sensitive fluorescent proteins. *Cell Calcium*, *38*(3-4), 213–222.

Demaurex, N., & Frieden, M. (2003). Measurements of the free luminal ER Ca(2+) concentration with targeted "cameleon" fluorescent proteins. *Cell Calcium*, *34*(2), 109–119.

Dhennin-Duthille, I., Gautier, M., Faouzi, M., Guilbert, A., Brevet, M., Vaudry, D., et al. (2011). High expression of transient receptor potential channels in human breast cancer epithelial cells and tissues: Correlation with pathological parameters. *Cellular Physiology and Biochemistry*, *28*(5), 813–822.

Dynes, J. L., Amcheslavsky, A., & Cahalan, M. D. (2016). Genetically targeted single-channel optical recording reveals multiple Orai1 gating states and oscillations in calcium influx. *Proceedings of the National Academy of Sciences of the United States of America*, *113*(2), 440–445.

Eikermann-Haerter, K., Arbel-Ornath, M., Yalcin, N., Yu, E. S., Kuchibhotla, K. V., Yuzawa, I., et al. (2015). Abnormal synaptic Ca(2+) homeostasis and morphology in cortical neurons of familial hemiplegic migraine type 1 mutant mice. *Annals of Neurology*, *78*(2), 193–210.

Ellenbroek, S. I., & van Rheenen, J. (2014). Imaging hallmarks of cancer in living mice. *Nature Reviews. Cancer*, *14*(6), 406–418.

Elliott, W. J., & Ram, C. V. (2011). Calcium channel blockers. *Journal of Clinical Hypertension (Greenwich, Conn.)*, *13*(9), 687–689.

Emery, E. C., Luiz, A. P., Sikandar, S., Magnusdottir, R., Dong, X., & Wood, J. N. (2016). In vivo characterization of distinct modality-specific subsets of somatosensory neurons using GCaMP. *Sciences Advances*, *2*(11), e1600990.

Faouzi, M., Hague, F., Potier, M., Ahidouch, A., Sevestre, H., & Ouadid-Ahidouch, H. (2011). Down-regulation of Orai3 arrests cell-cycle progression and induces apoptosis in breast cancer cells but not in normal breast epithelial cells. *Journal of Cellular Physiology*, *226*(2), 542–551.

Fearnley, C. J., Roderick, H. L., & Bootman, M. D. (2011). Calcium signaling in cardiac myocytes. *Cold Spring Harbor Perspectives in Biology*, *3*(11), a004242.

Fixemer, T., Wissenbach, U., Flockerzi, V., & Bonkhoff, H. (2003). Expression of the Ca^{2+} -selective cation channel TRPV6 in human prostate cancer: A novel prognostic marker for tumor progression. *Oncogene*, *22*(49), 7858–7861.

Giorgi, C., Bonora, M., Missiroli, S., Poletti, F., Ramirez, F. G., Morciano, G., et al. (2015). Intravital imaging reveals p53-dependent cancer cell death induced by phototherapy via calcium signaling. *Oncotarget*, *6*(3), 1435–1445.

GlaxoSmithKline. (2000). *A study to evaluate the effect of the transient receptor potential vanilloid 4 (TRPV4) channel blocker, GSK2798745, on pulmonary gas transfer and respiration in patients with congestive heart failure. In ClinicalTrials.gov NLM Identifier: NCT02497937 (Internet).* Bethesda (MD): National Library of Medicine (US), Available from https://clinicaltrials.gov/show/NCT02497937 (cited 11.11.2016).

Go, L. O., Moschella, M. C., Watras, J., Handa, K. K., Fyfe, B. S., & Marks, A. R. (1995). Differential regulation of two types of intracellular calcium release channels during end-stage heart failure. *Journal of Clinical Investigation*, *95*(2), 888–894.

Godfraind, T. (2014). Calcium channel blockers in cardiovascular pharmacotherapy. *Journal of Cardiovascular Pharmacology and Therapeutics*, *19*(6), 501–515.

Grynkiewicz, G., Poenie, M., & Tsien, R. Y. (1985). A new generation of Ca2+ indicators with greatly improved fluorescence properties. *Journal of Biological Chemistry*, *260*(6), 3440–3450.

Guilbert, A., Gautier, M., Dhennin-Duthille, I., Haren, N., Sevestre, H., & Ouadid-Ahidouch, H. (2009). Evidence that TRPM7 is required for breast cancer cell proliferation. *American Journal of Physiology. Cell Physiology*, *297*(3), C493–C502.

Hanahan, D., & Weinberg, R. A. (2011). Hallmarks of cancer: The next generation. *Cell*, *144*(5), 646–674.

Harzheim, D., Movassagh, M., Foo, R. S., Ritter, O., Tashfeen, A., Conway, S. J., et al. (2009). Increased InsP3Rs in the junctional sarcoplasmic reticulum augment Ca2+ transients and arrhythmias associated with cardiac hypertrophy. *Proceedings of the National Academy of Sciences of the United States of America*, *106*(27), 11406–11411.

Hasan, M. T., Friedrich, R. W., Euler, T., Larkum, M. E., Giese, G., Both, M., et al. (2004). Functional fluorescent Ca2+ indicator proteins in transgenic mice under TET control. *PLoS Biology*, *2*(6), e163.

Hasson, S. A., Kane, L. A., Yamano, K., Huang, C. H., Sliter, D. A., Buehler, E., et al. (2013). High-content genome-wide RNAi screens identify regulators of parkin upstream of mitophagy. *Nature*, *504*(7479), 291–295.

Heim, N., & Griesbeck, O. (2004). Genetically encoded indicators of cellular calcium dynamics based on troponin C and green fluorescent protein. *Journal of Biological Chemistry*, *279*(14), 14280–14286.

Helmchen, F., Svoboda, K., Denk, W., & Tank, D. W. (1999). In vivo dendritic calcium dynamics in deep-layer cortical pyramidal neurons. *Nature Neuroscience*, *2*(11), 989–996.

Helmchen, F., & Waters, J. (2002). Ca2+ imaging in the mammalian brain in vivo. *European Journal of Pharmacology*, *447*(2-3), 119–129.

Herington, J. L., Swale, D. R., Brown, N., Shelton, E. L., Choi, H., Williams, C. H., et al. (2015). High-throughput screening of myometrial calcium-mobilization to identify modulators of uterine contractility. *PloS One*, *10*(11), e0143243.

Hill, J. M., De Stefani, D., Jones, A. W., Ruiz, A., Rizzuto, R., & Szabadkai, G. (2014). Measuring baseline Ca(2+) levels in subcellular compartments using genetically engineered fluorescent indicators. *Methods in Enzymology*, *543*, 47–72.

Hinckley, C. A., & Pfaff, S. L. (2013). Imaging spinal neuron ensembles active during locomotion with genetically encoded calcium indicators. *Annals of the New York Academy of Sciences*, *1279*, 71–79.

Hoi, H., Matsuda, T., Nagai, T., & Campbell, R. E. (2013). Highlightable Ca2+ indicators for live cell imaging. *Journal of the American Chemical Society*, *135*(1), 46–49.

Homolya, L., Hollo, Z., Germann, U. A., Pastan, I., Gottesman, M. M., & Sarkadi, B. (1993). Fluorescent cellular indicators are extruded by the multidrug resistance protein. *Journal of Biological Chemistry*, *268*(29), 21493–21496.

Honarnejad, K., Daschner, A., Giese, A., Zall, A., Schmidt, B., Szybinska, A., et al. (2013). Development and implementation of a high-throughput compound screening assay for targeting disrupted ER calcium homeostasis in Alzheimer's disease. *PloS One*, *8*(11), e80645.
Horikawa, K., Yamada, Y., Matsuda, T., Kobayashi, K., Hashimoto, M., Matsu-ura, T., et al. (2010). Spontaneous network activity visualized by ultrasensitive Ca(2+) indicators, yellow Cameleon-Nano. *Nature Methods*, 7(9), 729–732.
Inoue, M., Takeuchi, A., Horigane, S., Ohkura, M., Gengyo-Ando, K., Fujii, H., et al. (2015). Rational design of a high-affinity, fast, red calcium indicator R-CaMP2. *Nature Methods*, *12*(1), 64–70.
Jackson, R. E., & Burrone, J. (2016). Visualizing presynaptic calcium dynamics and vesicle fusion with a single genetically encoded reporter at individual synapses. *Frontiers in Synaptic Neuroscience*, *8*, 21.
Kaestner, L., Scholz, A., Tian, Q., Ruppenthal, S., Tabellion, W., Wiesen, K., et al. (2014). Genetically encoded Ca2+ indicators in cardiac myocytes. *Circulation Research*, *114*(10), 1623–1639.
Karreman, M. A., Hyenne, V., Schwab, Y., & Goetz, J. G. (2016). Intravital correlative microscopy: Imaging life at the nanoscale. *Trends in Cell Biology*, *26*(11), 848–863.
Kuchibhotla, K. V., Goldman, S. T., Lattarulo, C. R., Wu, H. Y., Hyman, B. T., & Bacskai, B. J. (2008). Abeta plaques lead to aberrant regulation of calcium homeostasis in vivo resulting in structural and functional disruption of neuronal networks. *Neuron*, *59*(2), 214–225.
Kuchibhotla, K. V., Lattarulo, C. R., Hyman, B. T., & Bacskai, B. J. (2009). Synchronous hyperactivity and intercellular calcium waves in astrocytes in Alzheimer mice. *Science*, *323*(5918), 1211–1215.
Lee, K. S., Huang, X., & Fitzpatrick, D. (2016). Topology of ON and OFF inputs in visual cortex enables an invariant columnar architecture. *Nature*, *533*(7601), 90–94.
Lee, W. J., Roberts-Thomson, S. J., & Monteith, G. R. (2005). Plasma membrane calcium-ATPase 2 and 4 in human breast cancer cell lines. *Biochemical and Biophysical Research Communications*, *337*(3), 779–783.
Lehen'kyi, V., Flourakis, M., Skryma, R., & Prevarskaya, N. (2007). TRPV6 channel controls prostate cancer cell proliferation via Ca(2+)/NFAT-dependent pathways. *Oncogene*, *26*(52), 7380–7385.
Li, H., Wang, X., Zhang, N., Gottipati, M. K., Parpura, V., & Ding, S. (2014). Imaging of mitochondrial Ca2+ dynamics in astrocytes using cell-specific mitochondria-targeted GCaMP5G/6s: Mitochondrial Ca2+ uptake and cytosolic Ca2+ availability via the endoplasmic reticulum store. *Cell Calcium*, *56*(6), 457–466.
Liebscher, S., Keller, G. B., Goltstein, P. M., Bonhoeffer, T., & Hubener, M. (2016). Selective persistence of sensorimotor mismatch signals in visual cortex of behaving Alzheimer's disease mice. *Current Biology*, *26*(7), 956–964.
Lissandron, V., Podini, P., Pizzo, P., & Pozzan, T. (2010). Unique characteristics of Ca2+ homeostasis of the trans-Golgi compartment. *Proceedings of the National Academy of Sciences of the United States of America*, *107*(20), 9198–9203.
Lock, J. T., Parker, I., & Smith, I. F. (2015). A comparison of fluorescent Ca^{2+} indicators for imaging local Ca^{2+} signals in cultured cells. *Cell Calcium*, *58*(6), 638–648.
Lutcke, H., Murayama, M., Hahn, T., Margolis, D. J., Astori, S., Zum Alten Borgloh, S. M., et al. (2010). Optical recording of neuronal activity with a genetically-encoded calcium indicator in anesthetized and freely moving mice. *Frontiers in Neural Circuits*, *4*, 9.
Mank, M., & Griesbeck, O. (2008). Genetically encoded calcium indicators. *Chemical Reviews*, *108*(5), 1550–1564.
Mank, M., Santos, A. F., Direnberger, S., Mrsic-Flogel, T. D., Hofer, S. B., Stein, V., et al. (2008). A genetically encoded calcium indicator for chronic in vivo two-photon imaging. *Nature Methods*, *5*(9), 805–811.

Mattiazzi Usaj, M., Styles, E. B., Verster, A. J., Friesen, H., Boone, C., & Andrews, B. J. (2016). High-content screening for quantitative cell biology. *Trends in Cell Biology*, *26*(8), 598–611.

Mattson, M. P., & Chan, S. L. (2003). Neuronal and glial calcium signaling in Alzheimer's disease. *Cell Calcium*, *34*(4-5), 385–397.

McAndrew, D., Grice, D. M., Peters, A. A., Davis, F. M., Stewart, T., Rice, M., et al. (2011). ORAI1-mediated calcium influx in lactation and in breast cancer. *Molecular Cancer Therapeutics*, *10*(3), 448–460.

Missiaen, L., Robberecht, W., van den Bosch, L., Callewaert, G., Parys, J. B., Wuytack, F., et al. (2000). Abnormal intracellular Ca(2+)homeostasis and disease. *Cell Calcium*, *28*(1), 1–21.

Miyawaki, A., Llopis, J., Heim, R., McCaffery, J. M., Adams, J. A., Ikura, M., et al. (1997). Fluorescent indicators for Ca2+ based on green fluorescent proteins and calmodulin. *Nature*, *388*(6645), 882–887.

Monteith, G. R., & Bird, G. S. (2005). Techniques: High-throughput measurement of intracellular Ca(2+)—Back to basics. *Trends in Pharmacological Sciences*, *26*(4), 218–223.

Monteith, G. R., Davis, F. M., & Roberts-Thomson, S. J. (2012). Calcium channels and pumps in cancer: Changes and consequences. *Journal of Biological Chemistry*, *287*(38), 31666–31673.

Monteith, G. R., McAndrew, D., Faddy, H. M., & Roberts-Thomson, S. J. (2007). Calcium and cancer: Targeting Ca2+ transport. *Nature Reviews Cancer*, 7(7), 519–530.

Montijn, J. S., Meijer, G. T., Lansink, C. S., & Pennartz, C. M. (2016). Population-level neural codes are robust to single-neuron variability from a multidimensional coding perspective. *Cell Reports*, *16*(9), 2486–2498.

Nagai, T., Yamada, S., Tominaga, T., Ichikawa, M., & Miyawaki, A. (2004). Expanded dynamic range of fluorescent indicators for Ca(2+) by circularly permuted yellow fluorescent proteins. *Proceedings of the National Academy of Sciences of the United States of America*, *101*(29), 10554–10559.

Nakai, J., Ohkura, M., & Imoto, K. (2001). A high signal-to-noise Ca(2+) probe composed of a single green fluorescent protein. *Nature Biotechnology*, *19*(2), 137–141.

Navas-Navarro, P., Rojo-Ruiz, J., Rodriguez-Prados, M., Ganfornina, M. D., Looger, L. L., Alonso, M. T., et al. (2016). GFP-aequorin protein sensor for ex vivo and in vivo imaging of Ca(2+) dynamics in high-Ca(2+) organelles. *Cell Chemical Biology*, *23*(6), 738–745.

O'Donnell, J. C., Jackson, J. G., & Robinson, M. B. (2016). Transient oxygen/glucose deprivation causes a delayed loss of mitochondria and increases spontaneous calcium signaling in astrocytic processes. *Journal of Neuroscience*, *36*(27), 7109–7127.

Oheim, M., van 't Hoff, M., Feltz, A., Zamaleeva, A., Mallet, J. M., & Collot, M. (2014). New red-fluorescent calcium indicators for optogenetics, photoactivation and multi-color imaging. *Biochimica et Biophysica Acta*, *1843*(10), 2284–2306.

Ohkura, M., Sasaki, T., Sadakari, J., Gengyo-Ando, K., Kagawa-Nagamura, Y., Kobayashi, C., et al. (2012). Genetically encoded green fluorescent Ca2+ indicators with improved detectability for neuronal Ca2+ signals. *PloS One*, 7(12), e51286.

Ottolini, D., Cali, T., & Brini, M. (2014). Methods to measure intracellular Ca(2+) fluxes with organelle-targeted aequorin-based probes. *Methods in Enzymology*, *543*, 21–45.

Palmer, A. E., Giacomello, M., Kortemme, T., Hires, S. A., Lev-Ram, V., Baker, D., et al. (2006). Ca2+ indicators based on computationally redesigned calmodulin-peptide pairs. *Chemistry and Biology*, *13*(5), 521–530.

Palmer, A. E., Jin, C., Reed, J. C., & Tsien, R. Y. (2004). Bcl-2-mediated alterations in endoplasmic reticulum Ca2+ analyzed with an improved genetically encoded fluorescent sensor. *Proceedings of the National Academy of Sciences of the United States of America*, *101*(50), 17404–17409.

Palmer, A. E., Qin, Y., Park, J. G., & McCombs, J. E. (2011). Design and application of genetically encoded biosensors. *Trends in Biotechnology*, *29*(3), 144–152.
Palmer, A. E., & Tsien, R. Y. (2006). Measuring calcium signaling using genetically targetable fluorescent indicators. *Nature Protocols*, *1*(3), 1057–1065.
Paredes, R. M., Etzler, J. C., Watts, L. T., Zheng, W., & Lechleiter, J. D. (2008). Chemical calcium indicators. *Methods*, *46*(3), 143–151.
Pendin, D., Greotti, E., Filadi, R., & Pozzan, T. (2015). Spying on organelle Ca2+ in living cells: The mitochondrial point of view. *Journal of Endocrinological Investigation*, *38*(1), 39–45.
Peng, J. B., Zhuang, L., Berger, U. V., Adam, R. M., Williams, B. J., Brown, E. M., et al. (2001). CaT1 expression correlates with tumor grade in prostate cancer. *Biochemical and Biophysical Research Communications*, *282*(3), 729–734.
Perez Koldenkova, V., & Nagai, T. (2013). Genetically encoded Ca(2+) indicators: Properties and evaluation. *Biochimica et Biophysica Acta*, *1833*(7), 1787–1797.
Perry, J. L., Ramachandran, N. K., Utama, B., & Hyser, J. M. (2015). Use of genetically-encoded calcium indicators for live cell calcium imaging and localization in virus-infected cells. *Methods*, *90*, 28–38.
Peters, A. A., Simpson, P. T., Bassett, J. J., Lee, J. M., Da Silva, L., Reid, L. E., et al. (2012). Calcium channel TRPV6 as a potential therapeutic target in estrogen receptor-negative breast cancer. *Molecular Cancer Therapeutics*, *11*(10), 2158–2168.
Petrou, S., Bowser, D. N., Nicholls, R. A., Panchal, R. G., Smart, M. L., Reilly, A. M., et al. (2000). Genetically targeted calcium sensors enhance the study of organelle function in living cells. *Clinical and Experimental Pharmacology and Physiology*, *27*(9), 738–744.
Pittet, M. J., & Weissleder, R. (2011). Intravital imaging. *Cell*, *147*(5), 983–991.
Pologruto, T. A., Yasuda, R., & Svoboda, K. (2004). Monitoring neural activity and [Ca2+] with genetically encoded Ca2+ indicators. *Journal of Neuroscience*, *24*(43), 9572–9579.
Prevarskaya, N., Ouadid-Ahidouch, H., Skryma, R., & Shuba, Y. (2014). Remodelling of Ca2+ transport in cancer: How it contributes to cancer hallmarks? *Philosophical Transactions of the Royal Society of London Series B: Biological Sciences*, *369*(1638), 20130097.
Prevarskaya, N., Zhang, L., & Barritt, G. (2007). TRP channels in cancer. *Biochimica et Biophysica Acta*, *1772*(8), 937–946.
Ravier, M. A., Daro, D., Roma, L. P., Jonas, J. C., Cheng-Xue, R., Schuit, F. C., et al. (2011). Mechanisms of control of the free Ca2+ concentration in the endoplasmic reticulum of mouse pancreatic beta-cells: Interplay with cell metabolism and [Ca2+]c and role of SERCA2b and SERCA3. *Diabetes*, *60*(10), 2533–2545.
Rizzuto, R., & Pozzan, T. (2006). Microdomains of intracellular Ca2+: Molecular determinants and functional consequences. *Physiological Reviews*, *86*(1), 369–408.
Robert, V., Pinton, P., Tosello, V., Rizzuto, R., & Pozzan, T. (2000). Recombinant aequorin as tool for monitoring calcium concentration in subcellular compartments. *Methods in Enzymology*, *327*, 440–456.
Roderick, H. L., & Cook, S. J. (2008). Ca2+ signalling checkpoints in cancer: Remodelling Ca2+ for cancer cell proliferation and survival. *Nature Reviews. Cancer*, *8*(5), 361–375.
Rodriguez, E. A., Campbell, R. E., Lin, J. Y., Lin, M. Z., Miyawaki, A., Palmer, A. E., et al. (2017). The growing and glowing toolbox of fluorescent and photoactive proteins. *Trends in Biochemical Sciences*, *42*(2), 111–129.
Rodriguez-Garcia, A., Rojo-Ruiz, J., Navas-Navarro, P., Aulestia, F. J., Gallego-Sandin, S., Garcia-Sancho, J., et al. (2014). GAP, an aequorin-based fluorescent indicator for imaging Ca2+ in organelles. *Proceedings of the National Academy of Sciences of the United States of America*, *111*(7), 2584–2589.
Rodriguez-Prados, M., Rojo-Ruiz, J., Aulestia, F. J., Garcia-Sancho, J., & Alonso, M. T. (2015). A new low-Ca^{2+} affinity GAP indicator to monitor high Ca^{2+} in organelles by luminescence. *Cell Calcium*, *58*(6), 558–564.

Romoser, V. A., Hinkle, P. M., & Persechini, A. (1997). Detection in living cells of Ca^{2+} -dependent changes in the fluorescence emission of an indicator composed of two green fluorescent protein variants linked by a calmodulin-binding sequence. A new class of fluorescent indicators. *Journal of Biological Chemistry*, *272*(20), 13270–13274.
Rose, T., Goltstein, P. M., Portugues, R., & Griesbeck, O. (2014). Putting a finishing touch on GECIs. *Frontiers in Molecular Neuroscience*, *7*, 88.
Rudolf, R., Mongillo, M., Rizzuto, R., & Pozzan, T. (2003). Looking forward to seeing calcium. *Nature Reviews. Molecular Cell Biology*, *4*(7), 579–586.
Santisakultarm, T. P., Kersbergen, C. J., Bandy, D. K., Ide, D. C., Choi, S. H., & Silva, A. C. (2016). Two-photon imaging of cerebral hemodynamics and neural activity in awake and anesthetized marmosets. *Journal of Neuroscience Methods*, *271*, 55–64.
Schmidtko, A., Lotsch, J., Freynhagen, R., & Geisslinger, G. (2010). Ziconotide for treatment of severe chronic pain. *Lancet*, *375*(9725), 1569–1577.
Shaner, N. C., Lin, M. Z., McKeown, M. R., Steinbach, P. A., Hazelwood, K. L., Davidson, M. W., et al. (2008). Improving the photostability of bright monomeric orange and red fluorescent proteins. *Nature Methods*, *5*(6), 545–551.
Shiba, Y., Fernandes, S., Zhu, W. Z., Filice, D., Muskheli, V., Kim, J., et al. (2012). Human ES-cell-derived cardiomyocytes electrically couple and suppress arrhythmias in injured hearts. *Nature*, *489*(7415), 322–325.
Shigetomi, E., Kracun, S., Sofroniew, M. V., & Khakh, B. S. (2010). A genetically targeted optical sensor to monitor calcium signals in astrocyte processes. *Nature Neuroscience*, *13*(6), 759–766.
Shimomura, O., Johnson, F. H., & Saiga, Y. (1962). Extraction, purification and properties of aequorin, a bioluminescent protein from the luminous hydromedusan, Aequorea. *Journal of Cellular and Comparative Physiology*, *59*, 223–239.
Shinnawi, R., Huber, I., Maizels, L., Shaheen, N., Gepstein, A., Arbel, G., et al. (2015). Monitoring human-induced pluripotent stem cell-derived cardiomyocytes with genetically encoded calcium and voltage fluorescent reporters. *Stem Cell Reports*, *5*(4), 582–596.
Sidik, S. M., Hortua Triana, M. A., Paul, A. S., El Bakkouri, M., Hackett, C. G., Tran, F., et al. (2016). Using a genetically encoded sensor to identify inhibitors of Toxoplasma gondii Ca2+ signaling. *Journal of Biological Chemistry*, *291*(18), 9566–9580.
Smetters, D., Majewska, A., & Yuste, R. (1999). Detecting action potentials in neuronal populations with calcium imaging. *Methods*, *18*(2), 215–221.
Stewart, T. A., Yapa, K. T., & Monteith, G. R. (2015). Altered calcium signaling in cancer cells. *Biochimica et Biophysica Acta*, *1848*(10), 2502–2511.
Stosiek, C., Garaschuk, O., Holthoff, K., & Konnerth, A. (2003). In vivo two-photon calcium imaging of neuronal networks. *Proceedings of the National Academy of Sciences of the United States of America*, *100*(12), 7319–7324.
Sun, X. R., Badura, A., Pacheco, D. A., Lynch, L. A., Schneider, E. R., Taylor, M. P., et al. (2013). Fast GCaMPs for improved tracking of neuronal activity. *Nature Communications*, *4*, 2170.
Suzuki, J., Kanemaru, K., & Iino, M. (2016). Genetically encoded fluorescent indicators for organellar calcium imaging. *Biophysical Journal*, *111*(6), 1119–1131.
Suzuki, J., Kanemaru, K., Ishii, K., Ohkura, M., Okubo, Y., & Iino, M. (2014). Imaging intraorganellar Ca2+ at subcellular resolution using CEPIA. *Nature Communications*, *5*, 4153.
Takahashi, A., Camacho, P., Lechleiter, J. D., & Herman, B. (1999). Measurement of intracellular calcium. *Physiological Reviews*, *79*(4), 1089–1125.
Tallini, Y. N., Ohkura, M., Choi, B. R., Ji, G., Imoto, K., Doran, R., et al. (2006). Imaging cellular signals in the heart in vivo: Cardiac expression of the high-signal Ca2+ indicator GCaMP2. *Proceedings of the National Academy of Sciences of the United States of America*, *103*(12), 4753–4758.

Theis, L., Berens, P., Froudarakis, E., Reimer, J., Roman Roson, M., Baden, T., et al. (2016). Benchmarking spike rate inference in population calcium imaging. *Neuron, 90*(3), 471–482.

Thestrup, T., Litzlbauer, J., Bartholomaus, I., Mues, M., Russo, L., Dana, H., et al. (2014). Optimized ratiometric calcium sensors for functional in vivo imaging of neurons and T lymphocytes. *Nature Methods, 11*(2), 175–182.

Thomas, D., Tovey, S. C., Collins, T. J., Bootman, M. D., Berridge, M. J., & Lipp, P. (2000). A comparison of fluorescent Ca2+ indicator properties and their use in measuring elementary and global Ca2+ signals. *Cell Calcium, 28*(4), 213–223.

Tian, L., Akerboom, J., Schreiter, E. R., & Looger, L. L. (2012). Neural activity imaging with genetically encoded calcium indicators. *Progress in Brain Research, 196*, 79–94.

Tian, L., Hires, S. A., & Looger, L. L. (2012). Imaging neuronal activity with genetically encoded calcium indicators. *Cold Spring Harbor Protocols, 2012*(6), 647–656.

Tian, L., Hires, S. A., Mao, T., Huber, D., Chiappe, M. E., Chalasani, S. H., et al. (2009). Imaging neural activity in worms, flies and mice with improved GCaMP calcium indicators. *Nature Methods, 6*(12), 875–881.

Tosatto, A., Sommaggio, R., Kummerow, C., Bentham, R. B., Blacker, T. S., Berecz, T., et al. (2016). The mitochondrial calcium uniporter regulates breast cancer progression via HIF-1alpha. *EMBO Molecular Medicine, 8*(5), 569–585.

Tsien, R. Y., Pozzan, T., & Rink, T. J. (1982). T-cell mitogens cause early changes in cytoplasmic free Ca2+ and membrane potential in lymphocytes. *Nature, 295*(5844), 68–71.

Vandecaetsbeek, I., Vangheluwe, P., Raeymaekers, L., Wuytack, F., & Vanoevelen, J. (2011). The Ca2+ pumps of the endoplasmic reticulum and golgi apparatus. *Cold Spring Harbor Perspectives in Biology, 3*(5), a004184.

Vinegoni, C., Aguirre, A. D., Lee, S., & Weissleder, R. (2015). Imaging the beating heart in the mouse using intravital microscopy techniques. *Nature Protocols, 10*(11), 1802–1819.

Wabnig, S., Liewald, J. F., Yu, S. C., & Gottschalk, A. (2015). High-throughput all-optical analysis of synaptic transmission and synaptic vesicle recycling in Caenorhabditis elegans. *PloS One, 10*(8), e0135584.

Wang, J., Zhu, L. Y., Liu, Q., Hentzer, M., Smith, G. P., & Wang, M. W. (2015). High-throughput screening of antagonists for the orphan G-protein coupled receptor GPR139. *Acta Pharmacologica Sinica, 36*(7), 874–878.

Whitaker, M. (2010). Genetically encoded probes for measurement of intracellular calcium. *Methods in Cell Biology, 99*, 153–182.

Williams, D. A., Monif, M., & Richardson, K. L. (2013). Compartmentalizing genetically encoded calcium sensors. *Methods in Molecular Biology, 937*, 307–326.

Woods, N. K., & Padmanabhan, J. (2012). Neuronal calcium signaling and Alzheimer's disease. *Advances in Experimental Medicine and Biology, 740*, 1193–1217.

Wu, J., Prole, D. L., Shen, Y., Lin, Z., Gnanasekaran, A., Liu, Y., et al. (2014). Red fluorescent genetically encoded Ca2+ indicators for use in mitochondria and endoplasmic reticulum. *Biochemical Journal, 464*(1), 13–22.

Zanella, F., Lorens, J. B., & Link, W. (2010). High content screening: Seeing is believing. *Trends in Biotechnology, 28*(5), 237–245.

Zhang, J., Campbell, R. E., Ting, A. Y., & Tsien, R. Y. (2002). Creating new fluorescent probes for cell biology. *Nature Reviews. Molecular Cell Biology, 3*(12), 906–918.

Zhao, Y., Araki, S., Wu, J., Teramoto, T., Chang, Y. F., Nakano, M., et al. (2011). An expanded palette of genetically encoded Ca^{2+} indicators. *Science, 333*(6051), 1888–1891.

CHAPTER SIX

TRPV1 Channels in Immune Cells and Hematological Malignancies

Sofia A. Omari, Murray J. Adams, Dominic P. Geraghty[1]
School of Health Sciences, University of Tasmania, Launceston, TAS, Australia
[1]Corresponding author: e-mail address: d.geraghty@utas.edu.au

Contents

Abstract

Transient receptor potential vanilloid-1 (TRPV1) is a member of the TRP family of channels that are responsible for nociceptive, thermal, and mechanical sensations. Originally associated exclusively with sensory neurons, TRPV1 is now known to be present in almost all organs, including cells of the immune system, where TRPV1 has been shown to play a pivotal role in inflammation and immunity. Monocytes, macrophages, and dendritic cells express TRPV1, with both mouse and human studies suggesting that TRPV1 activation protects against endotoxin-induced inflammation. In contrast, TRPV1 (and other TRP channels) appears to be required for T-cell receptor activation by mitogens. Additionally, studies in cell lines derived from hematological and other

Advances in Pharmacology, Volume 79
ISSN 1054-3589
http://dx.doi.org/10.1016/bs.apha.2017.01.002

malignancies suggest altered expression/function of TRPV1 might serve as a target for novel cytotoxic therapies.

ABBREVIATIONS

ATL adult T-cell leukemia
Bax Bcl-2-associated X
Bcl-2 B-cell lymphoma-2 protein
Bcl-xL B-cell lymphoma-extra large
CaM calmodulin
CAP capsaicin
CDK cyclin-dependent kinases
DC dendritic cell
MM multiple myeloma
NADA *N*-arachidonoyldopamine
NFAT nuclear factor of activated T-cells
NF-κB nuclear factor kappa-light-chain-enhancer of activated B-cells
NGF nerve growth factor
NK natural killer
PIP_2 phosphatidyl-inositol-4,5-bisphosphate
ROS reactive oxygen species
RTX resiniferatoxin
STAT signal transducer and activator of transcription
TRPV1 transient receptor potential vanilloid-1

1. INTRODUCTION

Natural compounds have been used for millennia to treat diseases and relieve symptoms, and indeed, form the basis of modern pharmacotherapy. Capsaicin (CAP), the main active ingredient of "hot chili peppers" (*Capsicum* species), was isolated to increasing degrees of purity by Bucholz (1816), Thresh (1878), and Micko (1898). However, the use of hot peppers for medicinal purposes can be traced back to the 14th century where they were employed by the Aztecs to cure cramps, diarrhea, and dyspepsia, and later as an appetite stimulant, a treatment of gastric ulcers, rheumatism, and alopecia (Szallasi, 1995).

The CAP receptor, transient receptor potential vanilloid-1 (TRPV1), while originally thought to be exclusively (sensory) neuronal, TRPV1, and its structural homolog TRPV2 are now recognized for their wide species and tissue distribution (Birder et al., 2001; Cortright & Szallasi, 2004; Gunthorpe, Benham, Randall, & Davis, 2002; Heiner, Eisfeld, &

Luckhoff, 2003; Matthews et al., 2004; Nagy, Santha, Jancso, & Urban, 2004; Nilius & Voets, 2005; Stokes, Wakano, Del Carmen, Koblana Huberson, & Turner, 2005).

TRPV1 expression has been demonstrated in nearly all types of mammalian immune cells—macrophages and dendritic cells (DCs), lymphocytes and monocytes, natural killer (NK) cells, and neutrophils (in detail later). As a result, the role of TRPV1 in the innate and adaptive immune systems has been the subject of considerable research focus, particularly over the last 15 years. TRPV1 knockout mice confirmed the pivotal role of TRPV1 in pain and inflammation (Caterina et al., 2000), with more recent studies in this model demonstrating that TRPV1 channels are intimately involved in *T-cell receptor (TCR)-mediated* Ca^{2+} *influx, TCR signaling*, and *T-cell activation* (Bertin et al., 2014). Moreover, the overexpression of TRPV1 in many types of nonhematological cancers and apparent increased susceptibility to the cytotoxic effects of CAP-like agents, suggest that immune cell TRPV1 may serve as a novel therapeutic target in hematological malignancies. The focus of this brief review is the expression, regulation, and potential function of TRPV1 in human immune cells and hematological malignancies.

2. OVERVIEW OF TRP CHANNELS

TRP channels and more specifically, TRPV1, are not only important in sensory systems, they appear to be crucial components for the function of epithelial, blood, and smooth muscle cells (Minke, 2006). The TRP superfamily consists of a number of nonselective cation channels that are seen as "universal biological sensors," detecting changes in the external and internal environments including nociception, temperature and mechanical sensation, renal Ca^{2+}/Mg^{2+} handling, lysosomal function, cardiovascular/blood pressure regulation, control of cell growth and proliferation, perception of pungent compounds (e.g., those found in chili, mustard, and garlic), taste perception, and smooth muscle tone (Christensen & Corey, 2007; Clapham, Montell, Schultz, & Julius, 2003; Ramsey, Delling, & Clapham, 2006).

The channels consist of six-transmembrane domains segments (S1–S6) and a pore region between S5 and S6, with intracellular carboxy (C-) and amino (N-) termini (Clapham, Julius, Montell, & Schultz, 2005; Minke, 2006). Despite the structural similarities between the TRPs and the voltage-gated K^+ channels, these groups of channels are distinctly different

(Clapham et al., 2005). At least 28 different TRP subunit genes have been identified in mammals, comprising six subfamilies, namely the classical or canonical TRPs, TRPV (vanilloid), TRPM (melastatin), TRPA (ankyrin), TRPP (polycystin), and TRPML (mucolipin). Each subfamily comprises several channel subtypes, which differ in their selectivity for Ca^{2+}, activation mechanisms, and interacting proteins (Clapham, 2007; Holzer, 2008; Nilius, 2007).

The group of thermo-TRP channels, such as TRPV1 and TRPM8, sense a wide spectrum of temperatures from painful heat to painful cold (≥43°C and <22–26°C, respectively) (Dhaka, Viswanath, & Patapoutian, 2006). Moreover, they are able to detect specific chemical entities including unpleasant and/or painful toxins, whereby TRP channels subserve chemesthesis, defined as the chemical sensibility of the skin and mucus membranes, which is distinct from taste and smell (Bandell, Macpherson, & Patapoutian, 2007). TRP channels are opened or closed by conformational changes in the channel protein (Bandell et al., 2007; Dhaka et al., 2006). The ion selectivity differs markedly among the same family of TRP channels. Most TRPs are nonselective cation channels, with relative permeability, P_{Ca}/P_{Na}, usually ≤ 5 (Owsianik, Talavera, Voets, & Nilius, 2006). TRPV1 ($P_{Ca}/P_{Na} \sim 10$) is relatively selective for Ca^{2+}, and TRPV5 and TRPV6 ($P_{Ca}/P_{Na} > 100$) are classed as Ca^{2+} selective (Clapham, 2003).

3. TRPV1

Interest in what eventually became known as TRPV1 has been attributed to Endre Hőgyes who first described the pharmacological effects of CAP (Hőgyes, 1878). CAP and other capsaicinoids, including dihydrocapsaicin (DHC), are responsible for the sensation of "hot" and "burning" when mucous membranes are exposed to chili peppers. CAP acts on primary afferent C- and Aδ-nociceptive neurons originating from the CNS (dorsal root and trigeminal ganglia) to produce these well-known effects (Himi et al., 2012; Julius & Basbaum, 2001; Schicho, Florian, Liebmann, Holzer, & Lippe, 2004). The selectivity of CAP's action on primary afferent neurons could only be explained by an action on a specific CAP receptor, which ultimately led to the discovery of the vanilloid receptor-1 (VR1), later renamed TRPV1 (Caterina et al., 1997; Nagy et al., 2004; Szolcsanyi, Jancso-Gabor, & Joo, 1975).

3.1 Structure

TRPV1 is composed of six-transmembrane domains with a pore-forming hydrophobic span between the fifth and sixth transmembrane domains (Caterina et al., 1997). Like many other TRP channels, TRPV1 has a long N-terminus containing three ankyrin repeat domains and a C-terminus containing a TRP domain close to the sixth transmembrane domain (Tominaga & Tominaga, 2005). The binding site present on the ankyrin repeat domain of TRPV1 has been reported to bind triphosphate nucleotides such as ATP and calmodulin (CaM) in the same site (Lishko, Procko, Jin, Phelps, & Gaudet, 2007; Rosenbaum, Gordon-Shaag, Munari, & Gordon, 2004). Upon binding, these molecules alter the sensitivity and regulate the function of TRPV1 (Phelps, Wang, Choo, & Gaudet, 2010). The intracellular domain of TRPV1 contains multiple binding sites for phosphatidyl-inositol-4,5-bisphosphate (PIP_2) on the N- and C-termini (Grycova et al., 2012), and two other sites for a protein kinase C and Ca^{2+}/CaM-dependent protein kinase II (CAM-kinase II), which are crucial for TRPV1 regulation (Ferrer-Montiel et al., 2004; Jeske et al., 2009).

3.2 TRPV1 Activation

TRPV1 is a polymodal nociceptor that is activated and/or allosterically modulated by a number of noxious agents (Holzer, 2008; Rosenbaum & Simon, 2007). In addition to capsaicinoids, TRPV1 channels are also activated/modulated by a variety of other plant-derived vanilloids including, camphor and resiniferatoxin (RTX), and putative endogenous vanilloids such as the endocannabinoid, anandamide (*N*-arachidonoylethanolamine or AEA), some lipoxygenase products of arachidonic acid such as 12-(*S*)- and 15-(*S*)-hydroperoxyeicosatetraenoic acid (12*S*- and 15*S*-HPETE), *N*-arachidonoyldopamine (NADA), and its congener, *N*-oleoyldopamine (Chu et al., 2003; Meotti, Lemos de Andrade, & Calixto, 2014; Van Der Stelt & Di Marzo, 2004; Xu, Blair, & Clapham, 2005).

Plant-derived vanilloids bind to intracellular sites on the TRPV1 channel, and the amino acids critical for CAP/RTX binding include Arg-91, Tyr-511, Ser-512, Ile 514, Val-518, and residue 547 (Met in rat and Leu in human), which are part of transmembrane segments 3 and 4 (Jordt & Julius, 2002). CAP is the prototypic TRPV1 agonist, which acts by lowering the heat threshold required to open the TRPV1 channel (Szallasi & Blumberg, 1999). The affinity of CAP for the human (neuronal) TRPV1 channel ranges from 7 to 30 nM determined from electrophysiological studies (Seabrook et al., 2002; Voets et al., 2004) to in excess of 2 μM from [^{125}I]-RTX-binding studies (Chou, Mtui, Gao, Kohler, & Middleton, 2004). However, CAP blocks K^+ channels in rats and humans with approximate IC_{50}s of 25–160 and 18 μM, respectively (Xing, Ma, Zhang, & Fan, 2010; Yang, Xiong, Liu, & Liu, 2014). In addition, because of their lipophilicity, CAP (and other vanilloids) may affect cellular function via a direct interaction with the cell due to their ability to cross the plasma membrane bilayer (Ziglioli et al., 2009).

Other activators of the TRPV1 channel include noxious heat (≥43°C) (Loyd, Chen, & Hargreaves, 2012), acidosis (pH ≤5.9) (Kaszas et al., 2012), mechanical stress (Inoue, Jian, & Kawarabayashi, 2009), and other chemesthetic (irritant) agents including vanillatoxins 1–3 (tarantula), ginger, and ethanol (Bandell et al., 2007; Dhaka et al., 2006; Loyd et al., 2012). The thermal sensitivity of TRPV1 is enhanced by several endogenous modulators such as bradykinin, ATP, nerve growth factor (NGF) (Chuang et al., 2001), and protease-activated receptor-2 agonists (Amadesi et al., 2004). NGF appears to act via phospholipase C to hydrolyze PIP_2, leading to inhibition of the channel (Chuang et al., 2001). Sustained exposure to agonists increases the Ca^{2+} permeability of TRPV1 and causes pore dilation (Chung, Guler, & Caterina, 2008). In addition, TRPV1 allows protons to enter the cell in an acidic environment, which results in intracellular acidification (Hellwig et al., 2004).

One of the early observations made by János Szolcsanyi was that CAP-responsive neurons exposed to CAP either in low doses chronically, or high doses acutely, became overloaded with Ca^{2+} resulting in mitochondrial swelling, long-lasting defunctionalization (desensitization), and ultimately cell death (Szoke, Seress, & Szolcsanyi, 2002; Szolcsanyi, 1993; Szolcsanyi et al., 1975). This observation in many ways prompted the subsequent research focusing on TRPV1 as a target for cancer treatment.

3.3 Expression and Overexpression of TRPV1

Once believed to be exclusively neuronal, molecular, immunohistochemical, and functional studies have subsequently reported TRPV1 expression in nonneuronal cells in almost all organs (Cortright & Szallasi, 2004; Fernandes, Fernandes, & Keeble, 2012). These include the urothelium (Avelino & Cruz, 2006; Birder et al., 2001), human smooth muscle, keratinocytes (Jaggar, Scott, James, & Rice, 2001), muscle layer, mucosa and epithelial cells of the gastrointestinal tract (Geppetti & Trevisani, 2004), epidermis and keratinocytes (Bode et al., 2009), airway epithelial cells (Reilly et al., 2003), human umbilical vein endothelial cells (Himi et al., 2012), and microglia (Kim, Kim, Oh, & Jin, 2006).

CAP is known to be cytotoxic in a number of cancer cell lines (reviewed by Basith, Cui, Hong, & Choi, 2016; Fattori, Hohmann, Rossaneis, Pinho-Ribeiro, & Verri, 2016; Prevarskaya, Zhang, & Barritt, 2007; Santoni, Farfariello, & Amantini, 2011; Sharma, Vij, & Sharma, 2013). There are conflicting reviews which elude to both cancer preventing and cancer promoting actions of CAP and other capsaicinoids (Bley, Boorman, Mohammad, McKenzie, & Babbar, 2012; Bode & Dong, 2011). However, a recent large-scale prospective cohort study (median follow-up, 7.4 years) of almost 490,000 Chinese men and women found that daily (6–7 days per week) consumption of spicy (chili based) foods was inversely associated with all-cause mortality, and specific cause mortality including cancer (Lv et al., 2015). Although fresh chili contains a number of beneficial (poly)phenolic compounds, the reduced mortality rate was attributed to the capsaicinoid content.

There is, however, evidence to suggest that CAP causes apoptotic and/or necrotic death of cell lines by both TRPV1-dependent and -independent mechanisms (refer Sharma et al., 2013). Nevertheless, TRPV1 is expressed in prostate cancer (Sánchez, Sánchez, Malagarie-Cazenave, Olea, & az-Laviada, 2006; Ziglioli et al., 2009), overexpressed in pancreatic cancer (Hartel et al., 2006; Mergler et al., 2012) and colon adenocarcinoma (Domotor et al., 2005), and "aberrantly" overexpressed in cervical cancer (Contassot, Tenan, Schnuriger, Pelte, & Dietrich, 2004), which would presumably confer increased susceptibility to the cytotoxic action of CAP and other vanilloids. TRPV1 expression declines as transitional cell carcinoma of the urinary bladder progresses (Lazzeri et al., 2005), but well-differentiated low-grade RT4 cells that overexpress TRPV1 (but not undifferentiated EJ and TCCSUP cells with low TRPV1 expression) are susceptible to CAP-induced cell death, which is blocked by capsazepine (Amantini et al., 2009).

4. TRPV1 EXPRESSION AND FUNCTION IN IMMUNE CELLS

4.1 Lymphocytes

As early as 2002, a variety of TRP channels, including TRPM4 and TRPC7, were known to be expressed in lymphocytes (Launay et al.,

2004; Lievremont et al., 2005; Mori et al., 2002). However, as Schwartz and colleagues noted, "messenger RNA but not protein expression was analyzed and cell lines but not primary human, or murine lymphocytes were used" in the majority of studies of immune cell TRPV1 (Schwarz et al., 2007).

TRPV1 message (RT-PCR) and protein (immunocytochemistry) were reported in a lymphocyte-enriched human peripheral blood mononuclear cell (PBMC) preparation (Saunders, Kunde, Crawford, & Geraghty, 2007), and subsequently vanilloid-induced PBMC death that was TRPV1-dependent was demonstrated (Saunders, Fassett, & Geraghty, 2009). Western blot, confocal microscopic, and/or flow cytometric studies from other groups confirmed that human NK cells (Kim et al., 2014), CD4 (Bertin et al., 2014; Samivel et al., 2016), and >99% of primary CD3 T-cells express TRPV1 (Majhi et al., 2015).

An increase in $[Ca^{2+}]_i$ is essential for lymphocyte activation, proliferation, and differentiation (Gallo, Cante-Barrett, & Crabtree, 2006). In B- and T-lymphocytes, the reaction between antigen and receptor results in a dual phase Ca^{2+} response, a transient increase in $[Ca^{2+}]_i$ due to Ca^{2+} release from endoplasmic reticulum stores, and a subsequent prolonged $[Ca^{2+}]_i$ increment through Ca^{2+} influx from the extracellular environment across the plasma membrane. Both phases lead to increased $[Ca^{2+}]_i$ and subsequently activation of many transcription factors such as nuclear factor of activated T-cells (NFAT) and nuclear factor kappa-light-chain-enhancer of activated B-cells (NF-κB). These in turn lead to cell proliferation and the production of various cytokines (Inada, Iida, & Tominaga, 2006). Interestingly, while CAP (50 μM) impedes the cytotoxicity of NK cells, this effect appears to be largely independent of TRPV1 activation since the antagonists, capsazepine (1 μM) and SB366791 (10 μM), did not inhibit the CAP-induced effect on cytotoxicity (Kim et al., 2014).

Substance P, an "indirect" TRPV1 activator which is released by TRPV1 stimulation, is involved in regulating the functions of lymphocytes. Its gene expression and receptor have been detected on human lymphocytes (Lai, Douglas, & Ho, 1998). CAP has been shown to have immunomodulatory effects through its ability to modulate lymphocyte proliferation and immunoglobulin A, E, and G production (Nilsson, Alving, & Ahlstedt, 1991; Takano et al., 2007). In addition, CAP inhibits T-helper cell cytokine production in cultured murine Peyer's patch (PP) cells in vitro, whereas oral injection of capsicum extract and CAP enhances the production of T-helper 1 cytokines such as IL-2 and interferon-gamma in response to the mitogen, concanavalin A (Takano et al., 2007). Furthermore, direct treatment of PP cells with 3 and 30 μM of CAP reduced cell viability (Takano et al., 2007). TRPV1 has been detected on T-lymphocytes in PP and mediates CAP-induced T-cell reduction which was partly inhibited by the antagonist capsazepine. Interestingly, if administered subcutaneously to neonatal rats, CAP causes a marked reduction in thymus weight and a lack of thymocyte differentiation by triggering apoptosis (Santoni et al., 2000). This indicates a negative effect of CAP on the thymus and lymphocytes, which contributes to apoptosis in these cells.

4.2 Macrophages

In contrast to lymphocytes where CAP, either through TRPV1 activation or indirectly, stimulate activity, the effect on macrophages appears to be primarily inhibitory. Reactive oxygen species (ROS) generated by activated macrophages play a crucial role in the initiation of inflammation and have harmful effects on neuroinflammatory diseases. Early animal studies showed that treating macrophages with CAP (10 μM) suppressed superoxide anion, hydrogen peroxide, and nitrite radical production completely in vitro (Joe & Lokesh, 1994). Furthermore, CAP inhibited store-operated Ca^{2+} entry in rat peritoneal macrophages (Joe & Lokesh, 1994). In the CNS, ROS production was substantially inhibited upon TRPV1 suppression in microglia, which function as macrophages in the CNS.

CAP does not inhibit all macrophage types. An elegant study by Nevius and colleagues found that a single oral dose (10 μg) of CAP selectively attenuated the proliferation of autoreactive T-cells in pancreatic lymph nodes of mice by enhancing a discrete population of macrophages and protected against the development of type-1 diabetes (Nevius, Srivastava, & Basu, 2012). This may explain, at least in part, the inverse association of daily spicy food consumption with death due to diabetes (Lv et al., 2015).

4.3 Dendritic Cells

DCs are widely distributed in all tissues, especially in those that interface with the external environment. They are potent antigen presenting cells that have the ability to stimulate T-cells and differentiate B-cells (Satthaporn & Eremin, 2001). The myeloid and lymphoid-derived subsets of DCs perform specific stimulatory functions. DCs secrete cytokines, migrate to lymph nodes after activation and activate lymphocytes (Shortman & Liu, 2002). The expression and role of TRPV1 in DCs is controversial. TRPV1 protein has been detected in murine (Basu & Srivastava, 2005) and human DCs derived from THP-1 cells (Toth et al., 2009). In mice, activation of TRPV1 leads to the activation and maturation of DCs. However, O'Connell, Pingle, and Ahern (2005) failed to detect TRPV1 mRNA in murine DCs and criticized the lack of reported controls and potential genomic contamination in the study by Basu and Srivastava. Toth et al. (2009) have subsequently shown that human THP-1 monocytes, as well as both immature and mature DCs, express functional TRPV1 using flow cytometry, Ca^{2+}-imaging and quantitative real-time PCR (Q-PCR). Furthermore, TRPV1 expression dramatically increased during cytokine-induced in vitro differentiation of monocytes to immature DCs. Finally, CAP has been reported to suppress phagocytosis by a TRPV1-mediated pathway, but did not induce apoptosis in immature DCs. In contrast to mouse DCs, CAP did not promote DC maturation in human DCs in the absence of cytokines (Toth et al., 2009). Taken together, the above strongly suggests that TRPV1 modulates DC maturation and function, although further human studies are obviously warranted to clarify the exact role of TRPV1 and/or the effects of CAP in DC.

4.4 Neutrophils

Neutrophils play a central role in the inflammatory response and comprise an essential part of the innate immune system (Wang et al., 2005). An increase in cytosolic $[Ca^{2+}]_i$ is attributed to the neutrophil response to chemoattractants (Krause, Campbell, Welsh, & Lew, 1990), and induces synthesis and release of prostaglandins (Krump, Pouliot, Naccache, & Borgeat, 1995). CAP affects neutrophil function and increases $[Ca^{2+}]_i$ in rat neutrophils by inducing extracellular Ca^{2+} influx and Ca^{2+} release from the internal Ca^{2+} pool (Wang et al., 2005). TRPV1 mRNA has been detected in human and rat neutrophils, and in the HL-60 (neutrophilic promyelocytic leukemia) cell line using RT-PCR. However, the role of TRPV1 in these cells remains poorly understood (Heiner, Eisfeld, Halaszovisch, et al., 2003; Wang et al., 2005).

5. TRPV1 IN HEMATOLOGICAL MALIGNANCIES

A limited number of studies have addressed the role of TRPV1 in hematological malignancies, and even fewer have combined gene (PCR) and protein expression (Western blot/flow cytometry) with functional and antagonist studies (Table 1). Additionally, the antagonist capsazepine, which is known to have nonselective actions (Gunthorpe et al., 2004)

Table 1 Summary of Studies Investigating the Role of TRPV1 in Hematological Malignancies

Hematological Cancer Cell Line	TRPV1 Expression	Vanilloid	$\sim EC_{50}$ (μM)	Growth/Apoptosis/ Necrosis	TRPV1-Mediated? (Antagonist)	References
Acute myeloid leukemia: Kasumi-1	Not determined	CAP	60	Apoptosis	Not determined	Ito et al. (2004)
Acute monocytic leukemia: THP-1	Yes	CAP	220	Apoptosis	No (SB452533)	Omari, Adams, Kunde, and Geraghty (2016)
THP-1	Yes	CAP	(1)[a]	Inhibition of differentiation	Yes (capsazepine)	Toth et al. (2009)
Acute lymphoid leukemia: HPB-ALL	Not determined	CAP	75	Apoptosis	Not determined	Zhang, Nagasaki, Tanaka, and Morikawa (2003)
Jurkat T	Not determined	CAP/ capsicum extracts	(25)[a]	Apoptosis	Not determined	Dou, Ahmad, Yang, and Sarkar (2011)
Jurkat T	Not determined	CAP, PPAHV	(200)[a]	Necrosis	Yes (capsazepine)	Macho et al. (2000)
Jurkat T: 5.1 clone (lacks TRPV1)	Not determined	Arvanil	20	Apoptosis	Not determined	Sancho et al. (2003)
Human promyelocytic leukemia: HL-60	Not determined	CAP	75	Apoptosis	Not determined	Tsou et al. (2006)

Continued

Table 1 Summary of Studies Investigating the Role of TRPV1 in Hematological Malignancies—cont'd

Hematological Cancer Cell Line	TRPV1 Expression	Vanilloid	$\sim EC_{50}$ (μM)	Growth/Apoptosis/ Necrosis	TRPV1-Mediated? (Antagonist)	References
HL-60	Not determined	CAP	500	Apoptosis	Not determined	Ito et al. (2004)
HL-60	Not determined	CAP	75	Apoptosis	Not determined	Roy, Chakraborty, Siddiqi, and Bhattacharya (2002)
Adult T-cell leukemia: HPB-ATL-T, HPB-CTL-I, HUT-102	Not determined	CAP	60[a] (200)	Growth inhibition Apoptosis	Not determined	Zhang et al. (2003)
Chronic myeloid leukemia: KU812, K562	Not determined	CAP	>100	Apoptosis	Not determined	Roy et al. (2002)
KU812, K562	Not determined	CAP	500	Apoptosis	Not determined	Ito et al. (2004)
Multiple myeloma: MM.1S	Not determined	CAP	(50)[a]	Apoptosis	Not determined	Bhutani et al. (2007)
U266B1	Yes	CAP	430	Apoptosis	No (SB452533)	Omari et al. (2016)
Lymphoma (hystiocytic): U937	Not determined	CAP	500	Apoptosis	Not determined	Ito et al. (2004)

U937	Not determined	AEA	(1)[a]	Apoptosis	Yes (capsazepine)	Maccarrone, Lorenzon, Bari, Melino, and Finazzi-Agro (2000)
U937	Yes	CAP	200	Apoptosis	No (SB452533)	Omari et al. (2016)
U937	Not determined	CAP, Nonivamide	(50)[a]	No	Not determined	Walker et al. (2016)

[a]EC_{50} not provided, numbers in parentheses are maximum concentration tested.
AEA, anandamide; *CAP*, capsaicin; *EC_{50}*, concentration of agent (vanilloid) producing half-maximal effect; *PPAHV*, phorbol 12-phenylacetate 13-acetate 20-homovanillate.

was employed in some studies to delineate TRPV1-dependent and -independent cytotoxic actions of vanilloids (primarily CAP). Interestingly, the mean concentration of vanilloid, predominantly CAP, that reduces cell line viability by 50% is ~215 μM (range 20–500 μM), which far exceeds the reported affinity of CAP for classical or neuronal-type TRPV1 channels, suggesting a "mixed" TRPV1-dependent and -independent mode of action (Table 1).

5.1 Leukemic Cell Lines

CAP has been reported to inhibit the release of inflammatory cytokines from cultured human promyelocytic leukemia cells (Han, Keum, Chun, & Surh, 2002). Two human transcription factors, NF-κB and activator protein 1, which are involved in many inflammatory diseases and apoptosis, were inhibited by CAP and RTX (Han et al., 2002; Portis, Harding, & Ratner, 2001; Sancho et al., 2002; Singh, Natarajan, & Aggarwal, 1996).

TRPV1 is expressed by the acute monocytic THP-1 leukemia cell line (Schilling & Eder, 2009). Activation of TRPV1 was shown to increase Ca^{2+} influx leading to strengthening of the adhesion between THP-1 cells and human umbilical vein epithelial cells, whereas the TRPV1 antagonist, SB366791, reduced adherence (Himi et al., 2012). In contrast, we have recently reported that CAP-induced THP-1 cell death is independent of TRPV1, or cannabinoid CB1/2 receptor activation (Omari et al., 2016).

Ito et al. (2004) reported that CAP suppressed the growth of the leukemic cell lines, Kasumi-1, UF-1, and NB4 cells, but not normal bone marrow mononuclear cells, via induction of G0–G1 phase cell cycle arrest and apoptosis. Apoptosis was associated with increased ROS production. They concluded that CAP-induced cell death signaling was mediated in part by a mitochondrial-dependent pathway (Ip et al., 2012; Ito et al., 2004).

The tumor suppressor protein, p53, is the main mediator of cell death (Ko & Prives, 1996). CAP promotes the activation of p53 through phosphorylation, since nullification of p53 expression significantly reduced CAP-induced cell cycle arrest. CAP-sensitive leukemic cells, such as NB4 and Kasumi-1, express wild-type p53 (Ito et al., 2004). The activation of p53 by CAP leads to the upregulation of some genes including the tumor suppression gene cyclin-dependent kinases (CDK) inhibitor ($p21^{WAF1/CIP1}$), and the proapoptotic Bcl-2-associated X (*Bax*) genes (Ito et al., 2004; Lakin & Jackson, 1999; Miyashita & Reed, 1995). This leads to the production of BAX protein, which in turn moves from the cytosol to the outer mitochondrial membrane, causing the release of cytochrome *c*, and caspases cascade activation leading to apoptosis (Green & Reed, 1998; Ito et al., 2004; Sarkaria et al., 1998). While cell cycle activation involves many molecules including cyclins, CDKs, and inhibitors, the upregulation of such molecules leads to cell cycle arrest. This concept has been considered in anticancerous drug studies (Paschka, Butler, & Young, 1998).

5.2 Adult T-Cell Leukemia

Adult T-cell leukemia (ATL) is an aggressive form of human T-cell malignancy caused by human T-cell leukemia virus type-1 (Hinuma et al., 1981). Induction of the apoptosis inhibitor, NF-κB, appears to play a crucial role in the pathogenesis of ATL (Arima et al., 1999; Portis et al., 2001). Exposure of ATL cells to CAP in vitro inhibited the activation of NF-κB and DNA synthesis by decreasing NF-κB-binding activity of p65, resulting in the suppression of ATL (Zhang et al., 2003). The growth-inhibitory potential of CAP on ATL cells was reported to be mainly due to G_1/cell cycle arrest, a common apoptosis mechanism of many anticancerous drugs (Choi, Choi, Lee, Rhee, & Park, 2001; Fukuoka et al., 2000).

In addition to the role of decreased NF-κB activity in CAP-induced apoptosis, downregulation of B-cell lymphoma-2 protein (Bcl-2) may also be responsible for apoptosis. In contrast to Bax, Bcl-2 and B-cell lymphoma-extra large (Bcl-xL) are essential factors, which act to protect the cell against apoptosis (Yang & Korsmeyer, 1996). Indeed, the Bcl-2/Bax ratio is considered to be an important determinant of apoptosis (Reed, Zha, Aime-Sempe, Takayama, & Wang, 1996). CAP has the ability to reduce the expression of Bcl-2 as well as the Bcl-2/Bax ratio, leading to apoptosis in ATL cell lines (Zhang et al., 2003).

5.3 Multiple Myeloma

Signal transducer and activator of transcription (STAT) is a well-known family, which regulates the expression of gene products (Darnell, 2002). Among the STATs, STAT3 is the member mostly related to tumorigenesis. It is constitutively active in tumor cells and can be activated by growth factors, such as interleukin-6 (IL-6), and oncogenic kinase such as Src. STAT3 regulates the expression of genes that mediate proliferation (e.g., c-myc and cyclin D1), suppress apoptosis (e.g., Bcl-xL), and encourage angiogenesis.

CAP has been reported to cause apoptosis in multiple myeloma (MM) cells through the inhibition of IL-6-inducible STAT3 activation (Bhutani et al., 2007). STAT3 has been shown to be linked to a chemoresistance and radioresistance; therefore, inhibition of STAT3 activation may play a role in the prevention and treatment of cancer (Aggarwal et al., 2006). More recently, Amachi and coworkers reported activation of the Jak2/STAT3, NF-κB, and JNK pathways in three MM cell lines (RPMI8226, INA6, and MM.1S) by acidic conditions (a feature of the MM environment) and upregulation of TRPV1 (Amachi et al., 2016). They proposed that TRPV1 upregulation maintains activation of the P13K-Akt (cell) survival pathway in MM cells, as phosphorylation of Akt was suppressed when cells were cultured in the presence of the TRPV1 antagonist, SB366791.

Velcade (PS341) and thalidomide are common therapeutic agents for the treatment of MM (Cavo, 2006). Prolonged exposure to these compounds is associated with toxicity and development of chemoresistance. Upregulation of different antiapoptotic proteins such as Bcl-2 and Bcl-xL has a critical role in the mechanism of chemoresistance (Chauhan et al., 2007; Mitsiades et al., 2002). Intriguingly, CAP was shown to enhance the apoptotic effect of velcade and thalidomide (Bhutani et al., 2007). However, the role of TRPV1 in the apparently synergistic action of CAP was not explored.

6. "CHILI" AND VANILLOIDS AS NOVEL CHEMOTHERAPEUTIC AGENTS FOR HEMATOLOGICAL MALIGNANCIES?

Given the high concentrations of CAP required to retard the growth of and/or kill cell lines in vitro, what dose of "chili"/vanilloid would be required to kill hematological malignant cells in vivo?

In the *Assessing Capsaicin as a Chemopreventive Agent for Prostate Cancer* trial (NCT02037464), the approved daily dose of cayenne pepper is 80,000 "Scoville units" per day, which is a CAP equivalent of only 5 mg. There is thus a perception that even low doses of capsaicinoids can be effective against some types of cancer cell in vivo.

When considering pharmacokinetics and bioavailability, it should be remembered that hot peppers/extracts contain in excess of 20 capsaicinoids, although CAP and DHC which have almost identical pharmacological profiles, account for 80%–90% of the total and are usually present in a 60:40 ratio (Cordell & Araujo, 1993; Garces-Claver, Arnedo-Andres, Abadia, Gil-Ortega, & Alvarez-Fernandez, 2006). Hence, at a minimum, the combined "dose," and subsequent blood levels of both CAP and DHC must be determined. That said, although there has been a number of capsaicinoid intervention studies, mostly focused on weight management and metabolism (reviewed by Whiting, Derbyshire, & Tiwari, 2012), there is a paucity of reports describing the pharmacokinetics of capsaicinoids following oral administration (reviewed by Rollyson et al., 2014). Chaiyasit and coworkers reported that plasma CAP peaked (~8.2 nM) 47 min after ingestion of 5 g of chili and had an estimated half-life of 25 min (*Capsicum frutescens*) (Chaiyasit, Khovidhunkit, & Wittayalertpanya, 2009). More recently, sera of predominantly Caucasian subjects who had ingested 30 g of chili paste (containing ~18 mg of CAP and DHC) for 4 weeks yielded a combined CAP/DHC concentration of ~85 nM (Ahuja, Robertson, Geraghty, & Ball, 2006; Hartley, Stevens, Ahuja, & Ball, 2013).

Although chronic delivery of CAP by transdermal patch for the treatment of various neuropathic pain syndromes is associated with a number of side effects (see Basith et al., 2016), the limited oral capsaicinoid intervention studies described earlier suggest nanomolar concentrations of capsaicinoids can be achieved with relatively low doses of chili preparations, and much higher doses are certainly achievable over extended periods without significant side effects. Indeed, in one intervention study, 32 subjects ingested 135 mg of CAP for 3 months (10 others reduced the dose by half due to mild gastrointestinal discomfort), with no reported adverse events (Lejeune, Kovacs, & Westerterp-Plantenga, 2003).

7. CONCLUSION

Given the critical role of Ca^{2+} in immune cell function, the functional expression of TRPV1 by almost all immune cell types and large number of molecules that activate/modulate TRPV1 Ca^{2+} influx, considerable attention will continue to be focused on the role of TRPV1 in inflammation and immunity. Malignant hematological cell lines appear to be susceptible to vanilloid (primarily CAP)-induced apoptosis. However, the role of TRPV1-dependent vs -independent cell death needs to be resolved. Furthermore, detailed TRPV1 expression and functional (vanilloid) studies in clinical populations, rather than in cell lines, will be critical in determining whether TRPV1 and vanilloids are therapeutic targets and therapies, respectively, for hematological malignancies.

CONFLICT OF INTEREST

The authors declare no conflicts of interest.

REFERENCES

Aggarwal, B. B., Sethi, G., Ahn, K. S., Sandur, S. K., Pandey, M. K., Kunnumakkara, A. B., et al. (2006). Targeting signal-transducer-and-activator-of-transcription-3 for prevention and therapy of cancer: Modern target but ancient solution. *Annals of the New York Academy of Science*, *1091*, 151–169.

Ahuja, K. D., Robertson, I. K., Geraghty, D. P., & Ball, M. J. (2006). Effects of chili consumption on postprandial glucose, insulin, and energy metabolism. *The American Journal of Clinical Nutrition*, *84*(1), 63–69.

Amachi, R., Hiasa, M., Teramachi, J., Harada, T., Oda, A., Nakamura, S., et al. (2016). A vicious cycle between acid sensing and survival signaling in myeloma cells: Acid-induced epigenetic alteration. *Oncotarget*, *7*, 70447–70461.

Amadesi, S., Nie, J., Vergnolle, N., Cottrell, G. S., Grady, E. F., Trevisani, M., et al. (2004). Protease-activated receptor 2 sensitizes the capsaicin receptor transient receptor potential vanilloid receptor 1 to induce hyperalgesia. *Journal of Neuroscience*, *24*(18), 4300–4312.

Amantini, C., Ballarini, P., Caprodossi, S., Nabissi, M., Morelli, M., Lucciarini, R., et al. (2009). Triggering of transient receptor potential vanilloid type 1 (TRPV1) by capsaicin induces Fas/CD95-mediated apoptosis of urothelial cancer cells in an ATM-dependent manner. *Carcinogenesis*, *30*(8), 1320.

Arima, N., Matsushita, K., Obata, H., Ohtsubo, H., Fujiwara, H., Arimura, K., et al. (1999). NF-kappaB involvement in the activation of primary adult T-cell leukemia cells and its clinical implications. *Experimental Hematology*, *27*(7), 1168–1175.

Avelino, A., & Cruz, F. (2006). TRPV1 (vanilloid receptor) in the urinary tract: Expression, function and clinical applications. *Naunyn Schmiedeberg's Archives of Pharmacology*, *373*(4), 287–299.

Bandell, M., Macpherson, L. J., & Patapoutian, A. (2007). From chills to chilis: Mechanisms for thermosensation and chemesthesis via thermoTRPs. *Current Opinion in Neurobiology*, *17*(4), 490–497.

Basith, S., Cui, M., Hong, S., & Choi, S. (2016). Harnessing the therapeutic potential of capsaicin and its analogues in pain and other diseases. *Molecules*, *21*(8), pii: E966.

Basu, S., & Srivastava, P. (2005). Immunological role of neuronal receptor vanilloid receptor 1 expressed on dendritic cells. *Proceedings of the National Academy of Sciences of the United States of America*, *102*(14), 5120–5125.

Bertin, S., Aoki-Nonaka, Y., de Jong, P. R., Nohara, L. L., Xu, H., Stanwood, S. R., et al. (2014). The ion channel TRPV1 regulates the activation and proinflammatory properties of CD4(+) T cells. *Nature Immunology*, *15*(11), 1055–1063.

Bhutani, M., Pathak, A. K., Nair, A. S., Kunnumakkara, A. B., Guha, S., Sethi, G., et al. (2007). Capsaicin is a novel blocker of constitutive and interleukin-6-inducible STAT3 activation. *Clinical Cancer Research*, *13*(10), 3024–3032.

Birder, L. A., Kanai, A. J., de Groat, W. C., Kiss, S., Nealen, M. L., Burke, N. E., et al. (2001). Vanilloid receptor expression suggests a sensory role for urinary bladder epithelial cells. *Proceedings of the National Academy of Sciences United States of America*, *98*(23), 13396–13401.

Bley, K., Boorman, G., Mohammad, B., McKenzie, D., & Babbar, S. (2012). A comprehensive review of the carcinogenic and anticarcinogenic potential of capsaicin. *Toxicologic Pathology*, *40*(6), 847–873.

Bode, A. M., Cho, Y. Y., Zheng, D., Zhu, F., Ericson, M. E., Ma, W. Y., et al. (2009). Transient receptor potential type vanilloid 1 suppresses skin carcinogenesis. *Cancer Research*, *69*(3), 905–913.

Bode, A. M., & Dong, Z. (2011). The two faces of capsaicin. *Cancer Research*, *71*(8), 2809–2814.

Bucholz, C. F. (1816). "Chemische Untersuchung der trockenen reifen spanischen Pfeffers" [Chemical investigation of dry, ripe Spanish peppers]. *Almanac or Pocket-book for Analysts (Chemists) and Apothecaries*, *37*, 1–30.
Caterina, M. J., Leffler, A., Malmberg, A. B., Martin, W. J., Trafton, J., Petersen-Zeitz, K. R., et al. (2000). Impaired nociception and pain sensation in mice lacking the capsaicin receptor. *Science*, *288*(5464), 306–313.
Caterina, M. J., Schumacher, M. A., Tominaga, M., Rosen, T. A., Levine, J. D., & Julius, D. (1997). The capsaicin receptor: A heat-activated ion channel in the pain pathway. *Nature*, *389*(6653), 816–824.
Cavo, M. (2006). Proteasome inhibitor bortezomib for the treatment of multiple myeloma. *Leukemia*, *20*(8), 1341–1352.
Chaiyasit, K., Khovidhunkit, W., & Wittayalertpanya, S. (2009). Pharmacokinetic and the effect of capsaicin in Capsicum frutescens on decreasing plasma glucose level. *Journal of the Medical Association of Thailand*, *92*(1), 108–113.
Chauhan, D., Velankar, M., Brahmandam, M., Hideshima, T., Podar, K., Richardson, P., et al. (2007). A novel Bcl-2/Bcl-X(L)/Bcl-w inhibitor ABT-737 as therapy in multiple myeloma. *Oncogene*, *26*(16), 2374–2380.
Choi, Y. H., Choi, B. T., Lee, W. H., Rhee, S. H., & Park, K. Y. (2001). Doenjang hexane fraction-induced G1 arrest is associated with the inhibition of pRB phosphorylation and induction of Cdk inhibitor p21 in human breast carcinoma MCF-7 cells. *Oncology Reports*, *8*(5), 1091–1096.
Chou, M. Z., Mtui, T., Gao, Y. D., Kohler, M., & Middleton, R. E. (2004). Resiniferatoxin binds to the capsaicin receptor (TRPV1) near the extracellular side of the S4 transmembrane domain. *Biochemistry*, *43*(9), 2501–2511.
Christensen, A. P., & Corey, D. P. (2007). TRP channels in mechanosensation: Direct or indirect activation? *Nature Reviews. Neuroscience*, *8*(7), 510–521.
Chu, C. J., Huang, S. M., De Petrocellis, L., Bisogno, T., Ewing, S. A., Miller, J. D., et al. (2003). N-oleoyldopamine, a novel endogenous capsaicin-like lipid that produces hyperalgesia. *Journal of Biological Chemistry*, *278*(16), 13633–13639.
Chuang, H. H., Prescott, E. D., Kong, H., Shields, S., Jordt, S. E., Basbaum, A. I., et al. (2001). Bradykinin and nerve growth factor release the capsaicin receptor from PtdIns (4,5)P2-mediated inhibition. *Nature*, *411*(6840), 957–962.
Chung, M. K., Guler, A. D., & Caterina, M. J. (2008). TRPV1 shows dynamic ionic selectivity during agonist stimulation. *Nature Neuroscience*, *11*(5), 555–564.
Clapham, D. E. (2003). TRP channels as cellular sensors. *Nature*, *426*(6966), 517–524.
Clapham, D. E. (2007). SnapShot: Mammalian TRP channels. *Cell*, *129*(1), 220.
Clapham, D. E., Julius, D., Montell, C., & Schultz, G. (2005). International Union of Pharmacology. XLIX. Nomenclature and structure-function relationships of transient receptor potential channels. *Pharmacological Reviews*, *57*(4), 427–450.
Clapham, D. E., Montell, C., Schultz, G., & Julius, D. (2003). International Union of Pharmacology. XLIII. Compendium of voltage-gated ion channels: Transient receptor potential channels. *Pharmacological Reviews*, *55*(4), 591–596.
Contassot, E., Tenan, M., Schnuriger, V., Pelte, M. F., & Dietrich, P. Y. (2004). Arachidonyl ethanolamide induces apoptosis of uterine cervix cancer cells via aberrantly expressed vanilloid receptor-1. *Gynecologic Oncology*, *93*(1), 182–188.
Cordell, G. A., & Araujo, O. E. (1993). Capsaicin: Identification, nomenclature, and pharmacotherapy. *The Annals of Pharmacotherapy*, *27*(3), 330–336.
Cortright, D. N., & Szallasi, A. (2004). Biochemical pharmacology of the vanilloid receptor TRPV1—An update. *European Journal of Biochemistry*, *271*(10), 1814–1819.
Darnell, J. E., Jr. (2002). Transcription factors as targets for cancer therapy. *Nature Reviews. Cancer*, *2*(10), 740–749.

Dhaka, A., Viswanath, V., & Patapoutian, A. (2006). Trp ion channels and temperature sensation. *Annual Review of Neuroscience*, *29*, 135–161.

Domotor, A., Peidl, Z., Vincze, A., Hunyady, B., Szolcsanyi, J., Kereskay, L., et al. (2005). Immunohistochemical distribution of vanilloid receptor, calcitonin-gene related peptide and substance P in gastrointestinal mucosa of patients with different gastrointestinal disorders. *Inflammopharmacology*, *13*(1–3), 161–177.

Dou, D., Ahmad, A., Yang, H., & Sarkar, F. H. (2011). Tumor cell growth inhibition is correlated with levels of capsaicin present in hot peppers. *Nutrition and Cancer*, *63*(2), 272–281.

Fattori, V., Hohmann, M. S., Rossaneis, A. C., Pinho-Ribeiro, F. A., & Verri, W. A. (2016). Capsaicin: Current understanding of its mechanisms and therapy of pain and other preclinical and clinical uses. *Molecules*, *21*(7), pii: E844.

Fernandes, E., Fernandes, M., & Keeble, J. (2012). The functions of TRPA1 and TRPV1: Moving away from sensory nerves. *British Journal of Pharmacology*, *166*(2), 510–521.

Ferrer-Montiel, A., Garcia-Martinez, C., Morenilla-Palao, C., Garcia-Sanz, N., Fernandez-Carvajal, A., Fernandez-Ballester, G., et al. (2004). Molecular architecture of the vanilloid receptor. Insights for drug design. *European Journal of Biochemistry*, *271*(10), 1820–1826.

Fukuoka, K., Yamagishi, T., Ichihara, T., Nakaike, S., Iguchi, K., Yamada, Y., et al. (2000). Mechanism of action of aragusterol a (YTA0040), a potent anti-tumor marine steroid targeting the G(1) phase of the cell cycle. *International Journal of Cancer*, *88*(5), 810–819.

Gallo, E. M., Cante-Barrett, K., & Crabtree, G. R. (2006). Lymphocyte calcium signaling from membrane to nucleus. *Nature Immunology*, 7(1), 25–32.

Garces-Claver, A., Arnedo-Andres, M. S., Abadia, J., Gil-Ortega, R., & Alvarez-Fernandez, A. (2006). Determination of capsaicin and dihydrocapsaicin in capsicum fruits by liquid chromatography-electrospray/time-of-flight mass spectrometry. *Journal of Agricultural and Food Chemistry*, *54*(25), 9303–9311.

Geppetti, P., & Trevisani, M. (2004). Activation and sensitisation of the vanilloid receptor: Role in gastrointestinal inflammation and function. *British Journal of Pharmacology*, *141*(8), 1313–1320.

Green, D. R., & Reed, J. C. (1998). Mitochondria and apoptosis. *Science*, *281*(5381), 1309–1312.

Grycova, L., Holendova, B., Bumba, L., Bily, J., Jirku, M., Lansky, Z., et al. (2012). Integrative binding sites within intracellular termini of TRPV1 receptor. *PloS One*, 7(10). e48437

Gunthorpe, M., Benham, C., Randall, A., & Davis, J. (2002). The diversity in the vanilloid (TRPV) receptor family of ion channels. *Trends in the Pharmacological Sciences*, *23*, 183–191.

Gunthorpe, M. J., Rami, H. K., Jerman, J. C., Smart, D., Gill, C. H., Soffin, E. M., et al. (2004). Identification and characterisation of SB-366791, a potent and selective vanilloid receptor (VR1/TRPV1) antagonist. *Neuropharmacology*, *46*(1), 133–149.

Han, S., Keum, Y., Chun, K., & Surh, Y. (2002). Suppression of phorbol ester-induced NF-B activation by capsaicin in cultured human promyelocytic leukemia cells. *Archives of Pharmacal Research*, *25*(4), 475–479.

Hartel, M., di Mola, F. F., Selvaggi, F., Mascetta, G., Wente, M. N., Felix, K., et al. (2006). Vanilloids in pancreatic cancer: Potential for chemotherapy and pain management. *Gut*, *55*(4), 519–528.

Hartley, T., Stevens, B., Ahuja, K. D. K., & Ball, M. J. (2013). Development and experimental application of an HPLC procedure for the determination of capsaicin and dihydrocapsaicin in serum samples from human subjects. *Indian Journal of Clinical Biochemistry*, *28*(4), 329–335.

Heiner, I., Eisfeld, J., Halaszovisch, C., Wehage, E., Jungling, E., Zitt, C., et al. (2003a). Expression profile of the transient receptor potential (TRP) family in neutrophil granulocytes: Evidence for currents through long TRP channel 2 induced by ADP-ribose and NAD. *Biochemistry Journal, 371*, 1045–1053.

Heiner, I., Eisfeld, J., & Luckhoff, A. (2003b). Role and regulation of TRP channels in neutrophil granulocytes. *Cell Calcium, 33*, 533–540.

Hellwig, N., Plant, T. D., Janson, W., Schafer, M., Schultz, G., & Schaefer, M. (2004). TRPV1 acts as proton channel to induce acidification in nociceptive neurons. *Journal of Biological Chemistry, 279*(33), 34553–34561.

Himi, N., Hamaguchi, A., Hashimoto, K., Koga, T., Narita, K., & Miyamoto, O. (2012). Calcium influx through the TRPV1 channel of endothelial cells (ECs) correlates with a stronger adhesion between monocytes and ECs. *Advances in Medical Sciences, 57*(2), 224–229.

Hinuma, Y., Nagata, K., Hanaoka, M., Nakai, M., Matsumoto, T., Kinoshita, K., et al. (1981). Adult T-cell leukemia: Antigen in an ATL cell line and detection of antibodies to the antigen in human sera. *Proceedings of the National Academy of Sciences United States of America, 78*(10), 6476.

Hőgyes, E. (1878). Beiträge zur physiologischen Wirkung der Bestandteile des Capsicum annuum. *Archiv for Experimentelle Pathologie und Pharmakologie, 9*, 117–130.

Holzer, P. (2008). The pharmacological challenge to tame the transient receptor potential vanilloid-1 (TRPV1) nocisensor. *British Journal of Pharmacology, 155*(8), 1145–1162.

Inada, H., Iida, T., & Tominaga, M. (2006). Different expression patterns of TRP genes in murine B and T lymphocytes. *Biochemical and Biophysical Research Communications, 350*(3), 762–767.

Inoue, R., Jian, Z., & Kawarabayashi, Y. (2009). Mechanosensitive TRP channels in cardiovascular pathophysiology. *Pharmacology and Therapeutics, 123*(3), 371–385.

Ip, S.-W., Lan, S.-H., Lu, H.-F., Huang, A.-C., Yang, J.-S., Lin, J.-P., et al. (2012). Capsaicin mediates apoptosis in human nasopharyngeal carcinoma NPC-TW 039 cells through mitochondrial depolarization and endoplasmic reticulum stress. *Human and Experimental Toxicology, 31*(6), 539–549.

Ito, K., Nakazato, T., Yamato, K., Miyakawa, Y., Yamada, T., Hozumi, N., et al. (2004). Induction of apoptosis in leukemic cells by homovanillic acid derivative, capsaicin, through oxidative stress: Implication of phosphorylation of p53 at Ser-15 residue by reactive oxygen species. *Cancer Research, 64*(3), 1071–1078.

Jaggar, S. I., Scott, H. C. F., James, I. F., & Rice, A. S. C. (2001). The capsaicin analogue SDZ249-665 attenuates the hyper-reflexia and referred hyperalgesia associated with inflammation of the rat urinary bladder. *Pain, 89*(2–3), 229–235.

Jeske, N. A., Patwardhan, A. M., Ruparel, N. B., Akopian, A. N., Shapiro, M. S., & Henry, M. A. (2009). A-kinase anchoring protein 150 controls protein kinase C-mediated phosphorylation and sensitization of TRPV1. *Pain, 146*(3), 301–307.

Joe, B., & Lokesh, B. R. (1994). Role of capsaicin, curcumin and dietary n-3 fatty acids in lowering the generation of reactive oxygen species in rat peritoneal macrophages. *Biochimica et Biophysica Acta, 1224*(2), 255–263.

Jordt, S. E., & Julius, D. (2002). Molecular basis for species-specific sensitivity to "hot" chili peppers. *Cell, 108*(3), 421–430.

Julius, D., & Basbaum, A. I. (2001). Molecular mechanisms of nociception. *Nature, 413*(6852), 203–210.

Kaszas, K., Keller, J. M., Coddou, C., Mishra, S. K., Hoon, M. A., Stojilkovic, S., et al. (2012). Small molecule positive allosteric modulation of TRPV1 activation by vanilloids and acidic pH. *Journal of Pharmacology and Experimental Therapeutics, 340*(1), 152–160.

Kim, S. R., Kim, S. U., Oh, U., & Jin, B. K. (2006). Transient receptor potential vanilloid subtype 1 mediates microglial cell death in vivo and in vitro via Ca2+-mediated mitochondrial damage and cytochrome c release. *Journal of Immunology*, *177*(7), 4322–4329.

Kim, H. S., Kwon, H. J., Kim, G. E., Cho, M. H., Yoon, S. Y., Davies, A. J., et al. (2014). Attenuation of natural killer cell functions by capsaicin through a direct and TRPV1-independent mechanism. *Carcinogenesis*, *35*(7), 1652–1660.

Ko, L., & Prives, C. (1996). p53: Puzzle and paradigm. *Genes and Development*, *10*(9), 1054–1072.

Krause, K. H., Campbell, K. P., Welsh, M. J., & Lew, D. P. (1990). The calcium signal and neutrophil activation. *Clinical Biochemistry*, *23*(2), 159–166.

Krump, E., Pouliot, M., Naccache, P. H., & Borgeat, P. (1995). Leukotriene synthesis in calcium-depleted human neutrophils: Arachidonic acid release correlates with calcium influx. *Biochemistry Journal*, *310*(Pt. 2), 681–688.

Lai, J. P., Douglas, S. D., & Ho, W. Z. (1998). Human lymphocytes express substance P and its receptor. *Journal of Neuroimmunology*, *86*(1), 80–86.

Lakin, N., & Jackson, S. (1999). Regulation of p53 in response to DNA damage. *Oncogene*, *18*(53), 7644.

Launay, P., Cheng, H., Srivatsan, S., Penner, R., Fleig, A., & Kinet, J. P. (2004). TRPM4 regulates calcium oscillations after T cell activation. *Science*, *306*(5700), 1374–1377.

Lazzeri, M., Vannucchi, M. G., Spinelli, M., Bizzoco, E., Beneforti, P., Turini, D., et al. (2005). Transient receptor potential vanilloid type 1 (TRPV1) expression changes from normal urothelium to transitional cell carcinoma of human bladder. *European Urology*, *48*(4), 691–698.

Lejeune, M. P., Kovacs, E. M., & Westerterp-Plantenga, M. S. (2003). Effect of capsaicin on substrate oxidation and weight maintenance after modest body-weight loss in human subjects. *The British Journal of Nutrition*, *90*(3), 651–659.

Lievremont, J. P., Numaga, T., Vazquez, G., Lemonnier, L., Hara, Y., Mori, E., et al. (2005). The role of canonical transient receptor potential 7 in B-cell receptor-activated channels. *Journal of Biological Chemistry*, *280*(42), 35346–35351.

Lishko, P. V., Procko, E., Jin, X., Phelps, C. B., & Gaudet, R. (2007). The ankyrin repeats of TRPV1 bind multiple ligands and modulate channel sensitivity. *Neuron*, *54*(6), 905–918.

Loyd, D. R., Chen, P. B., & Hargreaves, K. M. (2012). Anti-hyperalgesic effects of anti-serotonergic compounds on serotonin-and capsaicin-evoked thermal hyperalgesia in the rat. *Neuroscience*, *203*, 207–215.

Lv, J., Qi, L., Yu, C., Yang, L., Guo, Y., Chen, Y., et al. (2015). Consumption of spicy foods and total and cause specific mortality: Population based cohort study. *BMJ*, *351*, h3942.

Maccarrone, M., Lorenzon, T., Bari, M., Melino, G., & Finazzi-Agro, A. (2000). Anandamide induces apoptosis in human cells via vanilloid receptors. Evidence for a protective role of cannabinoid receptors. *Journal of Biological Chemistry*, *275*(41), 31938–31945.

Macho, A., Lucena, C., Calzado, M. A., Blanco, M., Donnay, I., Appendino, G., et al. (2000). Phorboid 20-homovanillates induce apoptosis through a VR1-independent mechanism. *Chemical Biology*, 7(7), 483–492.

Majhi, R. K., Sahoo, S. S., Yadav, M., Pratheek, B. M., Chattopadhyay, S., & Goswami, C. (2015). Functional expression of TRPV channels in T cells and their implications in immune regulation. *The FEBS Journal*, *282*(14), 2661–2681.

Matthews, P. J., Aziz, Q., Facer, P., Davis, J. B., Thompson, D. G., & Anand, P. (2004). Increased capsaicin receptor TRPV1 nerve fibres in the inflamed human oesophagus. *European Journal of Gastroenterology and Hepatology*, *16*(9), 897–902.

Meotti, F. C., Lemos de Andrade, E., & Calixto, J. B. (2014). TRP modulation by natural compounds. *Handbook of Experimental Pharmacology*, *223*, 1177–1238.

Mergler, S., Skrzypski, M., Sassek, M., Pietrzak, P., Pucci, C., Wiedenmann, B., et al. (2012). Thermo-sensitive transient receptor potential vanilloid channel-1 regulates intracellular calcium and triggers chromogranin A secretion in pancreatic neuroendocrine BON-1 tumor cells. *Cellular Signalling*, *24*(1), 233–246.

Micko, K. (1898). "Zur Kenntniss des Capsaïcins" [On our knowledge of capsaicin]. *Journal for the Investigation of Necessities and Luxuries*, *1*, 818–829.

Minke, B. (2006). TRP channels and Ca^{2+} signaling. *Cell Calcium*, *40*(3), 261–275.

Mitsiades, N., Mitsiades, C. S., Poulaki, V., Chauhan, D., Fanourakis, G., Gu, X., et al. (2002). Molecular sequelae of proteasome inhibition in human multiple myeloma cells. *Proceedings of the National Academy of Sciences United States of America*, *99*(22), 14374–14379.

Miyashita, T., & Reed, J. (1995). Tumor suppressor p53 is a direct transcriptional activator of the human bax gene. *Cell*, *80*(2), 293–299.

Mori, Y., Wakamori, M., Miyakawa, T., Hermosura, M., Hara, Y., Nishida, M., et al. (2002). Transient receptor potential 1 regulates capacitative Ca(2+) entry and Ca(2+) release from endoplasmic reticulum in B lymphocytes. *Journal of Experimental Medicine*, *195*(6), 673–681.

Nagy, I., Santha, P., Jancso, G., & Urban, L. (2004). The role of the vanilloid (capsaicin) receptor (TRPV1) in physiology and pathology. *European Journal of Pharmacology*, *500*(1–3), 351–369.

Nevius, E., Srivastava, P. K., & Basu, S. (2012). Oral ingestion of Capsaicin, the pungent component of chili pepper, enhances a discreet population of macrophages and confers protection from autoimmune diabetes. *Mucosal Immunology*, *5*(1), 76–86.

Nilius, B. (2007). TRP channels in disease. *Biochimica et Biophysica Acta—Molecular Basis of Disease*, *1772*(8), 805–812.

Nilius, B., & Voets, T. (2005). TRP channels: A TR(I)P through a world of multifunctional cation channels. *Pflugers Archives—European Journal of Physiology*, *451*(1), 1–10.

Nilsson, G., Alving, K., & Ahlstedt, S. (1991). Effects on immune responses in rats after neuromanipulation with capsaicin. *International Journal of Immunopharmacology*, *13*(1), 21–26.

O'Connell, P. J., Pingle, S. C., & Ahern, G. P. (2005). Dendritic cells do not transduce inflammatory stimuli via the capsaicin receptor TRPV1. *FEBS Letters*, *579*(23), 5135–5139.

Omari, S. A., Adams, M. J., Kunde, D. A., & Geraghty, D. P. (2016). Capsaicin-induced death of human haematological malignant cell lines is independent of TRPV1 activation. *Pharmacology*, *98*(1–2), 79–86.

Owsianik, G., Talavera, K., Voets, T., & Nilius, B. (2006). Permeation and selectivity of TRP channels. *Annual Review of Physiology*, *68*, 685–717.

Paschka, A. G., Butler, R., & Young, C. Y. F. (1998). Induction of apoptosis in prostate cancer cell lines by the green tea component, (-)-epigallocatechin-3-gallate. *Cancer Letters*, *130*(1–2), 1–7.

Phelps, C. B., Wang, R. R., Choo, S. S., & Gaudet, R. (2010). Differential regulation of TRPV1, TRPV3, and TRPV4 sensitivity through a conserved binding site on the ankyrin repeat domain. *Journal of Biological Chemistry*, *285*(1), 731–740.

Portis, T., Harding, J. C., & Ratner, L. (2001). The contribution of NF-kappa B activity to spontaneous proliferation and resistance to apoptosis in human T-cell leukemia virus type 1 Tax-induced tumors. *Blood*, *98*(4), 1200–1208.

Prevarskaya, N., Zhang, L., & Barritt, G. (2007). TRP channels in cancer. *Biochimica et Biophysica Acta*, *1772*(8), 937–946.

Ramsey, I. S., Delling, M., & Clapham, D. E. (2006). An introduction to TRP channels. *Annual Review of Physiology*, *68*, 619–647.

Reed, J. C., Zha, H., Aime-Sempe, C., Takayama, S., & Wang, H. G. (1996). Structure-function analysis of Bcl-2 family proteins. Regulators of programmed cell death. *Advances in Experimental Medicine and Biology*, *406*, 99–112.

Reilly, C. A., Taylor, J. L., Lanza, D. L., Carr, B. A., Crouch, D. J., & Yost, G. S. (2003). Capsaicinoids cause inflammation and epithelial cell death through activation of vanilloid receptors. *Toxicological Sciences*, *73*(1), 170–181.

Rollyson, W. D., Stover, C. A., Brown, K. C., Perry, H. E., Stevenson, C. D., McNees, C. A., et al. (2014). Bioavailability of capsaicin and its implications for drug delivery. *Journal of Controlled Release*, *196*, 96–105.

Rosenbaum, T., Gordon-Shaag, A., Munari, M., & Gordon, S. E. (2004). Ca^{2+}/calmodulin modulates TRPV1 activation by capsaicin. *Journal of General Physiology*, *123*(1), 53–62.

Rosenbaum, T., & Simon, S. A. (2007). TRPV1 receptors and signal transduction. In W. B. Liedtke & S. Heller (Eds.), *TRP Ion channel function in sensory transduction and cellular signaling cascades*. Boca Raton, FL: CRC Press/Taylor & Francis Group, LLC.

Roy, M., Chakraborty, S., Siddiqi, M., & Bhattacharya, R. K. (2002). Induction of apoptosis in tumor cells by natural phenolic compounds. *Asian Pacific Journal of Cancer Prevention*, *3*(1), 61–67.

Samivel, R., Kim, D. W., Son, H. R., Rhee, Y. H., Kim, E. H., Kim, J. H., et al. (2016). The role of TRPV1 in the CD4+ T cell-mediated inflammatory response of allergic rhinitis. *Oncotarget*, 7(1), 148–160.

Sánchez, A., Sánchez, M., Malagarie-Cazenave, S., Olea, N., & Díaz-Laviada, I. (2006). Induction of apoptosis in prostate tumor PC-3 cells and inhibition of xenograft prostate tumor growth by the vanilloid capsaicin. *Apoptosis*, *11*, 89–99.

Sancho, R., de la Vega, L., Appendino, G., Di Marzo, V., Macho, A., & Munoz, E. (2003). The CB1/VR1 agonist arvanil induces apoptosis through an FADD/caspase-8-dependent pathway. *British Journal of Pharmacology*, *140*(6), 1035–1044.

Sancho, R., Lucena, C., Macho, A., Calzado, M., Blanco-Molina, M., Minassi, A., et al. (2002). Immunosuppressive activity of capsaicinoids: Capsiate derived from sweet peppers inhibits NF-kB activation and is a potent anti-inflammatory compound in vivo. *European Journal of Immunology*, *32*, 1753–1763.

Santoni, G., Farfariello, V., & Amantini, C. (2011). TRPV channels in tumor growth and progression. *Advances in Experimental Medicine and Biology*, *704*, 947–967.

Santoni, G., Perfumi, M., Pompei, P., Spreghini, E., Lucciarini, R., Martarelli, D., et al. (2000). Impairment of rat thymocyte differentiation and functions by neonatal capsaicin treatment is associated with induction of apoptosis. *Journal of Neuroimmunology*, *104*(1), 37–46.

Sarkaria, J. N., Tibbetts, R. S., Busby, E. C., Kennedy, A. P., Hill, D. E., & Abraham, R. T. (1998). Inhibition of phosphoinositide 3-kinase related kinases by the radiosensitizing agent wortmannin. *Cancer Research*, *58*(19), 4375–4382.

Satthaporn, S., & Eremin, O. (2001). Dendritic cells (I): Biological functions. *Journal of the Royal College of Surgeons of Edinburgh*, *46*(1), 9–19.

Saunders, C. I., Fassett, R. G., & Geraghty, D. P. (2009). Up-regulation of TRPV1 in mononuclear cells of end-stage kidney disease patients increases susceptibility to N-arachidonoyl-dopamine (NADA)-induced cell death. *Biochimica et Biophysica Acta*, *1792*(10), 1019–1026.

Saunders, C. I. M., Kunde, D. A., Crawford, A., & Geraghty, D. P. (2007). Expression of transient receptor potential vanilloid 1 (TRPV1) and 2 (TRPV2) in human peripheral blood. *Molecular Immunology*, *44*(6), 1429–1435.

Schicho, R., Florian, W., Liebmann, I., Holzer, P., & Lippe, I. T. (2004). Increased expression of TRPV1 receptor in dorsal root ganglia by acid insult of the rat gastric mucosa. *European Journal of Neuroscience*, *19*(7), 1811–1818.

Schilling, T., & Eder, C. (2009). Non-selective cation channel activity is required for lysophosphatidylcholine-induced monocyte migration. *Journal of Cellular Physiology*, *221*(2), 325–334.

Schwarz, E. C., Wolfs, M. J., Tonner, S., Wenning, A. S., Quintana, A., Griesemer, D., et al. (2007). TRP channels in lymphocytes. *Handbook of Experimental Pharmacology, 179*, 445–456.

Seabrook, G. R., Sutton, K. G., Jarolimek, W., Hollingworth, G. J., Teague, S., Webb, J., et al. (2002). Functional properties of the high-affinity TRPV1 (VR1) vanilloid receptor antagonist (4-hydroxy-5-iodo-3-methoxyphenylacetate ester) iodo-resiniferatoxin. *The Journal of Pharmacology and Experimental Therapeutics, 303*(3), 1052–1060.

Sharma, S. K., Vij, A. S., & Sharma, M. (2013). Mechanisms and clinical uses of capsaicin. *European Journal of Pharmacology, 720*(1–3), 55–62.

Shortman, K., & Liu, Y. J. (2002). Mouse and human dendritic cell subtypes. *Nature Reviews. Immunology, 2*(3), 151–161.

Singh, S., Natarajan, K., & Aggarwal, B. (1996). Capsaicin (8-methyl-N-vanillyl-6-nonenamide) is a potent inhibitor of nuclear transcription factor-kappa B activation by diverse agents. *Journal of Immunology, 157*(10), 4412.

Stokes, A., Wakano, C., Del Carmen, K., Koblana Huberson, M., & Turner, H. (2005). Formation of a physiological complex between TRPV2 and RGA protein promotes cell surface expression of TRPV2. *Journal of Cellular Biochemistry, 94*, 669–683.

Szallasi, A. (1995). Autoradiographic visualization and pharmacological characterization of vanilloid (capsaicin) receptors in several species, including man. *Acta Physiologica Scandinavica, 155*, 1–68.

Szallasi, A., & Blumberg, P. M. (1999). Vanilloid (capsaicin) receptors and mechanisms. *Pharmacological Reviews, 51*(2), 159–212.

Szoke, E., Seress, L., & Szolcsanyi, J. (2002). Neonatal capsaicin treatment results in prolonged mitochondrial damage and delayed cell death of B cells in the rat trigeminal ganglia. *Neuroscience, 113*(4), 925–937.

Szolcsanyi, J. (1993). *Capsaicin in the study of pain*. London: Academic Press.

Szolcsanyi, J., Jancso-Gabor, A., & Joo, F. (1975). Functional and fine structural characteristics of the sensory neuron blocking effect of capsaicin. *Naunyn Schmiedeberg's Archives of Pharmacology, 287*(2), 157–169.

Takano, F., Yamaguchi, M., Takada, S., Shoda, S., Yahagi, N., Takahashi, T., et al. (2007). Capsicum ethanol extracts and capsaicin enhance interleukin-2 and interferon-gamma production in cultured murine Peyer's patch cells ex vivo. *Life Sciences, 80*(17), 1553–1563.

Thresh, J. C. (1878). Isolation of capsaicin. *The Pharmaceutical Journal and Transactions*, 7(3), 21.

Tominaga, M., & Tominaga, T. (2005). Structure and function of TRPV1. *Pflugers Arch—European Journal of Physiology, 451*(1), 143–150.

Toth, B. I., Benko, S., Szollosi, A. G., Kovacs, L., Rajnavolgyi, E., & Biro, T. (2009). Transient receptor potential vanilloid-1 signaling inhibits differentiation and activation of human dendritic cells. *FEBS Letters, 583*(10), 1619–1624.

Tsou, M.-F., Lu, H.-F., Chen, S.-C., Wu, L.-T., Chen, Y.-S., Kuo, H.-M., et al. (2006). Involvement of Bax, Bcl-2, Ca^{2+} and Caspase-3 in capsaicin-induced apoptosis of human leukemia HL-60 cells. *Anticancer Research, 26*(3A), 1965–1971.

Van Der Stelt, M., & Di Marzo, V. (2004). Endovanilloids. Putative endogenous ligands of transient receptor potential vanilloid 1 channels. *European Journal of Biochemistry, 271*(10), 1827–1834.

Voets, T., Droogmans, G., Wissenbach, U., Janssens, A., Flockerzi, V., & Nilius, B. (2004). The principle of temperature-dependent gating in cold- and heat-sensitive TRP channels. *Nature, 430*(7001), 748–754.

Walker, J., Ley, J. P., Schwerzler, J., Lieder, B., Beltran, L., Ziemba, P. M., et al. (2016). Nonivamide, a capsaicin analogue, exhibits anti-inflammatory properties in peripheral blood mononuclear cells and U-937 macrophages. *Molecular Nutrition & Food Research, 61*(2), 1600474.

Wang, J. P., Tseng, C. S., Sun, S. P., Chen, Y. S., Tsai, C. R., & Hsu, M. F. (2005). Capsaicin stimulates the non-store-operated Ca^{2+} entry but inhibits the store-operated Ca^{2+} entry in neutrophils. *Toxicology and Applied Pharmacology*, *209*(2), 134–144.
Whiting, S., Derbyshire, E., & Tiwari, B. K. (2012). Capsaicinoids and capsinoids. A potential role for weight management? A systematic review of the evidence. *Appetite*, *59*(2), 341–348.
Xing, J., Ma, J., Zhang, P., & Fan, X. (2010). Block effect of capsaicin on hERG potassium currents is enhanced by S6 mutation at Y652. *European Journal of Pharmacology*, *630*(1–3), 1–9.
Xu, H., Blair, N. T., & Clapham, D. E. (2005). Camphor activates and strongly desensitizes the transient receptor potential vanilloid subtype 1 channel in a vanilloid-independent mechanism. *Journal of Neuroscience*, *25*(39), 8924–8937.
Yang, E., & Korsmeyer, S. J. (1996). Molecular thanatopsis: A discourse on the BCL2 family and cell death. *Blood*, *88*(2), 386–401.
Yang, R., Xiong, Z., Liu, C., & Liu, L. (2014). Inhibitory effects of capsaicin on voltage-gated potassium channels by TRPV1-independent pathway. *Cellular and Molecular Neurobiology*, *34*(4), 565–576.
Zhang, J., Nagasaki, M., Tanaka, Y., & Morikawa, S. (2003). Capsaicin inhibits growth of adult T-cell leukemia cells. *Leukemia Research*, *27*(3), 275–283.
Ziglioli, F., Frattini, A., Maestroni, U., Dinale, F., Ciufifeda, M., & Cortellini, P. (2009). Vanilloid-mediated apoptosis in prostate cancer cells through a TRPV-1 dependent and a TRPV-1-independent mechanism. *Acta Biomedica*, *80*(1), 13–20.

CHAPTER SEVEN

Modulation of Ion Channels by Cysteine-Rich Peptides: From Sequence to Structure

Mehdi Mobli*,[1], Eivind A.B. Undheim*, Lachlan D. Rash[†]
*Centre for Advanced Imaging, St Lucia, QLD, Australia
[†]School of Biomedical Sciences, The University of Queensland, St Lucia, QLD, Australia
[1]Corresponding author: e-mail address: m.mobli@uq.edu.au

Contents

Abstract

Venom peptides are natural ligands of ion channels and have been used extensively in pharmacological characterization of various ion channels and receptors. In this chapter, we survey all known venom peptide ion-channel modulators. Our survey reveals that the majority of venom peptides characterized to date target voltage-gated sodium or potassium channels. We further find that the majority of these peptides are found in scorpion and spider venoms. We discuss the influence of the pharmacological tools available in biasing discovery and the classical "toxin-to-sequence" approach to venom peptide biodiscovery. The impact of high-throughput sequencing on the existing discovery framework is likely to be significant and we propose here an alternative "sequence-to-toxin" approach to peptide screening, relying more on recently developed high-throughput methods. Methods for production and characterization of disulfide rich toxins in a high-throughput setting are then described, focusing on bacterial protein expression and solution state structural characterization by NMR spectroscopy.

Advances in Pharmacology, Volume 79
ISSN 1054-3589
http://dx.doi.org/10.1016/bs.apha.2017.03.001

Finally, the role of X-ray crystallography and cryo-EM are highlighted by discussing the currently known channel-peptide complexes.

1. INTRODUCTION

Venoms are a natural source of potent ion-channel modulators, and as such have found widespread use as pharmacological tools. Venoms, however, constitute a complex mix of various types of channel modulators, including salts and small molecules that can directly influence neurotransmission, peptides, and pore-forming proteins that can indirectly influence channel function by disrupting the cell membrane as well as disulfide-rich peptides (DRPs) that can directly block or modulate channel function (Lewis & Garcia, 2003; Mellor & Usherwood, 2004; Mouhat, Jouirou, Mosbah, De Waard, & Sabatier, 2004; Ushkaryov, Volynski, & Ashton, 2004). In this chapter, we will focus on DRPs as a source of ion-channel modulators. Short peptides typically form unstructured motifs that are readily broken down by proteases; it is therefore remarkable to find that DRPs exhibit great structural diversity and excellent stability. These unusual properties are due to the multiple covalent bonds formed between the sidechain thiols of cysteine residues that are distal in sequence space. These disulfide bonds force the protein into a compact globular fold with a very small hydrophobic core—sometimes encompassing only the cysteines themselves (Undheim, Mobli, & King, 2016). Indeed, without these cross braces, the protein would likely not fold and would rapidly degrade.

Table 1 summarizes all known venom peptides that have been experimentally verified as ion-channel modulators (based on Uniprot annotations—accessed December 2016). The peptides in the table are all DRPs and demonstrate the taxonomical and pharmacological distribution of this class of molecules. The average and median sequence lengths show that ion channel modulating DRPs are typically between 40–60 amino acids long. Although it is tempting to draw conclusions about the taxonomical distribution of different ion-channel modulators, such as their paucity in the relatively well-studied venoms of snakes, we note that this must take into account the availability of suitable assays in the laboratories where the molecules were discovered. For example, it may be that the groups that focus on cone snail venoms also have a particular interest in finding modulators of nicotinic acetylcholine receptors (nAChR), etc. It is, however, clear that scorpion

Table 1 Protein Sequences Annotated as Having Experimentally Determined Ion-Channels Activity

	Number of Peptides	**Average Sequence Length**	**Median Sequence Length**
Na_V	**407**	**63**	**65**
Scorpion	*182*		
Spider	116		
Anemone	55		
Cone snail	46		
Hymenoptera	3		
Snake	2		
Nemertean worm	2		
Centipede	1		
K_V	**278**	**52**	**42**
Scorpion	*167*		
Spider	49		
Snake	21		
Anemone	20		
Cone snail	16		
Hymenoptera	4		
Centipede	1		
Lizard	1		
nAChR	**134**	**59**	**63**
Snake	*74*		
Cone snail	59		
Spider	1		
Ca_V	**98**	**57**	**58**
Spider	*50*		
Cone snail	28		
Scorpion	6		

Continued

Table 1 Protein Sequences Annotated as Having Experimentally Determined Ion-Channels Activity—cont'd

	Number of Peptides	Average Sequence Length	Median Sequence Length
Snake	6		
Bug	2		
Centipede	2		
Hymenoptera	1		
Beetle	1		
Fly	1		
Lizard	1		
RYR	**14**	**106**	**69**
Scorpion	*11*		
Snake	2		
Lizard	1		
ASIC	**9**	**78**	**57**
Snake	*5*		
Anemone	3		
Spider	1		
TRP	**7**	**53**	**56**
Spider	*4*		
Anemone	3		
Centipede	1		
ClC	**7**	**45**	**36**
Scorpion	7		
Total	954		

venom peptides are the most broadly studied, with 421 characterized ion-channel modulators accounting for nearly half of all peptides studied. Spiders are a distant second with 221 peptides. It is also clear that these numbers are very modest, considering that a single venom may contain hundreds of DRPs (Escoubas, Quinton, & Nicholson, 2008).

The functional data summarized in Table 1 constitutes a significant amount of effort from the toxinology community over several decades. The majority of work to date has followed a similar approach that can be summarized in the following "toxin to sequence" steps:

(1) Venom extraction
(2) Functional screening
(3) Venom fractionation
(4) Rescreening
(5) Sequence determination
(6) Peptide production (when possible/necessary)
(7) Functional/structural validation of synthetic molecule (when possible/necessary)
(8) Structural characterization (when possible/necessary)

This classical approach is still the gold standard in the field but does suffer from low throughput, evident in the number sequences that have to date been characterized functionally (<3000 toxins with known function since the 1980s, average rate of ~100 per year). The low throughput of the classical approach lies primarily in the sensitivity of current methods of characterization leading to the following weaknesses: (i) sufficient quantities of a peptide of interest must be isolated to produce a reliable output in the functional assay of choice; (ii) substantial amount of material is required if de novo sequencing is attempted by mass spectrometry or Edman sequencing; (iii) if several components overlap during the chromatographic step, the wrong sequence may be elucidated; and (iv) there are no guarantees that the same venom expression profile may be found if additional material is required.

In addition to the above weaknesses in functional characterization, further restrictions apply if the peptide is produced synthetically. Historically, synthetic material has been rigorously scrutinized to ensure that the isolated natural product is chemically and geometrically equivalent to the synthesized versions, commonly through a combination of mass spectrometry, coelution in HPLC chromatograms, and by biochemical, biophysical, and functional assays—a process that imposes additional requirements on the minimal amount of natural peptide required for its characterization. Nevertheless, this foundational work has allowed for the structural characterization of a large number DRP folds, providing an excellent overview of the structural landscape of venom peptides. From this work two things have become clear. First, that the disulfide connectivities direct the fold to such an extent that if these are known the structural class of the peptide can be readily predicted. Second, that the disulfide bond connectivities can in the majority of cases be predicted based on the cysteine spacing (Lavergne, Alewood, Mobli, & King, 2015).

In parallel to the painstaking work of manual sequencing of venom peptides, there has been a revolution in gene sequencing technology. This has resulted in a staggering increase in the number of datasets in Sequence Reads Archive (SRA). There are currently ~350 datasets annotated with "toxin" and "venom" in the SRA and even a modest (based on the experience of the authors) estimate of ~200 toxin-like sequences per dataset would amount to 70,000 unique sequences. Indeed, a search of the transcriptome shotgun assembly for sequences containing the words toxin and venom (from animals only) results in ~110,000 sequences. This sequence data has accumulated largely since 2011. A similar search of Uniprot shows that in the same period, ~700 sequences have been deposited using the classical toxin-to-sequence approach (toxin sequences with experimental evidence at protein level).

The impact of these high-throughput sequencing methods is evident and has led to an ever-increasing gap between known DRP sequences and those that are experimentally detected and functionally characterized. To address this gap, pharmacological characterization of DRPs is likely to require a paradigm shift. This is indeed emerging with advances in parallelization of recombinant protein production and high-throughput structural characterization that allow the production of sufficient material for functional testing in high-throughput assays. In light of these advances, we are adopting a different strategy:

(1) Venom gland RNA extraction and sequencing (or data mining of available transcripts)
(2) Sequence analysis to identify peptides of interest (based on homology to known proteins of interest, sequence uniqueness, or transcript abundance)
(3) Validation of the presence of the sequence in the venom by mass identification (when possible)
(4) High-throughput gene synthesis
(5) Small-scale, parallel protein expression in multiple hosts
(6) Large-scale protein expression in suitable host
(7) Structural and functional characterization

Given the wealth of knowledge that has accumulated over the years in defining DRP scaffolds, it will be possible to validate that the protein adheres to the predicated class through high-throughput structural characterization. Of course, the above "sequence-to-toxin" approach has its own weaknesses and should be considered complementary to the classical toxin-to-sequence approach rather than its replacement. For example, it will be difficult to predict posttranslational modifications (PTMs), in particular if step 3 of the above is not possible. In this case, however, the traditional "toxin to sequence" approach may actually be completely unfeasible, if step 3 is due to lack of obtainable venom (in sufficient quantities). Similarly, unless the peptide of interest can also be isolated from the venom it will be difficult to validate novel structural classes if these have not been detected. Finally, we note that since the sequences are not extracted due to function (as in the toxin-to-sequence approach) it may be that the ultimate product does not have the desired activity and in cases where a particular activity is sought this should be carried out prior to costly large-scale expression and structural characterization. We note that a similar problem arises in the toxin-to-sequence approach where the isolated peptide is incorrectly assigned the function of an impurity (Zhang et al., 2007). In Fig. 1, the

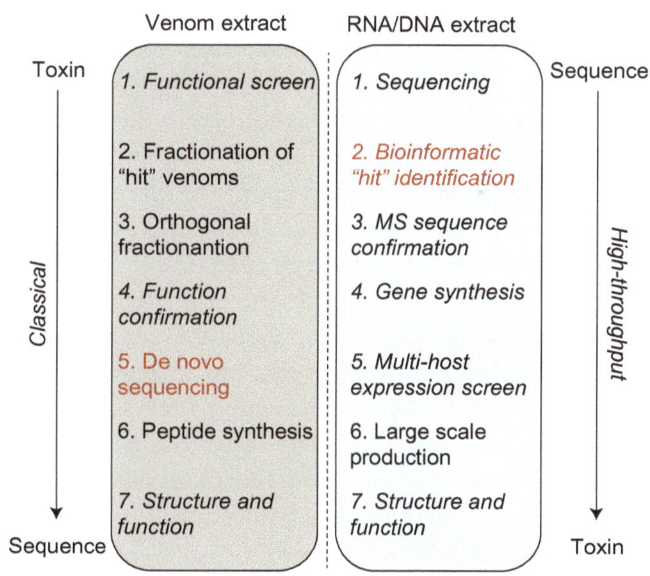

Fig. 1 Venom-based biodiscovery. *Left*: The classical approach starts from a venom extract and functional screening is performed to identify hits that are further purified and when possible sequenced using a variety of methods. *Right*: High-throughput methods have resulted in a rapid expansion of toxin sequences mined from transcriptomic or genomic data. A new approach is to couple this with other high-throughput methods to more rapidly survey the ever growing sequence space. For both methods, the step that is most challenging is highlighted in *red* and steps that are amenable to high-throughput methods are shown in *italics*.

two approaches are summarized, and it can be seen that they have different weaknesses and it may be that until sufficient manual data has been accumulated to improve bioinformatics analysis a hybrid approach will be most appropriate.

The above discussion is solely focused on functional characterization of DRPs, and any insights into the molecular details of this function have largely been restricted to structure–activity relationship studies that rely on extensive mutagenesis. The difficulty in directly visualizing interactions between DRPs and ion channels has largely been due to our inability to study the structure of the often membrane bound or embedded channels. However, recent improvements in structural biology approaches are providing hope that we can slowly start to explore structural models of channel-peptide complexes more efficiently. This is indeed an area at the forefront of structural biology evidenced by the presence of only a handful of peptide-ion-channel complexes solved to date.

In Sections 2 and 3 of this book chapter, we will discuss critical components (5 and 6) in the sequence-to-toxin approach described earlier. These two components are currently the most time-consuming steps and areas where progress is being actively made, motivating the sequence-to-toxin approach. This will be exemplified by high-throughput recombinant production and isotope labeling of venom peptides in *Escherichia coli* and recent advances in rapid structural characterization by high-throughput nuclear magnetic resonance (NMR) spectroscopy methods.

In both approaches shown in Fig. 1, the ultimate aim is to arrive at a deeper understanding of the mechanism of channel function, hence paving the way for rational design of molecules that can address medical conditions associated with distinct channel states. In Section 4, we will discuss the handful of experimentally determined peptide-ion-channel complex structures reported to date and discuss the emerging role of cryo-electron microscopy (cryo-EM) and the need for integrated structural biology approaches in future studies of toxin–channel complexes.

2. HIGH-THROUGHPUT PRODUCTION OF DRPS

Production of DRPs poses a particular challenge in that only one configuration of the disulfide bond connectivities will yield the natively folded peptides. The problem becomes more vexing as the number of disulfide bonds increases, by roughly one order of magnitude per disulfide bond according to:

$$\text{Isoforms} = \frac{(2n_{\text{dsb}})!}{2^{n_{\text{dsb}}}(n_{\text{dsb}})!} \tag{1}$$

where n_{dsb} is the number of disulfide bonds and where all cysteines are assumed to be oxidized and forming intramolecular disulfide bonds. From Eq. (1), we can calculate that 3, 4, 5, and 6 disulfide bonds yield 15, 105, 945, and 10,395 possible isoforms, respectively. As can be seen, the complexity increases steeply and any method of DRP production must address the issue of disulfide bond formation. The two broad categories for production of peptides are either by solid-phase peptide synthesis or through recombinant expression in a heterologous host. The synthetic route is particularly attractive for short peptides (<20 amino acids) with few disulfide bonds (de Araujo et al., 2014). These can be produced with orthogonal protecting groups that can be used to direct the correct folding of the peptide (Dekan et al., 2014). For larger peptides with more than four disulfide bonds, this approach becomes increasingly unfeasible due to excessive costs and reduced yields. Although advances in high-throughput peptide synthesis have been made, these typically preclude the use of orthogonal protecting groups, thus in general requiring a refolding step for DRPs. This currently makes peptide synthesis a poor candidate for high-throughput production of DRPs of arbitrary length and number of disulfide bonds.

The alternative approach of recombinant expression can itself be further broken down into different approaches depending on the choice of heterologous expression host. Bacterial, yeast, insect, and mammalian cells are typically used with the listed order, indicating decreasing yield and increasing cost. The order also denotes the complexity of the protein production machinery available and these are particularly important in proteins requiring extensive PTMs. Fortunately, disulfide bonds are commonly the only PTM encountered in venom peptides. Other PTMs such as C-terminal amidation or hydroxylation of prolines are present in some toxins, but can generally be ignored, as they typically do not significantly alter the function of the peptide.

For a general sequence-to-toxin strategy, the ideal approach would be to perform multihost parallel expression tests. Gene synthesis costs have reduced dramatically in recent years, and commercial services now offer this in addition to subcloning into multihost vectors, providing a rapid high-throughput method to identify a suitable expression vector (Berrow et al., 2007). These multihost vectors are typically designed with common solubility and purification tags such that scale-up can be done rapidly and using standard biochemical purification methods. In the majority of cases DRP expression can be achieved with minor modifications in *E. coli*, which is the simplest and also the cheapest expression vector (Klint et al., 2013). It should be noted that cell free expression is likely to be the least suited recombinant method for DRP production. This may be overcome by introduction of folding chaperons and disulfide isomerases, but such methods have not been applied to DRPs to date. In this chapter, we will focus only on bacterial expression, as it is the most common method, but we note that the procedures described can be modified for other expression hosts.

Heterologous proteins are generally expressed in the cytoplasm of *E. coli* as it offers the advantage of high protein yields and simple plasmid constructs. However, a major challenge with intracellular expression of DRPs in *E. coli* are the low yields of correctly folded (native) protein due to the reducing environment in the intracellular space (Makrides, 1996). The native fold can be recovered using denaturant-induced solubilization, followed by optimization of refolding conditions (Rudolph & Lilie, 1996). This is often a laborious process and finding a folding condition that will produce high yield of the native fold is not guaranteed. This issue can be overcome using two different approaches.

The first approach is to ensure that the nascent protein is secreted into the periplasm of the bacterium, where the protein machinery for disulfide bond formation is located (Baneyx & Mujacic, 2004; Choi & Lee, 2004; Heras et al., 2009). In essence, this allows one to hijack the existing *E. coli* refolding machinery in order to produce heterologous peptides with their native disulfide bond arrangement.

The second approach involves using engineered bacteria where the reducing cytoplasm is made more oxidizing and additionally has the expression of proteins that promote disulfide bond formation directed to the cytoplasm. SHuffle and Origami are strains that have been engineered by introducing mutations into the genes encoding glutathione reductase (gor) and thioredoxin reductase (trxB) (Origami™ strains) and by introducing a cytoplasmic disulfide isomerase protein (DsbC) to enhance disulfide bond formation (Shuffle™ strain) (Lobstein et al., 2012).

Typically, one of the above two strategies will lead to the production of soluble DRPs with native disulfide bond arrangement. In cases where these approaches fail, the more complex expression hosts can be explored (yeast, insect and mammalian cells). In our experience ~80% of all toxins with less than five disulfide bonds can be produced in *E. coli* (Klint et al., 2013). Beyond the obvious advantage of low production costs, bacterial expression is particularly attractive as it allows for incorporation of isotope labels, which allows for application of high-throughput structural characterization by NMR spectroscopy. This can be utilized in studying the structure and dynamics of the toxin in solution as well as allowing for studies of toxin: channel or toxin:membrane interactions. These aspects are discussed in the following sections.

3. HIGH-THROUGHPUT TOXIN STRUCTURE DETERMINATION

NMR spectroscopy has historically been the method of choice for structural characterization of DRPs. Indeed, the first protein NMR structure was of a proteinase inhibitor, containing six cysteine residues and folding into a Kazal-like fold (Williamson, Havel, & Wüthrich, 1985). Crystallography has typically not been applied to toxins, in particular those that have disordered regions, where presumably sufficient stable crystal contacts cannot be achieved. The flexible loops and tails of DRPs constitute a much larger percentage of the surface area of the toxins compared to large globular proteins, and this is likely one of the reasons for the dominance of NMR in structural elucidation for these molecules. An EM structure of an individual DRP has not been reported, as their size is substantially below the resolving power of the current generation of detectors. Nevertheless, EM structures of toxin:channel complexes have emerged recently and the application of EM in such studies is likely to become dominant in the future (Cao, Liao, Cheng, & Julius, 2013).

The early NMR studies of DRPs utilized homonuclear NMR where resonance assignments and distance restraints rely on ^{1}H atoms only. For small DRPs up to ~4 kDa, this approach still yields well-resolved structures of good quality. However, for proteins >8 kDa, the approach becomes increasingly difficult to apply as spectral crowding in the 2D homonuclear (^{1}H—^{1}H) leads to overlap of signals that introduce ambiguity in the structure determination process, ultimately leading to poorly resolved structures. The homonuclear approach has an additional disadvantage in that manual analysis is required and even for small ~4 kDa DRPs, it would be nearly impossible to achieve automated resonance assignment and structure determination. Thus, homonuclear NMR is poorly suited as a component in a high-throughput sequence-to-toxin approach as described earlier. In the classical toxin-to-sequence approach, however, homonuclear NMR remains a central and critical component.

In a high-throughput setting, modern multidimensional heteronuclear NMR methods are far more applicable. The heteronuclear approach utilizes through-bond correlations between ^{1}H, ^{13}C, and ^{15}N nuclei to yield unambiguous connectivities. This, of course, requires production of toxins uniformly labeled with ^{13}C and ^{15}N isotopes (Atreya, 2012). The isotope-labeled sample is used to acquire multiple 2D, 3D, and 4D NMR experiments. These multidimensional experiments contain far less information than the 2D homonuclear experiments, as they are filtered to show very specific correlations (like a 2D gel). Thus, analysis can be time consuming, not because the data is complex or difficult to interpret, but rather because signals must be identified in vast empty regions of multiple 3D experiments. This procedure is fortunately highly amenable to automation through spectral analysis software (Lee, Petit, Cornilescu, Stark, & Markley, 2016). The NMR experiments used for heteronuclear structural analysis are summarized in Table 2.

The general procedure is to first achieve resonance assignment, which is done by acquisition of two experiments that identify the correlation between the resonances of backbone atoms of two adjacent residues. This is referred to sequential backbone resonance assignment. Once this is achieved a series of 3D NMR experiments are used to correlate the nuclear frequencies of sidechain ^{1}H, ^{13}C atoms and ^{15}N atoms. Once complete resonance assignment is achieved, a number of 3D experiments are acquired that correlate ^{1}H atoms that are close in space. The atoms are further resolved through correlation of one of the ^{1}H atoms to its covalently attached ^{13}C or ^{15}N atom. Typically a few thousand distances are measured in these experiments, which are subsequently used to determine the structure of the protein by a computational method.

When coupled to spectral analysis software, the entire procedure can be fully automated. A universal platform for achieving this is being developed by the NMR community called NMRbox (https://www.nmrbox.org/), which is a virtual box that contains all necessary tools for automated structure determination. These approaches are an area of intense research and it is likely that such automation will become routine in the near future.

An aspect of the heteronuclear NMR approach that makes it ill suited for high-throughput applications is the time requirement of the many multidimensional NMR experiments required. Furthermore, the success of the

Table 2 Triple Resonance Experiments Used to Solve Proteins Structures by Heteronuclear NMR

	Dimensionality	Experiment	Scans	Linear (time/h)	NUS (time/h)
Backbone assignment	2D	*^1H–^{15}N HSQC*	2	0.1	*0.1*
	3D	*HNCO*	2	4	*0.5*
	3D	HN(CA)CO	8	16	4
	3D	*CBCA(CO)NH*	8	16	*4*
	3D	*HNCACB*	16	32	*8*
	3D	HNCA	8	16	4
	3D	HN(CO)CA	8	16	4
	3D	H(C)CH	8	40	12
	3D	(H)CCH	8	40	12
Sidechain assignment	2D	*$H(CC_{AR})$-(CG) CB*	16	1	*1*
	3D	*HBHA(CO)NH*	8	16	*6*
	3D	H(CC)(CO)NH	16	40	12
	3D	(H)CC(CO)NH	16	40	12
	4D	*HCC(CO)NH*	8	582	*20*
NOEs restraints	3D	*^{15}N NOESY*	8	*18*	9
	3D	*^{13}C $NOESY_{ALI}$*	8	*30*	15
	3D	*^{13}C $NOESY_{ARO}$*	8	*16*	8

The experiments are divided into backbone, sidechain, and NOE experiments, describing the purpose of the experiment. Pairs of experiments for backbone assignment are given together without a gap, similarly paired 3D sidechain experiments providing C or H correlations are shown without a gap. The experiments given in *italics* are those used in the ASAP-NMR method shown in Fig. 2. "NUS" (nonuniform sampling) and "Linear" refer to the acquisition mode and "Scans" is the number repetition of the experiment required to provide sufficient resolution.

automation will critically depend on the resolution and signal to noise. The relationship between the time requirement and resolution increases as the power of the dimensionality. An 8-h 2D experiment thus becomes a 64-h 3D experiment and a 4096-h 4D experiment. It is therefore not uncommon that time requirements for data acquisition to solve the structure of a single protein can run into several weeks if not months. This would

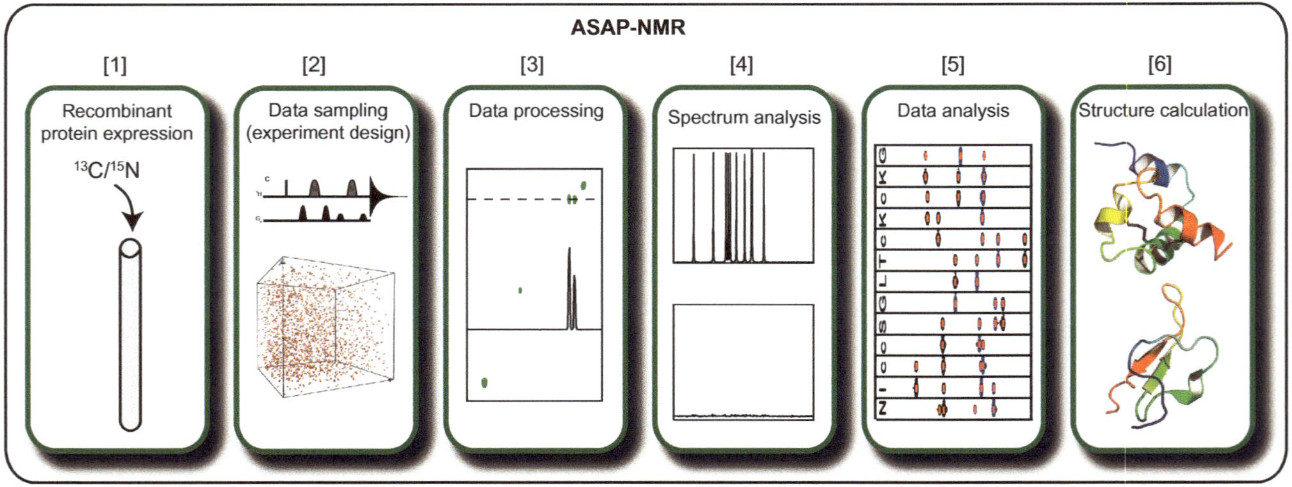

Fig. 2 Automated structural analysis of proteins by NMR (ASAP-NMR) established by one of the authors (M.M.). The steps of protein structure determination are broken down into six components and each is optimized for high-throughput and automation. Nonuniform sampling enables rapid data acquisition (step 2), automated maximum entropy generates highly resolved spectra with reduced noise level (step 3), these spectra are analyzed automatically by an automated spectral fitting procedure (step 4), the extracted information is automatically assigned to the protein sequence through automated algorithms and finally used to produce a structure by automated NOE assignments and structure calculation. The entire pipeline (2–6) requires less than 1 week for a toxin.

certainly be stretching the definition of high throughput. Fortunately, the majority of multidimensional heteronuclear NMR spectra are largely empty, containing information in a few percent of the spectrum. Statistically, it may then be possibly to extract this information without the heavy time burden imposed by the Fourier transform in traditional NMR data acquisition. The problem is very similar to how very large raw images can be compressed into tiny files by compression methods such as JPEG. The same compression philosophy can be implemented in NMR and it has been shown that 3D and 4D NMR data can be acquired in the same amount of time that would traditionally be required for a 2D NMR spectrum (Mobli, 2015; Mobli & Hoch, 2014; Mobli, Stern, Bermel, King, & Hoch, 2010). Using these advanced statistical methods of spectral reconstruction from nonuniformly sampled (NUS) multidimensional NMR data, it is then possible to reduce the weeks of NMR time typically required to less than 1 week. In theory, it is possible to reduce this time even further if optimal sampling can be achieved. Currently, such optimized sampling methods have not emerged but it if the full potential of NUS can be achieved it is likely that fully automated DRP structure determination will be achieved in the near future in a few hours of acquisition time for concentrated samples (>2 mM), and in a few days for dilute samples. Thus, currently a fully occupied NMR magnet can be used to solve ~50 DRP structures per year, but we anticipate that this number can increased to anywhere between 100 and 500. The relatively low throughput of current structural characterization methods therefore requires prioritization of peptides to be analyzed, which can be guided based on preliminary functional studies.

In the research group of one of the authors, a pipeline for automated DRP structure determination called ASAP-NMR is being developed. In its current form, isotopically labeled proteins are used to acquire multidimensional heteronuclear NMR data at high field (900 MHz NMR spectrometer at UQ is typically used). The following 3D datasets are acquired using NUS and used for backbone resonance assignment: 3D HNCO, 3D CBCA(CO)NH, and 3D HNCACB. In general, 5–10% of a very high-resolution "master" dataset is sampled. These three 3D experiments require ~12 h of NMR time in total (see also Table 2). A 4D HCC(CO)NH experiment is then collected using NUS to assign aliphatic sidechain atoms; this experiment requires ~1 day of NMR time (Mobli et al., 2010). Three NOESY datasets are collected: one 3D ^{15}N-edited NOESY-HSQC experiment as well as two ^{13}C-edited HSQC-NOESY experiment focused on the aliphatic and aromatic regions, respectively.

These 3D experiments are currently acquired using traditional uniform sampling, primarily because these experiments are not as sparse as the experiments used for resonance assignment, and in the absence of optimal sampling only modest time savings can be achieved through NUS. The NOESY data requires a total of 3 days, resulting in a total data acquisition time of ~4 days per toxin. NUS datasets are automatically processed using MaxEnt, while the traditional NOESY datasets are processed by Fourier transformation (Mobli, Maciejewski, Gryk, & Hoch, 2007). Peak information is automatically extracted from the spectra using in house software (PEAKY). This software performs peak picking followed by line-shape fitting using the Levenberg–Marquardt algorithm and is applicable to spectra with up to four dimensions. Automated sequence-specific resonance assignment is achieved using the FLYA algorithm (Lopez-Mendez & Guntert, 2006). Backbone dihedral angles are determined from chemical shifts using TALOS (Cornilescu, Delaglio, & Bax, 1999; Shen, Delaglio, Cornilescu, & Bax, 2009), and automated NOESY assignment and structure calculation performed using CYANA (Güntert, 2004). Structure calculations are currently manually supervised and amended until all inconsistencies have been rectified. This final step generally requires 1 day of manual work. So far, we have used this approach to obtain complete NMR resonance assignments for >20 toxins and have obtained near complete assignment (~90%) for several larger proteins (10–15 kDa) (Casey et al., 2016; Klint, Chin, & Mobli, 2015; Lau, King, & Mobli, 2016).

4. STRUCTURE OF CHANNEL:TOXIN COMPLEXES

In this section, we will survey the few toxin:channel complexes that have been solved experimentally. To date, only six such structures have been reported to our knowledge, summarized in Table 3. The table highlights that NMR, X-ray crystallography, and EM have all been utilized in this field, and we will here highlight a number of these structures to illustrate common themes. First, we will discuss the structure of the KcsA:CTX and KvAP:VSD complexes to highlight the differences in the NMR methods used. Next, we will discuss the DkTx:TRPV1 structures which have been solved both in amphipoles and nanodiscs, providing additional insight into lipid binding. Finally, we will look at the cocrystal structures of PcTx1 and MitTx in complex with chicken ASIC1, solved by X-ray crystallography, and represent two different channel states.

Table 3 A Summary of Toxin-Ion Channel Structures Derived From Experimental Measurements

Ion channel	Toxin	PDB ID	Method	Comment
ASIC	PcTx1	4FZ0, 3S3X	X-ray	Binds to soluble domain
ASIC	MiTx	4NTX	X-ray	
KcsA	ChTX	2A9H, 4JTA	NMR	KcsA/Shaker chimera
KvAP	VsTx1	N/A	NMR	VSD domain, based on chemical shift changes
TRPV1	DkTx	3J5Q, 5IRX	Cryo-EM	In nanodiscs
nAChR	PnIa	2BR8	X-ray	AChBP homolog of nAChR
nAChR	Cbtx	1YI5	X-ray	AChBP homolog of nAChR

The modest number of structures in Table 3 is largely due to the difficulties associated with the production, purification, and structural characterization of membrane proteins. Until recently, high-resolution structures of membrane proteins were exceedingly rare. Improvements in membrane protein solubilizing and stabilizing agents coupled with advances in experimental techniques, notably in cryo-EM, have all contributed to a recent increase in momentum in this field.

A common theme of all of the structures in Table 3 is that they describe the binding of the toxin to a particular state of the channel, relatively stable in solution in the absence of the toxin, with toxin binding leading to only modest conformational changes. Ion channels are highly dynamic and in most cases only a few of the many functional states of the channel have be captured in vitro. Notably, the resting state of voltage-gated ion channels in the presence of a membrane voltage remains elusive. Consequently, there are currently no structures of any toxin:channel complexes that stabilize this state. Future work will be required to determine conditions that allow access to channel states that are poorly populated in solution.

4.1 KcsA:ChTX (Fig. 3A)

Charybdotoxin was isolated from scorpion venom and adheres to the classical cysteine-stabilized α/β-fold and blocks voltage-gated potassium channels by binding to closed state of the channel (Miller, Moczydlowski, Latorre, & Phillips, 1985). KcsA is a homotetrameric bacterial potassium channel that shares high homology to eukaryotic voltage-gated potassium

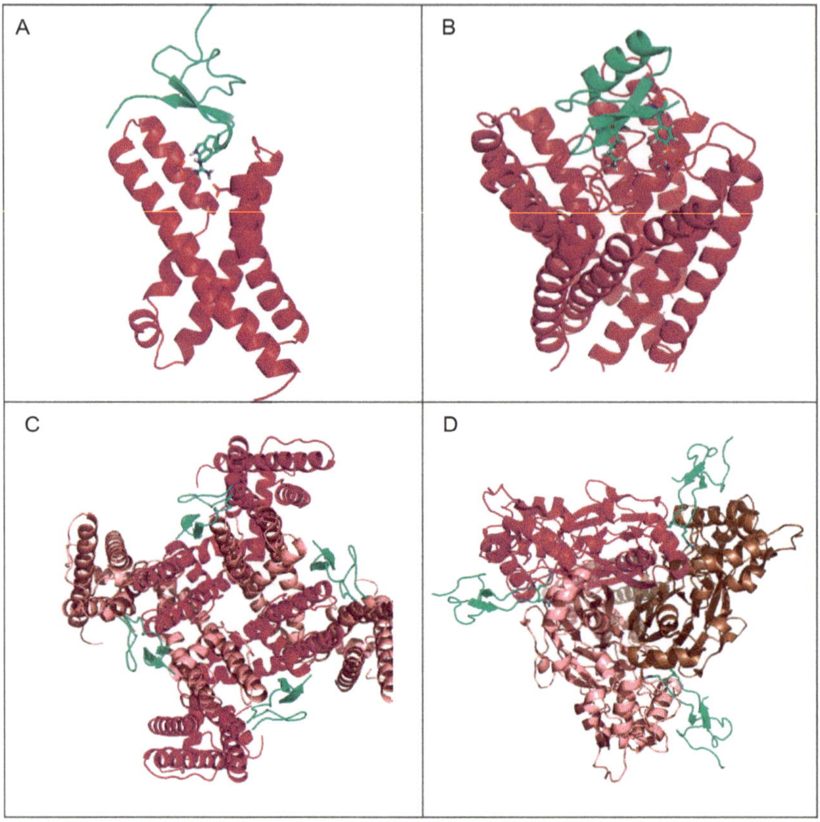

Fig. 3 Diversity of toxin: channel interactions. Toxins are shown in *cyan* and channels in shades of magenta. (A) The interaction of a scorpion venom peptide (ChTX) with the pore of a potassium channel. (B) The interaction of a spider venom peptide (VSTx1) with the VSD of a voltage-gated potassium channel. (C) The interaction of a spider venom peptide (DkTx) at the domain interfaces of the pore region of a heat sensitive TRPV1 channel (alternate domains are shown in *different shades* to denote the domain interface). (D) The interaction of a spider venom peptide with the ligand-binding site of an acid-sensing ion channel (alternate domains are shown in *different shades* to denote the domain interface).

channels in the pore region, but in contrast to its eukaryote counterparts lacks a voltage-sensing domain (VSD). The simpler architecture of this channel made it very attractive in early structural studies of ion channels and by some fortunate twist of fate, the channel is able to bind to the toxin in both closed and open conformations.

The structure reported by Yu et al. (2005) remains the only NMR structure of a toxin:channel complex solved by unambiguous intermolecular

NOEs. In many ways, the study was ahead of its time with complex methods of resonance assignment combined with the use of deuterated detergents to allow for these measurements. The nature of the structure determination process allowed the investigators to also examine the pH sensitivity of the channel. They found that neither the structure of the channel nor the binding of toxin was sensitive to pH down to ∼4.5. The structure revealed several very interesting features, the first is that the crucial lysine residue in the peptide does not engage a negative charge but instead binds to backbone carbonyl atoms that otherwise coordinate a potassium ion in the selectivity filter. Further stabilizing interactions were found to be largely hydrophobic including π-stacking of tyrosine residues from the two molecules. The authors further found that although computational models based solely on mutational data were largely supported by the 3D structure, several mutations led to weakening of the tetramer structure, highlighting the importance of and difficulties in dissecting functionally and structurally important residues in protein–protein interactions. Overall, the binding surface is extensive, covering much of the exposed surface of the pore. This structure was later also shown to be consistent with an X-ray crystal structure of a similar complex with a eukaryotic potassium channel (Banerjee, Lee, Campbell, & MacKinnon, 2013).

4.2 KvAP$_{VSD}$:VSTx1 (Fig. 3B)

VSTx1 is a spider venom peptide that folds into the classical inhibitor cysteine knot (ICK) fold. KvAP is a voltage-gated potassium channel from a thermophilic archaebacterium. This channel protein much like KcsA has been an important and complementary model system as, in contrast to KcsA, it has a VSD and shares high homology to its mammalian counterparts. The protein is homotetrameric with four identical VSDs positioned around the central pore (Jiang, Ruta, Chen, Lee, & MacKinnon, 2003). VSTx1 binds to the channel in a nonion-conducting, inactivated state, in the absence of membrane voltage. This prohibits the channel from returning to its resting closed state, thereby indirectly blocking the channel. Early structural studies of KvAP showed that the VSD was an autonomous domain that retained its fold in the absence of the pore domain (Butterwick & MacKinnon, 2010; Jiang et al., 2003; Shenkarev et al., 2010).

The structural model of the VSTx1 binding to the VSD of KvAP (KvAP$_{VSD}$) was based on indirect evidence from chemical shift perturbation data in lipid micelles and supported by mutagenesis. This remains the only high-resolution structure of a gating modifier toxin bound to the VSD of an ion channel. The slow progress in this field has been largely due to the weak interaction of the peptide with the VSD, which in vitro is ~300 μM, in stark contrast to in vivo measurements of nanomolar inhibition. The discrepancy has been attributed to the compounding effect of peptide–lipid interactions in addition to peptide–channel interactions. VSTx1 has indeed been to shown to partition into bilayers of lipids containing negatively charged head groups. In the absence of interatomic NOEs, the model of the peptide remains to be confirmed with competing models also being proposed (Ozawa et al., 2015).

The model proposed by Lau et al. places the toxin in the center of the helices that make up the VSD, and as in the ChTX structure, this results in a very large protein–protein interface (Lau et al., 2016). Similar to ChTX, VSTx1 has a critical basic residue, R25, which protrudes into the central, solvent exposed vestibule of the VSD. In contrast to KcsA, the VSD of KvAP does not contain ion-coordinating carbonyls, instead the central cavity contains a number negatively charged residues that counter balance positive charges in the voltage-sensing S4 helix. The model shows that R25 from the toxin binds to these negatively charged residues, trapping the channel in the inactivated state (Fig. 3B).

It is most likely that a peptide:VSD complex will only be stabilized sufficiently for high-resolution structural studies in a lipid bilayer system such as a lipid nanodisc (Shenkarev et al., 2014). Another challenge in the studies of peptide:VSD complexes is that the majority of venom peptides bind to the resting state of the channel in the presence of membrane voltage. It is unclear if the presence of a toxin alone in the absence of sufficient membrane potential will be capable of stabilizing this state in vitro and structural studies of the resting state of voltage-gated ion channels remain elusive.

4.3 TRPV1:DkTx (Fig. 3C)

DkTx is an unusual spider toxin in that it contains two ICK motifs in tandem. This architecture provides the toxin with very high avidity against its receptor. TRPV1 is a heat-sensitive tetrameric ion channel. It has a similar architecture to voltage-gated ion channels, containing a pore domain surrounded by four VSDs. Curiously, the VSDs do not seem to function as voltage sensors and the channel is instead gated by either temperature or ligands such as capsaicin commonly found in hot chilies (Cao et al., 2013; Gao, Cao, Julius, & Cheng, 2016). DkTx binds to the open state of TRPV1, a state that is stabilized by the allosteric modulator resiniferatoxin (RTX).

Under conditions for structural analysis, DkTx alone does not appear to be able to drive the conformational change to the open state and requires the presence of the very potent agonist RTX.

The cryo-EM structures of TRPV1 represent a landmark study and marked the entry of this method in providing important structural information of ion-channel structure and function. The initial study stabilized the protein in amphipols that are amphipathic polymers designed to stabilize membrane proteins (Cao et al., 2013). In the case of TRPV1, the structure showed the presence of several stable interactions between the amphipols and the channel; however, the nonphysiological nature of these interactions made their interpretation difficult. More recently, the same group revisited the structure of this complex, with the important difference that TRPV1 was now instead solubilized in a bilayer composed of soybean lipid extracts held together by a membrane scaffolding protein in a nanodisc (Gao et al., 2016). The overall structure is nearly identical to the original one, although it has higher resolution. The increased level of detail apparent in the second complex revealed that the linker between the two ICK moieties of DkTx forms a stable structure. Furthermore, the DkTx molecule was found to make contacts with both the channel and nearby lipids. This study further highlights the importance of the lipid:toxin:channel paradigm and suggests that insight into membrane embedded receptors will not be complete in the absence of lipids.

Another interesting aspect of this structure is that the channel is bound to two copies of DkTx. Thus, a total of four ICKs are present at any one time. This is an interesting observation as many channels are homo- or heteromeric and it maybe that domain duplication has evolved as a means of targeting the natural symmetry in ion channels. Each ICK sits at the interface of two monomers of the channel trapping it in the activated state (Fig. 3C).

4.4 ASIC1a:PcTx1/MiTx (PcTx1 in Fig. 3D)

PcTx1 is a spider venom peptide that folds into a similar ICK motif as the isolated domains of DkTx and of VSTx1. In contrast, MitTx was isolated from snake venom and has a more exotic fold, consisting of two domains that are noncovalently bound. The two domains fold into a Kunitz-type and PLA2-type motif, both of which are commonly encountered in venoms. PcTx1 stabilizes the desensitized state of the channel while MitTx stabilizes the open state of the channel (Baconguis, Bohlen, Goehring,

Julius, & Gouaux, 2014; Dawson et al., 2012). Acid-sensing ion channels are trimeric proton-gated ion channels that respond to changes in the extracellular pH. The binding of the two toxins is mutually exclusive which is interesting considering they stabilize different states of the channel. Indeed PcTx1 is analgesic while MitTx has been shown to induce pain.

The two cocrystal structures reveal that there is indeed substantial overlap between the binding sites of the two toxins. In particular, both PcTx1 and the PLA2-like β-subunit of MitTx make multiple contacts with the alpha-helix 5 of ASIC1 (especially residue F350) on the lower side of the proton binding acidic pocket of the channel. However, the nature of this interaction is quite different with PcTx1 protruding deep into the pocket. PcTx1's substantial interaction surface spans the interface of two channel subunits thus explaining the selectivity of the peptide for the homotrimeric ASIC1a channel (Fig. 3D). The insertion of PcTx1's positively charged R27 and R28 into the acidic pocket mimics protonation of the channel and stabilizes the desensitized state, thereby locking the channel in a non-conducting state.

In contrast, β-MitTx makes interactions with residues closer to the surface of the acidic pocket whilst the Kunitz-like α-MitTx binds below the acidic pocket with an extended interaction interface along the entire length of the thumb domain as well as making interactions with the top of transmembrane region 1 of the channel some 60 Å away. This large surface locks the two toxin subunits together on the same channel monomer and traps it in the open conformation causing the observed pharmacological response. The interactions of MitTx are, however, confined to a single subunit, making the toxin also active on heterotrimeric ASIC channels.

4.5 Summary

The four case studies here show a few trends. First, the interaction surface between the toxin and the channel is extensive in all cases and often involves a key electrostatic interaction together with numerous hydrophobic contacts. This underlies the high potency of these molecules, and in some cases confers substantial selectivity. Second, for membrane embedded ion channels, lipid interactions can be critical for high affinity toxin:channel complex formation. Finally, we note that the peptides bind to preconfigured forms of the channel, trapping the channel in that state by increasing the energetic requirements for departing from that state.

5. CONCLUSION

Venom peptides have long been used to characterize ion-channel pharmacology, and similarly ion-channel function has allowed the classification of venom peptides. In this chapter, we have provided an overview of how venom peptides have been mined for this purpose and how they may be mined in the future in light of the revolution in sequencing technologies. In this context, we have provided an overview of high-throughput toxin production and structural characterization methods that will form important components of future toxin characterization studies.

Finally, we have surveyed the majority of toxin-channel structures available, highlighting the unique structural determinants of channel inhibitions by toxins. With the advent of novel membrane mimetics suitable for structural characterization of ion channels and the improvements in biophysical structural characterization, in particular in cryo-EM, the future looks bright for understanding the structural basis of ion-channel modulation by toxins at the atomic level.

CONFLICT OF INTEREST

The authors declare no conflicts of interest.

ACKNOWLEDGMENTS

M.M. and E.A.B.U. are supported by research funding from the Australian Research Council (Fellowships and Discovery Projects), and M.M. and L.D.R. are supported by the Australian National Health and Medical Research Council (Project Grants).

REFERENCES

Atreya, H. S. (2012). *Isotope labeling in biomolecular NMR, Vol. 992*. Springer.

Baconguis, I., Bohlen, C. J., Goehring, A., Julius, D., & Gouaux, E. (2014). X-ray structure of acid-sensing ion channel 1–snake toxin complex reveals open state of a Na^+-selective channel. *Cell, 156*(4), 717–729.

Banerjee, A., Lee, A., Campbell, E., & MacKinnon, R. (2013). Structure of a pore-blocking toxin in complex with a eukaryotic voltage-dependent K^+ channel. *eLife, 2*, e00594.

Baneyx, F., & Mujacic, M. (2004). Recombinant protein folding and misfolding in *Escherichia coli*. *Nature Biotechnology, 22*(11), 1399–1408.

Berrow, N. S., Alderton, D., Sainsbury, S., Nettleship, J., Assenberg, R., Rahman, N., et al. (2007). A versatile ligation-independent cloning method suitable for high-throughput expression screening applications. *Nucleic Acids Research, 35*(6), e45.

Butterwick, J. A., & MacKinnon, R. (2010). Solution structure and phospholipid interactions of the isolated voltage-sensor domain from KvAP. *Journal of Molecular Biology, 403*(4), 591–606.

Cao, E., Liao, M., Cheng, Y., & Julius, D. (2013). TRPV1 structures in distinct conformations reveal activation mechanisms. *Nature*, *504*(7478), 113–118.

Casey, L. W., Lavrencic, P., Bentham, A. R., Cesari, S., Ericsson, D. J., Croll, T., et al. (2016). The CC domain structure from the wheat stem rust resistance protein Sr33 challenges paradigms for dimerization in plant NLR proteins. *Proceedings of the National Academy of Sciences*, *113*(45), 12856–12861.

Choi, J. H., & Lee, S. Y. (2004). Secretory and extracellular production of recombinant proteins using *Escherichia coli*. *Applied Microbiology and Biotechnology*, *64*(5), 625–635.

Cornilescu, G., Delaglio, F., & Bax, A. (1999). Protein backbone angle restraints from searching a database for chemical shift and sequence homology. *Journal of Biomolecular NMR*, *13*(3), 289–302.

Dawson, R. J. P., Benz, J., Stohler, P., Tetaz, T., Joseph, C., Huber, S., et al. (2012). Structure of the acid-sensing ion channel 1 in complex with the gating modifier psalmotoxin 1. *Nature Communications*, *3*, 936.

de Araujo, A. D., Mobli, M., Castro, J., Harrington, A. M., Vetter, I., Dekan, Z., et al. (2014). Selenoether oxytocin analogues have analgesic properties in a mouse model of chronic abdominal pain. *Nature Communications*, *5*.

Dekan, Z., Mobli, M., Pennington, M. W., Fung, E., Nemeth, E., & Alewood, P. F. (2014). Total synthesis of human hepcidin through regioselective disulfide-bond formation by using the safety-catch cysteine protecting group 4,4′-dimethylsulfinylbenzhydryl. *Angewandte Chemie International Edition*, *53*, 2931–2934.

Escoubas, P., Quinton, L., & Nicholson, G. M. (2008). Venomics: Unravelling the complexity of animal venoms with mass spectrometry. *Journal of Mass Spectrometry*, *43*(3), 279–295.

Gao, Y., Cao, E., Julius, D., & Cheng, Y. (2016). TRPV1 structures in nanodiscs reveal mechanisms of ligand and lipid action. *Nature*, *534*(7607), 347–351.

Güntert, P. (2004). Automated NMR structure calculation with CYANA. *Methods in Molecular Biology*, *278*, 353–378.

Heras, B., Shouldice, S. R., Totsika, M., Scanlon, M. J., Schembri, M. A., & Martin, J. L. (2009). DSB proteins and bacterial pathogenicity. *Nature Reviews. Microbiology*, *7*(3), 215–225.

Jiang, Y., Ruta, V., Chen, J., Lee, A., & MacKinnon, R. (2003). The principle of gating charge movement in a voltage-dependent K^+ channel. *Nature*, *423*(6935), 42–48.

Klint, J. K., Chin, Y. K. Y., & Mobli, M. (2015). Rational engineering defines a molecular switch that is essential for activity of spider-venom peptides against the analgesics target NaV1.7. *Molecular Pharmacology*, *88*(6), 1002–1010.

Klint, J. K., Senff, S., Saez, N. J., Seshadri, R., Lau, H. Y., Bende, N. S., et al. (2013). Production of recombinant disulfide-rich venom peptides for structurale and functional analysis via expression in the periplasm of *E. coli*. *PloS One*, *8*(5), e63865.

Lau, C. H. Y., King, G. F., & Mobli, M. (2016). Molecular basis of the interaction between gating modifier spider toxins and the voltage sensor of voltage-gated ion channels. *Scientific Reports*, *6*, 34333.

Lavergne, V., Alewood, P. F., Mobli, M., & King, G. F. (2015). The structural universe of disulfide-rich venom peptides. In *Venoms to drugs: Venom as a source for the development of human therapeutics*, (Vol. 37). London, UK: Royal Society of Chemistry.

Lee, W., Petit, C. M., Cornilescu, G., Stark, J. L., & Markley, J. L. (2016). The AUDANA algorithm for automated protein 3D structure determination from NMR NOE data. *Journal of Biomolecular NMR*, *65*, 51–57.

Lewis, R. J., & Garcia, M. L. (2003). Therapeutic potential of venom peptides. *Nature Reviews in Drug Discovery*, *2*(10), 790–802.

Lobstein, J., Emrich, C. A., Jeans, C., Faulkner, M., Riggs, P., & Berkmen, M. (2012). SHuffle, a novel Escherichia coli protein expression strain capable of correctly folding disulfide bonded proteins in its cytoplasm. *Microbial Cell Factories*, *11*, 56.

Lopez-Mendez, B., & Guntert, P. (2006). Automated protein structure determination from NMR spectra. *Journal of the American Chemical Society, 128*(40), 13112–13122.
Makrides, S. C. (1996). Strategies for achieving high-level expression of genes in *Escherichia coli. Microbiological Reviews, 60*(3), 512–538.
Mellor, I. R., & Usherwood, P. N. R. (2004). Targeting ionotropic receptors with polyamine-containing toxins☆. *Toxicon, 43*(5), 493–508.
Miller, C., Moczydlowski, E., Latorre, R., & Phillips, M. (1985). Charybdotoxin, a protein inhibitor of single Ca^{2+}-activated K^{+} channels from mammalian skeletal muscle. *Nature, 313*(6000), 316–318.
Mobli, M. (2015). Reducing seed dependent variability of non-uniformly sampled multidimensional NMR data. *Journal of Magnetic Resonance, 256*, 60–69.
Mobli, M., & Hoch, J. C. (2014). Nonuniform sampling and non-Fourier signal processing methods in multidimensional NMR. *Progress in Nuclear Magnetic Resonance Spectroscopy, 83*, 21–41.
Mobli, M., Maciejewski, M. W., Gryk, M. R., & Hoch, J. C. (2007). An automated tool for maximum entropy reconstruction of biomolecular NMR spectra. *Nature Methods, 4*(6), 467–468.
Mobli, M., Stern, A. S., Bermel, W., King, G. F., & Hoch, J. C. (2010). A non-uniformly sampled 4D HCC(CO)NH-TOCSY experiment processed using maximum entropy for rapid protein sidechain assignment. *Journal of Magnetic Resonance, 204*(1), 160–164.
Mouhat, S., Jouirou, B., Mosbah, A., De Waard, M., & Sabatier, J.-M. (2004). Diversity of folds in animal toxins acting on ion channels. *Biochemical Journal, 378*(3), 717–726.
Ozawa, S.-I., Kimura, T., Nozaki, T., Harada, H., Shimada, I., & Osawa, M. (2015). Structural basis for the inhibition of voltage-dependent K+ channel by gating modifier toxin. *Scientific Reports, 5*, 14226.
Rudolph, R., & Lilie, H. (1996). In vitro folding of inclusion body proteins. *The FASEB Journal, 10*(1), 49–56.
Shen, Y., Delaglio, F., Cornilescu, G., & Bax, A. (2009). TALOS+: A hybrid method for predicting protein backbone torsion angles from NMR chemical shifts. *Journal of Biomolecular NMR, 44*(4), 213–223.
Shenkarev, Z. O., Lyukmanova, E. N., Paramonov, A. S., Panteleev, P. V., Balandin, S. V., Shulepko, M. A., et al. (2014). Lipid-protein nanodiscs offer new perspectives for structural and functional studies of water-soluble membrane-active peptides. *Acta Naturae, 6*(2), 84–94.
Shenkarev, Z. O., Paramonov, A. S., Lyukmanova, E. N., Shingarova, L. N., Yakimov, S. A., Dubinnyi, M. A., et al. (2010). NMR structural and dynamical investigation of the isolated voltage-sensing domain of the potassium channel KvAP: Implications for voltage gating. *Journal of the American Chemical Society, 132*(16), 5630–5637.
Undheim, E. A. B., Mobli, M., & King, G. F. (2016). Toxin structures as evolutionary tools: Using conserved 3D folds to study the evolution of rapidly evolving peptides. *BioEssays, 38*(6), 539–548.
Ushkaryov, Y. A., Volynski, K. E., & Ashton, A. C. (2004). The multiple actions of black widow spider toxins and their selective use in neurosecretion studies. *Toxicon, 43*(5), 527–542.
Williamson, M. P., Havel, T. F., & Wüthrich, K. (1985). Solution conformation of proteinase inhibitor IIA from bull seminal plasma by 1H nuclear magnetic resonance and distance geometry. *Journal of Molecular Biology, 182*(2), 295–315.
Yu, L., Sun, C., Song, D., Shen, J., Xu, N., Gunasekera, A., et al. (2005). Nuclear magnetic resonance structural studies of a potassium channel – charybdotoxin complex. *Biochemistry, 44*(48), 15834–15841.
Zhang, J. V., Klein, C., Ren, P.-G., Kass, S., Donck, L. V., Moechars, D., et al. (2007). Response to comment on "obestatin, a peptide encoded by the ghrelin gene, opposes Ghrelin's effects on food intake". *Science, 315*(5813), 766.

CHAPTER EIGHT

Glycine Receptor Drug Discovery

Joseph W. Lynch*,†,1, Yan Zhang*, Sahil Talwar*, Argel Estrada-Mondragon*

*Queensland Brain Institute, University of Queensland, Brisbane, QLD, Australia
†School of Biomedical Sciences, University of Queensland, Brisbane, QLD, Australia
[1]Corresponding author: e-mail address: j.lynch@uq.edu.au

Contents

Abstract

Postsynaptic glycine receptor (GlyR) chloride channels mediate inhibitory neurotransmission in the spinal cord and brain stem, although presynaptic and extrasynaptic GlyRs are expressed more widely throughout the brain. In humans, GlyRs are assembled as

Advances in Pharmacology, Volume 79
ISSN 1054-3589
http://dx.doi.org/10.1016/bs.apha.2017.01.003

homo- or heteromeric pentamers of α1–3 and β subunits. GlyR malfunctions have been linked to a range of neurological disorders including hyperekplexia, temporal lobe epilepsy, autism, breathing disorders, and chronic inflammatory pain. Although it is possible that GlyRs may eventually be clinically targeted for a variety of neurological disorders, most research to date has focused on developing GlyR-targeted treatments for chronic pain. Inflammatory pain sensitization is caused by inflammatory mediators downregulating the magnitude of α3 GlyR-mediated inhibitory postsynaptic currents in spinal nociceptive neurons. Consistent with this paradigm, it is now well established that the selective enhancement of α3 GlyR current magnitude is effective in alleviating inflammatory pain. In this review, we briefly describe the physiological roles and pharmacological properties of GlyRs. We then outline the methods commonly used to discover new GlyR-active compounds and review recent progress, in our laboratory and elsewhere, in developing GlyR-targeted analgesics. We conclude that the eventual development of an α3 GlyR-targeted analgesic is an eminently feasible goal. However, in selecting or designing new therapeutic leads, we caution against the automatic exclusion of compounds with potentiating effects on α1 GlyRs. Also, as GlyRs are strongly potentiated by Zn^{2+} at nanomolar concentrations, we also caution against the identification of false positives caused by contaminating Zn^{2+} in otherwise pure compound samples.

ABBREVIATIONS

2,6-DTBP 2,6-di-*tert*-butylphenol
5-HT$_3$R 5-hydroxytryptamine type 3 receptor
ASD autism spectrum disorder
FMP fluorescent membrane potential
GABA$_A$R type-A γ-aminobutyric acid receptor
GlyR glycine receptor
IPSC inhibitory postsynaptic current
nAChR nicotinic acetylcholine receptor
PKA protein kinase A
pLGIC pentameric ligand-gated ion channel
THC Δ9-tetrahydrocannabinol
YFP yellow fluorescent protein

1. INTRODUCTION

Glycine receptor (GlyR) chloride channels are abundantly expressed throughout the central nervous system. Postsynaptic GlyRs play a critical role in mediating fast inhibitory neurotransmission in the human adult spinal cord, brain stem, and retina. GlyRs are also found in presynaptic terminals and they play an important role in modulating neurotransmitter release at glutamatergic and glycinergic synapses (Dutertre, Becker, & Betz, 2012; Lynch, 2009). In addition, extrasynaptic GlyRs play an important role in neurodevelopment (Avila, Nguyen, & Rigo, 2013).

GlyRs belong to the superfamily of pentameric ligand-gated ion channels (pLGICs), which also includes the nicotinic acetylcholine receptor (nAChR), the serotonin 5-hydroxytryptamine type 3 receptor (5-HT_3R), and the type-A γ-aminobutyric acid receptor ($GABA_AR$). There are four known GlyR α subunits (α1–α4) and a single β subunit in vertebrates. Functional GlyRs assemble as homopentamers of α subunits, or as heteropentamers of α and β subunits. Heteromeric GlyRs comprise either three α and two β or two α and three β subunits (Durisic et al., 2012; Yang, Taran, Webb, & Lynch, 2012). Each transmembrane subunit is composed of an extracellular domain harboring a ligand-binding site, a transmembrane domain made of four α-helical domains (TM1–TM4), and a large intracellular loop domain connecting the TM3 and TM4 that influences the ion conductance (Carland et al., 2009) and mediates interaction with intracellular proteins (Del Pino et al., 2014; Kim et al., 2006). Recent reports have revealed the molecular structures of the α1 GlyR in complex with its competitive antagonist, strychnine, and the agonists, glycine and ivermectin (Du, Lu, Wu, Cheng, & Gouaux, 2015), and of the α3 GlyR in complex with strychnine, glycine, and AM-3607, a novel analgesic potentiator (Huang, Chen, Michelsen, Schneider, & Shaffer, 2015; Huang et al., 2017). A structural model of the α3 GlyR based on the crystal structure as determined by Huang et al. (2015, 2017) is shown in Fig. 1A and B. The locations of the binding sites for strychnine, glycine, and AM-3607 within this structure are shown in Fig. 1C.

Fast quantal (<1 ms) and high concentration (1–3 mM) release of glycine from the presynaptic terminal triggers the opening of the GlyR channel gate (Beato, 2008; Legendre, 1998), resulting in a flux of anions through the channel pore that causes a rapid hyperpolarization and inhibition of the postsynaptic neurons. Glycinergic inhibition is important in many physiological processes including regulation of muscle tone, motor control, and sensory processing (Lynch, 2009).

GlyR malfunctions have been directly linked to a range of neurological disorders including hyperekplexia, temporal lobe epilepsy, and, most importantly, chronic inflammatory pain. However, GlyRs are not clinically targeted by any currently available therapeutic. In this review, we describe the neurological disorders that are linked to defective GlyR function, outline our current knowledge of GlyR pharmacology, and describe

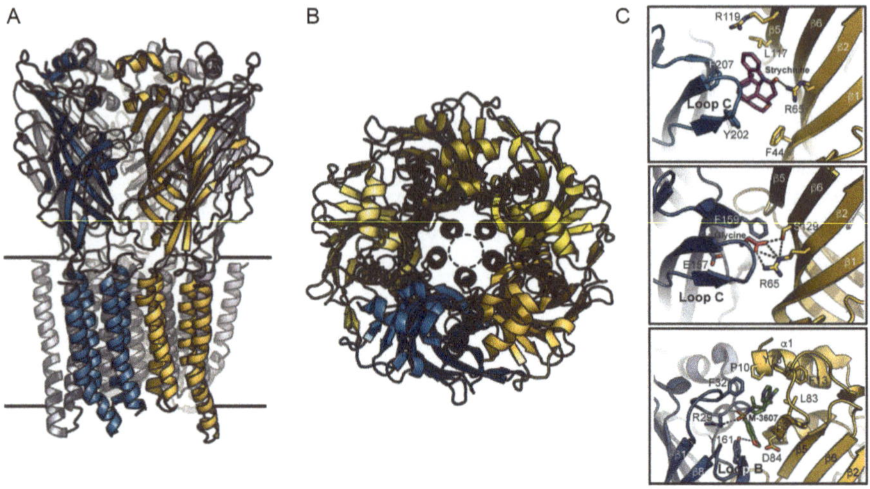

Fig. 1 Molecular structure of the human α3 GlyR. (A) View of the pentameric receptor from within the membrane, highlighting two subunits facing each other. (B) View of the pentamer from the outside of the membrane, showing the central ion-conducting pore. One subunit is highlighted on a *darker color*, delineating its position in the structure. (C) Strychnine-binding site (*upper panel*), glycine-binding site (*center panel*), and AM-3607-binding site (*lower panel*). The loop C, loop B, and other secondary structures as well as important residues for interactions are shown. The representations were created using PyMOL from PDB files: 5CFB and 5TIO.

recent progress in developing new therapeutics for treating chronic inflammatory pain.

2. GlyR SUBUNITS

The four α subunits generally share a >90% amino acid sequence homology with each other. Their gene expression profiles are developmentally and regionally regulated. In the embryonic state, α2 transcripts are abundantly and widely expressed in all layers of the cerebral cortex, diencephalon, hippocampus, thalamus, cerebellum, spinal cord, and brain stem (Avila et al., 2013; Kuhse et al., 1991; Malosio, Marqueze-Pouey, Kuhse, & Betz, 1991). During the developmental period, there is a switch from α2 homomeric GlyRs to α1β heteromeric GlyRs (Lynch, 2009). Nonetheless, reduced densities of α2 mRNA are still present in adult hippocampus, cerebral cortex, and thalamus (Lynch, 2004; Malosio et al., 1991; Sato, Kiyama, & Tohyama, 1992). After birth, α1 and α3 expression becomes more abundant. In situ hybridization studies reveal that α1 is prominently expressed in the spinal cord, brain stem cerebellar deep nuclei, hypothalamus, and colliculi (Greferath et al., 1994; Malosio et al., 1991). α3 subunit expression is relatively lower than α1 subunit at all developmental stages and in adults is restricted to superficial laminae of the dorsal horn and respiratory network of the brain stem (Harvey et al., 2004; Malosio et al., 1991; Manzke et al., 2010). α4 has been described as an embryonic GlyR subunit isoform, which in chick is only expressed in the spinal cord, lumbosacral sympathetic ganglia, and dorsal root ganglia (Harvey et al., 2000), but is presumed to be a pseudogene in humans due to a premature stop codon upstream of the final TM4 domain. In contrast, the β subunit gene is transcribed at all developmental stages but cannot form functional receptors when expressed alone. β Subunit mRNA is widely and abundantly distributed in the spinal cord and brain (Fujita et al., 1991; Grenningloh et al., 1990). This pattern of distribution overlaps with, but is broader than, the distribution of α1 subunit mRNA. β Subunit is considered to be indispensable for synaptic clustering by interacting with the receptor-anchoring protein gephyrin (Meyer, Kirsch, Betz, & Langosch, 1995); therefore, it is generally assumed that the α1β isoform of the GlyR dominates at synapses in the adult spinal cord and brain stem (Singer, Talley, Bayliss, & Berger, 1998).

3. GyRs AND DISEASE

3.1 Hyperekplexia

Loss of glycinergic synaptic signaling has been implicated in a rare human hereditary neurological disorder, known as hyperekplexia or startle disease. Hyperekplexia is characterized by neonatal hypertonia and an exaggerated startle reflex in response to sudden, unexpected stimuli (Bakker, van Dijk, van den Maagdenberg, & Tijssen, 2006). Mutations in the *GLRA1* or *GLRB* genes, which encode the α1 and β GlyR subunits, respectively, are the major causes of hyperekplexia (Bode & Lynch, 2014; Harvey, Topf, Harvey, & Rees, 2008). To date, more than 50 *GLRA* mutations and 18 *GLRB* mutations have been identified in humans (Bode & Lynch, 2014). The vast majority of these mutations are loss of function in that they reduce the ability of GlyRs to flux chloride. Recessive hyperekplexia mutations generally result in the loss of α1 or β GlyR protein expression at the cell surface, whereas dominant mutations usually allow strong surface expression but impair channel function via reduced open probability, single-channel conductance, or glycine sensitivity. Given that inhibitory glycinergic synapses on spinal motor neurons are responsible for limiting their excitability, it is evident that the loss of this inhibition will chronically increase the level of excitation of these neurons. Patients generally develop compensatory mechanisms to counteract this enhanced excitability, although they are not able to cope with the increased inhibitory demand that results from unexpected excitatory commands. Thus, patients generally exhibit normal movement patterns but exhibit strong hypertonia when startled.

Several gain-of-function GlyR hyperekplexia mutations to both α and β subunits have recently been shown to result in spontaneous GlyR channel activity (Bode & Lynch, 2013; Chung et al., 2010; James et al., 2013; Zhang, Bode, Nguyen, Keramidas, & Lynch, 2016). When these subunits are incorporated into glycinergic synapses, they prolong the decay time course of glycinergic inhibitory postsynaptic currents (IPSCs) (Zhang, Bode, et al., 2016). It seems paradoxical that both gain- and loss-of-function mutations can cause exactly the same disease phenotype. An attempt was recently made to characterize the mechanism by which gain-of-function mutations cause hyperekplexia. The authors concluded that aberrant spontaneous GlyR activity throughout nervous system development would preclude the formation of α1β glycinergic synapses in adults (Zhang, Bode, et al., 2016).

All genetic forms of hyperekplexia are successfully treated with the benzodiazepine, clonazepam (Bakker et al., 2006; Thomas et al., 2013), which acts by enhancing GABAergic synaptic transmission. Since hyperekplexia is a very rare disorder with an effective treatment, the development of new therapeutics is not considered a high priority.

3.2 Autism

Autism spectrum disorders (ASDs) are a group of heterogeneous neurodevelopmental disorders characterized by deficits in social interaction and communication. ASD is a highly prevalent neurodevelopmental disorder with an estimated incidence of 1 in 68 births (Sztainberg & Zoghbi, 2016). The cost of supporting an individual with ASD throughout their lifetime was estimated at >$US2 million in the United States and the United Kingdom in 2014 (Buescher, Cidav, Knapp, & Mandell, 2014). There is thus an enormous economic and social imperative to develop biomarkers and therapeutics for this devastating disorder.

ASD is thought to result from dysfunctional development of multiple brain areas and to be associated with perturbed excitatory and inhibitory balance. Neuroligins are postsynaptic cell-adhesion molecules that are essential for synapse maturation and specification. Mutations in the human neuroligin genes *NLGN3* and *NLGN4* were detected in patients with ASDs (Mackowiak, Mordalska, & Wedzony, 2014). Because neuroligins are also responsible for glycinergic synaptogenesis (Hoon et al., 2009, 2011; Poulopoulos et al., 2009; Zhang, Dixon, Keramidas, & Lynch, 2015), these findings potentially implicate GlyRs in autism. Moreover, autism is also known to be caused by hereditary mutations to gephyrin (Lionel et al., 2013), another protein which is responsible for clustering GlyRs at synapses.

GlyRs containing α2 subunits exert excitatory effects in immature neurons, and α2 GlyR activity has been shown to modulate the rate of neuronal migration and synapse formation during neurodevelopment (Avila et al., 2013). Microdeletions and missense mutations in *GLYA*2 gene, encoding the GlyR α2 subunit, have been reported to represent a rare cause of ASDs (Pilorge et al., 2015; Piton et al., 2011). A recent study demonstrated that *GLYA2* mutations associated with ASD cause reduced surface expression and glycine sensitivity, as well as an aberrant plasticity in the prefrontal cortex that resulted from altered glycinergic transmission (Pilorge et al., 2015). Further investigation of the precise link between *GLYRA2* dysfunction and neuronal migration abnormalities related to ASDs may provide essential insights into the underlying molecular mechanisms of these disorders.

Since disruption to α2 GlyR function is only one of many causes of ASD, it seems likely that pharmacological potentiation of α2 GlyR function may correct only those ASD phenotypes caused by α2 GlyR disruption. However, this raises two questions. First, will such a drug be effective only if applied at the appropriate (prenatal) developmental time point? If so, this would require prenatal diagnosis and drug delivery in utero. Second, would such a drug be able to treat ASD phenotypes caused by other factors? Addressing these questions are important priorities for the field.

3.3 Chronic Inflammatory Pain

Nociceptors located in the skin, deep tissues, and viscera signal the presence of noxious stimuli and transmit this information to nociceptive neurons in laminae I and II (the outermost strata) of the spinal cord dorsal horn (Zeilhofer, Wildner, & Yevenes, 2012). In lamina I neurons, synaptic inhibition is almost exclusively mediated by glycine (Chery & de Koninck, 1999).

Inflammation often leads to exaggerated pain sensation as a result of an increase in responsiveness of peripheral nociceptors (hyperalgesia) or by conversion of nonpainful into painful stimuli (allodynia). It is well established that inflammatory pain is mediated in part by the production of prostaglandins both in peripheral tissues and in the spinal cord (Vanegas & Schaible, 2001). Electrophysiological studies have identified PGE_2 as the most active prostaglandin in the spinal cord (Zeilhofer, 2005). PGE_2 was found to specifically inhibit glycinergic IPSCs in lamina I and II nociceptive neurons (Ahmadi, Lippross, Neuhuber, & Zeilhofer, 2002). This effect, mediated via activation of prostaglandin E_2 receptor, involved the activation of a cholera toxin-sensitive G protein and a cAMP-dependent protein kinase A (PKA). This important finding implied that chronic inflammatory pain sensitization is mediated, at least in part, by an inhibition of spinal glycinergic IPSCs.

Evidence to date indicates that GlyR α1 and α3 subunits are equally represented at glycinergic synapses in lamina I and II neurons (Harvey et al., 2004). The same study also showed that recombinantly expressed α3 GlyRs were inhibited by PGE_2 via PKA-dependent phosphorylation (Harvey et al., 2004). However, α1 GlyRs, which do not have PKA phosphorylation sites, were not affected. This prompted the hypothesis that the α3 subunit was specifically modulated by inflammatory stimuli. A GlyR α3 knockout mouse was generated to test this theory further. Although GlyR $\alpha3^{-/-}$ mice displayed no overt behavioral phenotype, the PGE_2-dependent decrease of lamina II glycinergic IPSCs was abolished in these mice (Harvey et al., 2004). Behaviorally, normal and knockout mice responded similarly to non-painful tactile stimuli and acute inflammatory pain stimuli. However, chronic peripheral inflammation produced pain sensitization in normal animals but not in the GlyR $\alpha3^{-/-}$ animals (Harvey et al., 2004). Satisfyingly, $EP_2^{-/-}$ mice exhibited identical behavior (Reinold et al., 2005). In addition, targeted ablation of spinal glycinergic interneurons has confirmed their important role in nociceptive and itch pathways (Foster et al., 2015). Together, these results show that currents carried by α3-containing GlyRs are specifically inhibited during chronic inflammation. Inhibition of α3 GlyRs reduces the inhibitory drive onto nociceptive projection neurons, thus increasing the transmission of nociceptive stimuli to the brain. A model detailing our understanding of the role of α3 GlyRs in chronic pain sensitization is shown in Fig. 2.

Agents that potentiate glycinergic currents should therefore be useful for treating chronic inflammatory pain. Because α1 and α3 GlyR subunits are both expressed in inhibitory synapses on nociceptive neurons, potentiation of either or both receptors should produce analgesia. The α3 GlyR is

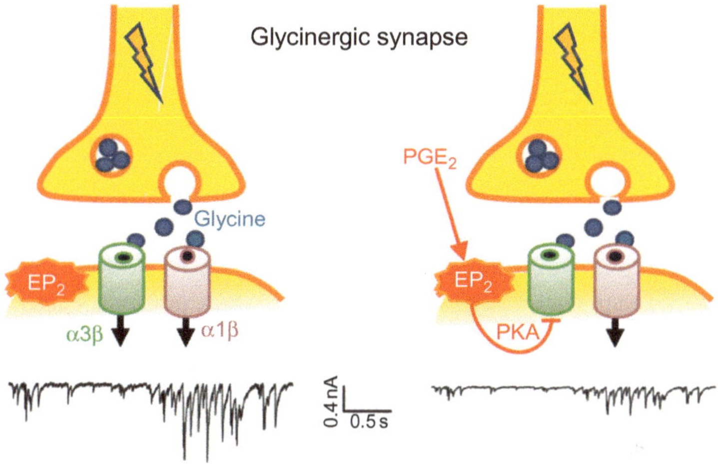

Fig. 2 Model of a glycinergic synapse onto a dorsal horn nociceptive neuron. The *left panel* shows the control (pain free) situation where Cl influx is mediated by both α1β and α3β GlyRs. The *right panel* shows the effect of PGE_2 on glycinergic signaling. PGE_2 activates EP_2 receptors which in turn phosphorylate α3 GlyRs in a PKA-dependent manner, thereby inhibiting Cl flux through α3β GlyRs. This leads to a downregulation in IPSC magnitude and the subsequent disinhibition of nociceptive neurons.

considered a more promising therapeutic target as its sparse distribution outside the dorsal horn implies a reduced risk of side effects (Lynch & Callister, 2006; Zeilhofer, 2005). However, the α1 GlyR should not be dismissed as a potential analgesic target for three reasons: (a) it may prove difficult to develop drugs that can overcome the strong inhibition caused by the phosphorylation of α3-containing GlyRs, (b) experiments to date indicate that potentiation of α1 GlyRs alleviates pain without impairing motor performance (Xiong et al., 2011), and (c) a clinical concentration (1 nM) of the well-tolerated antinausea drug, tropisetron, potentiates α1β GlyR-mediated IPSCs without causing movement or other side effects (Zhang, Bode, et al., 2016). Given that α1 GlyRs mediate inhibitory transmission spinal motor reflex arcs (Lynch, 2009), impairment of motor performance should be one of the major visible consequences of inappropriate α1 GlyR modulation. Given these considerations, we conclude that potentiation of α1 GlyRs is not a strong criterion by which to exclude compounds as potential treatments for chronic inflammatory pain. Although GlyRs have so far been formally implicated as targets for chronic inflammatory pain only, GlyR-potentiating drugs are also successful at treating neuropathic pain (Bregman et al., 2017; Xiong et al., 2011; Xiong, Cui, et al., 2012).

It is estimated that ~20% of adult Australians suffer chronic pain in any 6-month period (Brennan, Carr, & Cousins, 2007). In 2012, the cost of chronic pain in the United States was estimated at $600 billion/year (Gaskin & Richard, 2012). Unfortunately, most currently available pain treatments exhibit limited analgesic efficacy and dose-limiting side effects. As noted in a recent review, "despite substantial financial investment by the pharmaceutical industry over several decades, there has been little progress in developing new efficacious and safe analgesics" (Woolf, 2010). New pain targets are therefore desperately needed, and the GlyR certainly provides a promising new therapeutic opportunity. It is thus not surprising that many academic and commercial laboratories are actively pursuing novel therapeutics targeting this receptor type.

3.4 Breathing Disorders

Inhibitory interactions between neurons of the brain stem respiratory network enable stable rhythmic breathing. A failure of glycinergic inhibitory transmission has been implicated in impairment of respiratory rhythm (Busselberg, Bischoff, Becker, Becker, & Richter, 2001; Pierrefiche, Schwarzacher, Bischoff, & Richter, 1998; Schmid, Bohmer, & Gebauer, 1991), which may lead to sudden death (Busselberg et al., 2001; Harvey et al., 2008; Markstahler, Kremer, Kimmina, Becker, & Richter, 2002). The rhythmic activity of this neuronal network is maintained by serotonin receptor type 1 receptor activation, which ensures that synaptic α3 GlyRs remain in a dephosphorylated, and thus maximally activated, state (Manzke et al., 2010). Thus, drugs that selectively potentiate α3 GlyRs should be useful for correcting breathing disturbances caused by hyperekplexia or opioid-induced apnea. However, this hypothesis has yet to be tested. Nevertheless, it seems possible that the α3 GlyR-specific potentiators that are currently being developed as treatments for chronic pain (see later) may have a secondary application as treatments for opioid-induced breathing depression.

3.5 Temporal Lobe Epilepsy

In addition to processing of nociceptive signals, extrasynaptic α3 GlyRs are also involved in the hippocampal pathophysiology of temporal lobe epilepsy (Eichler et al., 2009, 2008; Meier et al., 2005). It has been demonstrated that posttranscriptional RNA editing produces a new gain-of-function GlyR α3 isoform, the GlyR $\alpha3^{P185L}$, that results from cytidine 554 deamination

(C554U) (Meier et al., 2005). The proline to leucine editing of GlyR α3 remarkably enhances sensitivity to glycine, and thus, these channels remain open for longer during each synaptic event (Dixon, Zhang, & Lynch, 2015; Legendre, Forstera, Juttner, & Meier, 2009; Meier et al., 2005). Additionally, RNA editing of GlyR α2 at the corresponding position (P192L) was found in patients with temporal lobe epilepsy, and this also produces receptors with increased agonist affinities (Eichler et al., 2008). These GlyRs are expressed extrasynaptically in both the cortex and the hippocampus.

It thus seems that the selective inhibition of RNA-edited high-affinity α2 or α3 GlyRs may provide a treatment for temporal lobe epilepsy. As the edited proline residue is located close to the glycine-binding site, the development of blockers specific for RNA-edited GlyRs should be feasible. However, it is yet to be determined whether such blockers would provide a generalized epilepsy treatment or whether they would be useful for only those patients with phenotypes caused by RNA-edited GlyRs.

3.6 Alcoholism

GlyRs mediate inhibition in the brain stem and in higher brain areas (e.g., nucleus accumbens) that are known to be sensitive to ethanol modulation (Molander & Soderpalm, 2005a, 2005b). GlyRs are positively modulated by ethanol at behaviorally relevant concentrations, and the ethanol-binding sites and molecular modulatory mechanisms of ethanol have been characterized intensively (Burgos, Munoz, Guzman, & Aguayo, 2015; Perkins, Trudell, Crawford, Alkana, & Davies, 2010). The involvement of GlyRs in the intoxicating effects of alcohol is supported by a variety of evidence from behavioral studies. For example, the loss-of-righting effects of ethanol in mice are antagonized by strychnine, a GlyR-specific antagonist (Williams, Ferko, Barbieri, & DiGregorio, 1995). Transgenic expression of the mutant $\alpha1^{S276Q}$ GlyR subunit that disrupts the ethanol-binding site also renders mice resistant to ethanol (Findlay et al., 2002). There is evidence that extrasynaptic GlyRs in the nucleus accumbens are involved in the initiation, maintenance, and relapse phases of alcohol addiction (Vengeliene, Bilbao, Molander, & Spanagel, 2008). Indeed, it has recently been proposed that accumbal GlyRs may also be involved in mediating the addictive effects of nicotine and tetrahydrocannabinol (Jonsson, Adermark, Ericson, & Soderpalm, 2014). Thus, the development of inhibitors that prevent the actions of ethanol on α1 and α2 GlyRs could provide a treatment for acute alcohol intoxication or addiction.

3.7 Motor Neuron Disease

Motor neuron disease or amyotrophic lateral sclerosis (ALS) is a fatal adult-onset neurological disease that results from the progressive degeneration of motor neurons. It has been shown that the glycinergic innervation of motor neurons in an ALS mouse model is deficient due to a reduction in surface expression of GlyRs (Chang & Martin, 2009, 2011). This would chronically enhance the excitability of motor neurons and could plausibly contribute to the pathogenesis of ALS. Therapies that increase the surface expression or pharmacologically enhance the activation of synaptic α1β GlyRs may thus provide a treatment for ALS. This possibility has yet to be investigated in animal models.

4. GlyR PHARMACOLOGY

4.1 Competitive Antagonist: Strychnine

GlyR channels are activated by the amino acid agonists, glycine, taurine, and β-alanine and efficiently antagonized by the plant alkaloid, strychnine. Strychnine inhibits the function of GlyRs in a competitive manner with a K_i near 20 nM (Akagi, Hirai, & Hishinuma, 1991; Brams et al., 2011). The binding site for both glycinergic agonists and strychnine is located in a pocket at the interface of adjacent subunits in the extracellular N-terminal domain (Fig. 1C). The core strychnine-binding residues are highly conserved across the GlyR subunits but not in other pLGIC members. This accounts for the high selectivity of strychnine for GlyRs over other receptor types. Strychnine is commonly used to pharmacologically separate glycinergic from GABAergic IPSCs in physiological experiments.

4.2 Allosteric Agonist: Ivermectin

Glutamate-gated chloride channel receptors (GluRs) are members of the pLGIC family that are found predominantly in nematodes and arthropods, but they are not found in any vertebrate species. GluRs are expressed in the neurons and muscle cells of parasitic nematodes (McCavera, Rogers, Yates, Woods, & Wolstenholme, 2009). Ivermectin, a naturally occurring macrocyclic lactone, potently activates the GluR. Because this efficiently paralyzes or kills many parasitic nematode and arthropod pests, ivermectin is commercially used as an antiparasitic agent in human medicine, agriculture, and veterinary practice (Omura, 2008). A previous study from our laboratory showed that ivermectin irreversibly activates α1-containing GlyRs with an EC_{50} of 0.39 μM (Shan, Haddrill, & Lynch, 2001). Substitution of the residue Ala-288 (in TM3) and Pro-230 (in TM1) profoundly disrupted GlyR sensitivity to ivermectin, suggesting that the transmembrane regions play a crucial role in influencing allosteric modulation by ivermectin (Lynagh, Webb, Dixon, Cromer, & Lynch, 2011). The molecular structure of the α1 GlyR with ivermectin docked has recently been published (Du et al., 2015), and this confirms that it binds in the pocket lined by Ala-288 and Pro-230. In addition, ivermectin was found to exert significant allosteric modulatory effects on other pLGICs, notably α7 nAChRs and $GABA_A$Rs (Krause et al., 1998; Krusek & Zemkova, 1994). Many ivermectin analogues and their aglyconic relatives, the milbemycins, are also potent irreversible agonists at GlyRs (Lynagh & Lynch, 2010; Lynagh et al., 2011).

4.3 Allosteric Modulators

A large number of small-molecule GlyR allosteric modulators have been identified. Examples of potent modulators that have been extensively characterized on different GlyR subtypes include cannabinoids (Hejazi et al., 2006; Xiong, Wu, et al., 2012; Yang et al., 2008; Yevenes & Zeilhofer, 2011b), cyanotriphenylborate (Rundstrom, Schmieden, Betz, Bormann, & Langosch, 1994), ethanol (Burgos et al., 2015; Perkins et al., 2010), dihydropyridines (Chen et al., 2009; Chesnoy-Marchais & Cathala, 2001), gelsemine (Lara et al., 2016), ginkgolides (Hawthorne, Cromer, Ng, Parker, & Lynch, 2006; Heads, Hawthorne, Lynagh, & Lynch, 2008; Jensen, Bergmann, Sander, & Balle, 2010; Kondratskaya, Betz, Krishtal, & Laube, 2005), ginkgolic acid (Maleeva, Buldakova, & Bregestovski, 2015), bilobalide (Lynch & Chen, 2008), lindane (Islam & Lynch, 2012), fipronil (Islam & Lynch, 2012), propofol (Acuna et al., 2016; Ahrens et al., 2004), and other anesthetics (Lobo & Harris, 2005; Olsen et al., 2014), glutamate (Liu, Wu, & Wang, 2010), neuroactive steroids (Maksay, Laube, & Betz, 2001), tropeines (Maksay, 1998; Maksay et al., 2009; Supplisson & Chesnoy-Marchais, 2000; Yang, Ney, et al., 2007), and picrotoxin (Hawthorne & Lynch, 2005; Pribilla, Takagi, Langosch, Bormann, & Betz, 1992; Yang, Cromer, Harvey, Parker, & Lynch, 2007). In most cases, these modulators display little specificity among different GlyR α subtypes, and many have potent effects on unrelated receptor types. Nevertheless, the studies listed earlier have defined a variety of druggable binding pockets in the GlyR. The discovery of highly potent, subtype-selective GlyR pharmacological inhibitors would be very useful in helping to define the physiological roles of specific GlyR isoforms in different regions of the mammalian brain.

Many other molecules are also known to modulate GlyRs. Examples of other modulators with relatively low-potency effects on GlyRs can be found in recent reviews (Betz & Laube, 2006; Webb & Lynch, 2007; Yevenes & Zeilhofer, 2011a). It is interesting to note that a recent study that performed a virtual screen of 1549 FDA-approved drugs against the α1 GlyR discovered 12 new molecules with strong potentiating effects (Wells et al., 2015). However, their binding sites and mechanisms of action have yet to be investigated. Compounds developed as novel analgesic lead candidates are described separately later.

4.4 Metals

Zn^{2+} ions allosterically modulate GlyRs in a dose-dependent manner. Low (20 nM to 10 μM) concentrations of Zn^{2+} potentiate glycine-activated currents, and higher concentrations (>10 μM) of Zn^{2+} inhibit glycine-evoked currents (Bloomenthal, Goldwater, Pritchett, & Harrison, 1994; Laube et al., 1995; Miller, Beato, Harvey, & Smart, 2005; Miller, Da Silva, & Smart, 2005). The locations of the potentiating and inhibitory sites have been characterized in detail (Grudzinska, Schumann, Schemm, Betz, & Laube, 2008; Lynch, Jacques, Pierce, & Schofield, 1998; Miller, Beato, et al., 2005; Miller, Da Silva, et al., 2005; Miller, Topf, & Smart, 2008; Nevin et al., 2003). Evidence has recently been presented for presynaptically released Zn^{2+} reaching a concentration of at least 1 μM in the glycinergic synaptic cleft following a single presynaptic stimulation (Zhang, Keramidas, & Lynch, 2016). This Zn^{2+} concentration significantly prolongs the IPSC decay time. No other metal is known to mimic the biphasic actions of Zn^{2+}. However, GlyRs are also potentiated by Pb^{2+}, La^{3+}, and Co^{2+} and inhibited by Ni^{2+} and Cu^{2+} (Lynch, 2004).

4.5 Zn^{2+}, a Potential Confound in GlyR Drug Discovery

Zn^{2+} is commonly used as a catalyst in chemical synthesis, and it is difficult to remove it from compound samples. This can create a problem whereby the presumed pharmacological effect of a compound may actually be due to the contaminating Zn^{2+}. One solution to this is to perform all drug screening experiments in the presence of a Zn^{2+} buffer such as tricine. However, as Zn^{2+} is present at low nanomolar concentrations in the cerebrospinal fluid (Frederickson et al., 2006) and at higher concentrations in the synapse

(Zhang, Keramidas, et al., 2016), excessive Zn^{2+} buffering would result in a nonphysiological receptor environment. It is possible, for example, that a potentially valuable drug may require a low concentration of Zn^{2+} as a coagonist. Indeed, evidence has been presented that this is the case: peptides, isoflurane, and ethanol all exert much weaker effects on GlyRs when Zn^{2+} is removed from the extracellular solution (Cornelison, Pflanz, Tipps, & Mihic, 2016; Kirson, Cornelison, Philpo, Todorovic, & Mihic, 2013; McCracken, Trudell, Goldstein, Harris, & Mihic, 2010). Rather than buffer Zn^{2+} to nonphysiologically low levels, we recommend quantifying the Zn^{2+} concentration in drug samples of interest via inductively coupled plasma mass spectroscopy. Providing the contaminating Zn^{2+} does not attain a concentration of >10 nM once dissolved into the perfusion solution, direct effects on the GlyR are highly unlikely.

5. TECHNOLOGIES FOR GlyR DRUG DISCOVERY

5.1 Fluorescence Assays

Fluorescence-based assays are commonly used for primary high-throughput drug screens because they allow many cells to be evaluated simultaneously. They are also relatively cheap, fast, and offer high signal-to-noise ratios. Although a range of fluorescence-based assays have been employed to screen GlyRs (Lynch, 2005), here we will consider only voltage-sensitive dyes and yellow fluorescent protein (YFP).

The fluorescent membrane potential (FMP) dye (molecular devices) has long been a voltage-sensitive dye of choice for primary drug screening at ligand-gated chloride channels (Jensen & Kristiansen, 2004). As an exogenously applied indicator, it involves a significant recurrent expense. Exogenously applied indicators often also require separate dye-loading and wash steps that increase the number of process steps. Another concern is that such dyes are taken up by all cells regardless of whether they express the GlyR isoform of interest. Thus, if 50% of cells do not express the GlyR, then the dynamic range of the fluorescence response is halved (assuming one is averaging the fluorescence response from all cells). Exogenous indicators, such as FMP, are therefore best suited to screening stably expressing cell lines.

YFP is quenched by halide anions and is thus suited to detecting anion influx into cells. We employ the YFP-I152L mutant (Galietta, Haggie, & Verkman, 2001), which is rapidly and potently quenched by iodide influx through open GlyRs. This assay has three advantages over the FMP assay.

First, the YFP assay is threefold faster in achieving a given percentage fluorescence change following GlyR activation (Kruger et al., 2005). Second, as a genetically encoded probe, it is inexpensive to propagate. Third, the simultaneous transfection of YFP and ion channel cDNAs in separate plasmid vectors results in a high rate of coexpression of YFP and the GlyR of interest in individual cells (Kruger et al., 2005). Thus, this assay does not require stably expressing cell lines to achieve its full dynamic range. A description of the custom-built fluorescence screening equipment we use for YFP-based assays has previously been presented (Kruger et al., 2005), along with descriptions of our cell transfection techniques, drug screening methodologies, and our image analysis techniques (Gilbert, Esmaeili, & Lynch, 2009; Gilbert, Islam, Lynagh, Lynch, & Webb, 2009; Gilbert, Meinhof, Pepperkok, & Runz, 2009; Talwar, Lynch, & Gilbert, 2013). Our laboratory employs YFP imaging in live cells for all preliminary drug screens.

5.2 Electrophysiology

Patch clamping is considered the "gold standard" for ion channel screening due to its unrivaled signal-to-noise ratio and temporal resolution. However, conventional patch clamping is far too laborious for high-throughput screening. Automated patch-clamp technologies have been steadily advancing over the past 15 years with several planar chip devices, including the Biolin Scientific/Sophion Qube (Chambers, Witton, Adams, Marrington, & Kammonen, 2016) and the Nanion Syncropatch 384PE (Obergrussberger et al., 2015), capable of high-throughput primary drug screening. However, these machines and the single-use planar chips they employ are expensive. We employ either a manual patch clamp or a Nanion Patchliner (Bruggemann, Stoelzle, George, Behrends, & Fertig, 2006) to confirm hits identified in the YFP-based assay. The Patchliner permits the simultaneous whole-cell recording from eight cells at once at a moderate cost. A major advantage of planar chip devices is that the extracellular solution can be exchanged with as little as 25 μL of new solution, which is useful when screening the minute quantities of compounds that are typically provided from natural product libraries.

5.3 Artificial Synapses

When evaluating drugs as potential therapeutic lead compounds at synaptic GlyRs, it is important to test their potency, efficacy, and subtype selectivity under realistic synaptic activation conditions. Although one option is to study the effects of drugs on glycinergic IPSCs in neurons, the interpretation of results is complicated by the presence of multiple unknown GlyR isoforms in neurons. These concerns can be addressed by testing drugs on IPSCs mediated by "artificial" glycinergic synapses that can be induced to form between glycinergic neurons and HEK293 cells that express the desired GlyR isoform (Dixon et al., 2015). This system has been validated by demonstrating that the rise and decay rates of IPSCs mediated by wild-type and mutant α1β, α2β, and α3β GlyRs in artificial synapses correspond closely to those mediated by the same isoforms in neurons (Dixon et al., 2015; Zhang et al., 2015). We consider drug screening in glycinergic artificial synapses to be an important part of the GlyR drug evaluation procedure.

5.4 Virtual Screening

As high-resolution molecular structures are now available for the α1 and α3 GlyRs in multiple conformations (Du et al., 2015; Huang et al., 2015, 2017), virtual screening technologies can now be used with a high level of confidence to discover new GlyR modulators. Indeed, as described earlier, this has already been successfully achieved (Wells et al., 2015). With the steady increase in the number of relevant pLGIC molecular structures and the rapid advances in virtual screening algorithms and computational power, computational screening is destined to play an increasingly important role in the GlyR drug discovery.

6. PROGRESS TOWARD DEVELOPING GlyR-TARGETED ANALGESICS

△9-tetrahydrocannabinol (THC), the main psychoactive component of marijuana, is well known to directly potentiate GlyRs (Hejazi et al., 2006; Yang et al., 2008). When the 1- and 5-hydroxy groups were individually removed from THC, the resulting compounds retained full potentiating efficacy at α1 and α3 GlyRs, although their ability to activate CB1 and CB2 G protein-coupled receptors was completely ablated (Xiong et al., 2011). In contrast, di-desoxy-THC did not potentiate GlyRs but rather antagonized the potentiating actions of 1- and 5-desoxy-THC on GlyRs. By comparing the effects of these compounds on pain-related behaviors in wild-type and $\alpha3^{-/-}$ knockout mice, the authors demonstrated that the analgesic effects of THC and 5-desoxy-THC are mediated by α3 GlyRs (Xiong et al., 2011). This provided the first demonstration that chronic inflammatory pain could be relieved via pharmacological enhancement of α3 GlyR currents. A follow-up publication from the same group demonstrated that THC potentiation of α3 GlyRs was also effective against neuropathic pain (Xiong, Cui, et al., 2012). Furthermore, although the THC derivatives also potentiated α1 GlyRs, this did not result in motor or other side effects.

The nonanesthetic propofol derivative, 2,6-di-*tert*-butylphenol (2,6-DTBP), has long been known to potentiate homomeric GlyRs (Ahrens et al., 2004). A recent study demonstrated that this compound does not potentiate heteromeric α3β GlyRs unless they have been phosphorylated (Acuna et al., 2016). This fits with an earlier observation that α3 GlyR phosphorylation induces a global conformational change throughout the receptor which may alter the structure of drug-binding pockets (Han, Talwar, Wang, Shan, & Lynch, 2013). In mouse models of inflammatory pain, 2,6-DTBP produced analgesia in an α3 GlyR-dependent manner (Acuna et al., 2016). This important result supports the idea of α3 GlyR phosphorylation underlying inflammatory pain sensitization.

A range of approaches have been applied to discovering novel classes of compounds with potentiating effects on α1 GlyRs. These include the development of RNA aptamers (Shalaly et al., 2015) and heptapeptides (Cornelison et al., 2016), as well as computational screening as described earlier (Wells et al., 2015). Although these studies made no attempt to identify α3-specific modulators and the potencies of identified drugs were generally low (EC_{50} values >0.3 μM), they have identified new structural scaffolds that may warrant further interest.

A team from Pfizer recently published the results of a high-throughput screen of a proprietary small-molecule, ion channel-targeted library of 56,558 compounds against α3 and α3β GlyRs (Stead et al., 2016). A first-round FMP assay identified 214 hits of which 147 were progressed to an automated patch-clamp assay. This second-round assay identified seven compounds as efficient α3 GlyR potentiators. The compound of most interest, 4-fluoro-*N*-(2-(quinolin-8-yloxy)ethyl)benzenesulfonamide, exhibited favorable physicochemical properties and highly efficacious potentiation in the 1–10 μM concentration range. Although it was selective for GlyRs over r $GABA_A$Rs, it was not selective for α3 GlyRs over α1 GlyRs (Stead et al., 2016).

A team from Amgen has recently reported the development of a series of novel GlyR potentiators as candidate analgesics (Bregman et al., 2017). An initial high-throughput screen led to the discovery of a tricyclic sulfonamide that potentiated α3 GlyRs, albeit with a low potency and a suboptimal pharmacokinetic profile. Extensive structure–activity investigations around this scaffold led to the development of a molecule, AM-1488, with greatly improved potency and pharmacokinetic properties. When delivered orally, this molecule successfully reversed tactile allodynia in a mouse model of neuropathic pain. A related compound with strong potentiating effects on α3 GlyRs, AM-3607, was cocrystallized with the human α3 GlyR and was found to bind in a novel pocket at the extracellular subunit interface just above the glycine-binding pocket (Bregman et al., 2017; Huang et al., 2017). Fig. 1E depicts AM-3607 docked into this site. Notably, none of the Amgen compounds appear to be selective for α3 over α1 GlyRs (Huang et al., 2017).

Our GlyR drug discovery program focussed initially on screening marine natural product libraries provided by our collaborator Prof. Rob Capon (Balansa et al., 2010; Balansa, Islam, Fontaine, et al., 2013; Balansa, Islam, Gilbert, et al., 2013). We originally screened >2500 marine fractions against both α1 and α3 GlyRs using the YFP assay and identified a total of 27 active fractions. Based on knowledge of the compound families present in the active fractions, we identified and screened an array of sesterterpene tetronic acids from three geographically distinct sponges of the family Irciniidae. These compounds showed potent subunit-selective GlyR modulation in an electrophysiological assay (Balansa et al., 2010). In addition, bioassay-guided fractionation of three southern Australian marine sponges of the genus *Psammocinia* yielded rare marine sesterterpenes such as (−)-ircinianin and (−)-ircinianin sulfate along with biosynthetically related metabolites (−)-iricinianin lactam and analogues. Several of these metabolites showed selective GlyR modulation with one of them showing strong selective potentiation of α3 over α1 GlyRs (Balansa, Islam, Fontaine, et al., 2013). Examples of the effects of this compound on α1 and α3 GlyRs are shown in Fig. 3A and B, with an averaged potentiating dose–response at α3 GlyRs presented in Fig. 3C.

Due to limited raw material availability and the presence of several chiral centers in the natural product molecules, the compounds were not ideal from a medicinal chemistry point of view. However, our collaborators have since synthesized novel synthetic molecules based on a de novo approach from the pharmacophores reported earlier to eliminate the chiral centers and to overcome the resupply limitation. This has resulted in the discovery of a highly potent α3 GlyR-preferring potentiator with favorable physicochemical properties, strong analgesic potency, and no effect on $GABA_ARs$ (unpublished results).

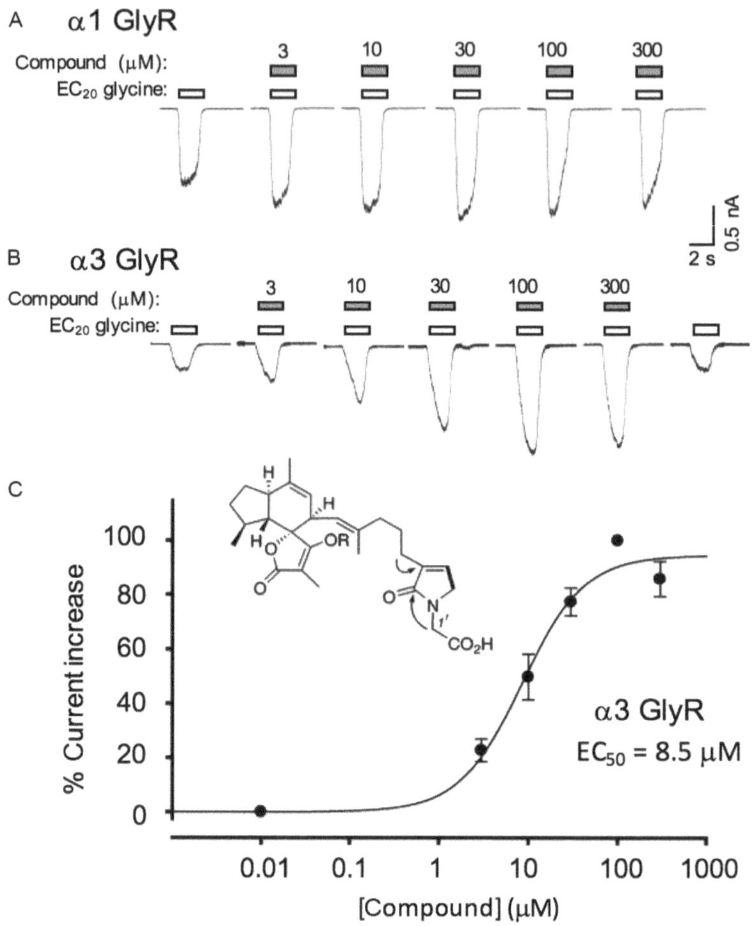

Fig. 3 Effects of the sesterterpene glycinyl-lactam, (−)-ircinianin lactam A, on glycine-activated currents in α1 and α3 GlyRs. Currents were activated by 2 s applications of an EC_{20} glycine concentration, applied either alone or together with the indicated concentration of compound. (A) The compound had no significant effect on α1 GlyRs. (B) The compound exhibited highly efficacious potentiation of α3 GlyRs. (C) Averaged dose–response relationship for the compound at α3 GlyRs. The compound structure is shown in the inset. See Balansa, Islam, Fontaine, et al. (2013) for full details of the methodology.

7. CONCLUSION

Although it is possible that GlyRs may eventually be clinically targeted to treat a variety of neurological disorders, most research to date has focused on developing GlyR-targeted treatments for chronic inflammatory pain. It is now well established that drugs that potentiate α3β GlyRs in vivo are effective in alleviating chronic pain. The eventual development of a GlyR-targeted analgesic thus appears feasible. In an attempt to facilitate these efforts, we reiterate two points. First, the question of possible Zn^{2+} contamination of drug samples must always be considered. Second, dogma has it that potentiation of α1-containing GlyRs should be avoided due to these receptors being more widespread in neural circuits outside the dorsal horn. In our experience, however, strict adherence to this rule would drastically reduce the number of compounds available for further development, and indeed, there is as yet no evidence that the modest potentiation of α1-containing GlyRs causes motor or other side effects. Thus, we consider that drugs that potentiate both α1- and α3-containing GlyRs are suitable as therapeutic candidates.

CONFLICT OF INTEREST STATEMENT

The authors have no conflicts of interest to declare.

ACKNOWLEDGMENTS

Funding for drug discovery research in the author's laboratory has been provided by the Australian Research Council (A09800748) and the National Health and Medical Research Council (301023, 569570, 1058542). We acknowledge the contributions of numerous colleagues to the research outlined in this review.

REFERENCES

Acuna, M. A., Yevenes, G. E., Ralvenius, W. T., Benke, D., Di Lio, A., Lara, C. O., et al. (2016). Phosphorylation state-dependent modulation of spinal glycine receptors alleviates inflammatory pain. *The Journal of Clinical Investigation*, *126*, 2547–2560.

Ahmadi, S., Lippross, S., Neuhuber, W. L., & Zeilhofer, H. U. (2002). PGE(2) selectively blocks inhibitory glycinergic neurotransmission onto rat superficial dorsal horn neurons. *Nature Neuroscience*, *5*, 34–40.

Ahrens, J., Haeseler, G., Leuwer, M., Mohammadi, B., Krampfl, K., Dengler, R., et al. (2004). 2,6-Di-tert-butylphenol, a nonanesthetic propofol analog, modulates alpha1beta glycine receptor function in a manner distinct from propofol. *Anesthésie et Analgésie*, *99*, 91–96.

Akagi, H., Hirai, K., & Hishinuma, F. (1991). Functional properties of strychnine-sensitive glycine receptors expressed in Xenopus oocytes injected with a single mRNA. *Neuroscience Research*, *11*, 28–40.

Avila, A., Nguyen, L., & Rigo, J. M. (2013). Glycine receptors and brain development. *Frontiers in Cellular Neuroscience*, *7*, 184.

Bakker, M. J., van Dijk, J. G., van den Maagdenberg, A. M., & Tijssen, M. A. (2006). Startle syndromes. *Lancet Neurology*, *5*, 513–524.

Balansa, W., Islam, R., Fontaine, F., Piggott, A. M., Zhang, H., Webb, T. I., et al. (2010). Ircinialactams: Subunit-selective glycine receptor modulators from Australian sponges of the family Irciniidae. *Bioorganic & Medicinal Chemistry*, *18*, 2912–2919.

Balansa, W., Islam, R., Fontaine, F., Piggott, A. M., Zhang, H., Xiao, X., et al. (2013a). Sesterterpene glycinyl-lactams: A new class of glycine receptor modulator from Australian marine sponges of the genus Psammocinia. *Organic & Biomolecular Chemistry, 11*, 4695–4701.

Balansa, W., Islam, R., Gilbert, D. F., Fontaine, F., Xiao, X., Zhang, H., et al. (2013b). Australian marine sponge alkaloids as a new class of glycine-gated chloride channel receptor modulator. *Bioorganic & Medicinal Chemistry, 21*, 4420–4425.

Beato, M. (2008). The time course of transmitter at glycinergic synapses onto motoneurons. *Journal of Neuroscience, 28*, 7412–7425.

Betz, H., & Laube, B. (2006). Glycine receptors: Recent insights into their structural organization and functional diversity. *Journal of Neurochemistry, 97*, 1600–1610.

Bloomenthal, A. B., Goldwater, E., Pritchett, D. B., & Harrison, N. L. (1994). Biphasic modulation of the strychnine-sensitive glycine receptor by Zn^{2+}. *Molecular Pharmacology, 46*, 1156–1159.

Bode, A., & Lynch, J. W. (2013). Analysis of hyperekplexia mutations identifies transmembrane domain rearrangements that mediate glycine receptor activation. *Journal of Biological Chemistry, 288*, 33760–33771.

Bode, A., & Lynch, J. W. (2014). The impact of human hyperekplexia mutations on glycine receptor structure and function. *Molecular Brain, 7*, 2.

Brams, M., Pandya, A., Kuzmin, D., van Elk, R., Krijnen, L., Yakel, J. L., et al. (2011). A structural and mutagenic blueprint for molecular recognition of strychnine and D-tubocurarine by different cys-loop receptors. *PLoS Biology, 9*, e1001034.

Bregman, H., Simard, J. R., Andrews, K. L., Ayube, S., Chen, H., Gunaydin, H., et al. (2017). The discovery and hit-to-lead optimization of tricyclic sulfonamides as potent and efficacious potentiators of glycine receptors. *Journal of Medicinal Chemistry, 60*, 1105–1125.

Brennan, F., Carr, D. B., & Cousins, M. (2007). Pain management: A fundamental human right. *Anesthésie et Analgésie, 105*, 205–221.

Bruggemann, A., Stoelzle, S., George, M., Behrends, J. C., & Fertig, N. (2006). Microchip technology for automated and parallel patch-clamp recording. *Small, 2*, 840–846.

Buescher, A. V., Cidav, Z., Knapp, M., & Mandell, D. S. (2014). Costs of autism spectrum disorders in the United Kingdom and the United States. *JAMA Pediatrics, 168*, 721–728.

Burgos, C. F., Munoz, B., Guzman, L., & Aguayo, L. G. (2015). Ethanol effects on glycinergic transmission: From molecular pharmacology to behavior responses. *Pharmacological Research, 101*, 18–29.

Busselberg, D., Bischoff, A. M., Becker, K., Becker, C. M., & Richter, D. W. (2001). The respiratory rhythm in mutant oscillator mice. *Neuroscience Letters, 316*, 99–102.

Carland, J. E., Cooper, M. A., Sugiharto, S., Jeong, H. J., Lewis, T. M., Barry, P. H., et al. (2009). Characterization of the effects of charged residues in the intracellular loop on ion permeation in alpha1 glycine receptor channels. *The Journal of Biological Chemistry, 284*, 2023–2030.

Chambers, C., Witton, I., Adams, C., Marrington, L., & Kammonen, J. (2016). High-throughput screening of Na(V)1.7 modulators using a giga-seal automated patch clamp instrument. *Assay and Drug Development Technologies, 14*, 93–108.

Chang, Q., & Martin, L. J. (2009). Glycinergic innervation of motoneurons is deficient in amyotrophic lateral sclerosis mice: A quantitative confocal analysis. *The American Journal of Pathology, 174*, 574–585.

Chang, Q., & Martin, L. J. (2011). Glycine receptor channels in spinal motoneurons are abnormal in a transgenic mouse model of amyotrophic lateral sclerosis. *The Journal of Neuroscience, 31*, 2815–2827.

Chen, X., Cromer, B., Webb, T. I., Yang, Z., Hantke, J., Harvey, R. J., et al. (2009). Dihydropyridine inhibition of the glycine receptor: Subunit selectivity and a molecular determinant of inhibition. *Neuropharmacology, 56*, 318–327.

Chery, N., & de Koninck, Y. (1999). Junctional versus extrajunctional glycine and GABA(A) receptor-mediated IPSCs in identified lamina I neurons of the adult rat spinal cord. *The Journal of Neuroscience, 19*, 7342–7355.

Chesnoy-Marchais, D., & Cathala, L. (2001). Modulation of glycine responses by dihydropyridines and verapamil in rat spinal neurons. *The European Journal of Neuroscience, 13*, 2195–2204.

Chung, S. K., Vanbellinghen, J. F., Mullins, J. G., Robinson, A., Hantke, J., Hammond, C. L., et al. (2010). Pathophysiological mechanisms of dominant and recessive GLRA1 mutations in hyperekplexia. *The Journal of Neuroscience, 30*, 9612–9620.

Cornelison, G. L., Pflanz, N. C., Tipps, M. E., & Mihic, S. J. (2016). Identification and characterization of heptapeptide modulators of the glycine receptor. *European Journal of Pharmacology, 780*, 252–259.

Del Pino, I., Koch, D., Schemm, R., Qualmann, B., Betz, H., & Paarmann, I. (2014). Proteomic analysis of glycine receptor beta subunit (GlyRbeta)-interacting proteins: Evidence for syndapin I regulating synaptic glycine receptors. *The Journal of Biological Chemistry, 289*, 11396–11409.

Dixon, C. L., Zhang, Y., & Lynch, J. W. (2015). Generation of functional inhibitory synapses incorporating defined combinations of GABA(a) or glycine receptor subunits. *Frontiers in Molecular Neuroscience, 8*, 80.

Du, J., Lu, W., Wu, S., Cheng, Y., & Gouaux, E. (2015). Glycine receptor mechanism elucidated by electron cryo-microscopy. *Nature, 526*, 224–229.

Durisic, N., Godin, A. G., Wever, C. M., Heyes, C. D., Lakadamyali, M., & Dent, J. A. (2012). Stoichiometry of the human glycine receptor revealed by direct subunit counting. *Journal of Neuroscience, 32*, 12915–12920.

Dutertre, S., Becker, C. M., & Betz, H. (2012). Inhibitory glycine receptors: An update. *The Journal of Biological Chemistry, 287*, 40216–40223.

Eichler, S. A., Forstera, B., Smolinsky, B., Juttner, R., Lehmann, T. N., Fahling, M., et al. (2009). Splice-specific roles of glycine receptor alpha3 in the hippocampus. *The European Journal of Neuroscience, 30*, 1077–1091.

Eichler, S. A., Kirischuk, S., Juttner, R., Schaefermeier, P. K., Legendre, P., Lehmann, T. N., et al. (2008). Glycinergic tonic inhibition of hippocampal neurons with depolarizing GABAergic transmission elicits histopathological signs of temporal lobe epilepsy. *Journal of Cellular and Molecular Medicine, 12*, 2848–2866.

Findlay, G. S., Wick, M. J., Mascia, M. P., Wallace, D., Miller, G. W., Harris, R. A., et al. (2002). Transgenic expression of a mutant glycine receptor decreases alcohol sensitivity of mice. *The Journal of Pharmacology and Experimental Therapeutics, 300*, 526–534.

Foster, E., Wildner, H., Tudeau, L., Haueter, S., Ralvenius, W. T., Jegen, M., et al. (2015). Targeted ablation, silencing, and activation establish glycinergic dorsal horn neurons as key components of a spinal gate for pain and itch. *Neuron, 85*, 1289–1304.

Frederickson, C. J., Giblin, L. J., Krezel, A., McAdoo, D. J., Mueller, R. N., Zeng, Y., et al. (2006). Concentrations of extracellular free zinc (pZn)e in the central nervous system during simple anesthetization, ischemia and reperfusion. *Experimental Neurology, 198*, 285–293.

Fujita, M., Sato, K., Sato, M., Inoue, T., Kozuka, T., & Tohyama, M. (1991). Regional distribution of the cells expressing glycine receptor beta subunit mRNA in the rat brain. *Brain Research, 560*, 23–37.

Galietta, L. J., Haggie, P. M., & Verkman, A. S. (2001). Green fluorescent protein-based halide indicators with improved chloride and iodide affinities. *FEBS Letters*, *499*, 220–224.

Gaskin, D. J., & Richard, P. (2012). The economic costs of pain in the United States. *The Journal of Pain*, *13*, 715–724.

Gilbert, D., Esmaeili, A., & Lynch, J. W. (2009). Optimizing the expression of recombinant alphabetagamma GABAA receptors in HEK293 cells for high-throughput screening. *Journal of Biomolecular Screening*, *14*, 86–91.

Gilbert, D. F., Islam, R., Lynagh, T., Lynch, J. W., & Webb, T. I. (2009). High throughput techniques for discovering new glycine receptor modulators and their binding sites. *Frontiers in Molecular Neuroscience*, *2*, 17.

Gilbert, D. F., Meinhof, T., Pepperkok, R., & Runz, H. (2009). DetecTiff: A novel image analysis routine for high-content screening microscopy. *Journal of Biomolecular Screening*, *14*, 944–955.

Greferath, U., Brandstatter, J. H., Wassle, H., Kirsch, J., Kuhse, J., & Grunert, U. (1994). Differential expression of glycine receptor subunits in the retina of the rat: A study using immunohistochemistry and in situ hybridization. *Visual Neuroscience*, *11*, 721–729.

Grenningloh, G., Pribilla, I., Prior, P., Multhaup, G., Beyreuther, K., Taleb, O., et al. (1990). Cloning and expression of the 58 kD beta subunit of the inhibitory glycine receptor. *Neuron*, *4*, 963–970.

Grudzinska, J., Schumann, T., Schemm, R., Betz, H., & Laube, B. (2008). Mutations within the agonist-binding site convert the homomeric alpha1 glycine receptor into a Zn^{2+}-activated chloride channel. *Channels (Austin, TX)*, *2*, 13–18.

Han, L., Talwar, S., Wang, Q., Shan, Q., & Lynch, J. W. (2013). Phosphorylation of alpha3 glycine receptors induces a conformational change in the glycine-binding site. *ACS Chemical Neuroscience*, *4*, 1361–1370.

Harvey, R. J., Depner, U. B., Wassle, H., Ahmadi, S., Heindl, C., Reinold, H., et al. (2004). GlyR alpha3: An essential target for spinal PGE2-mediated inflammatory pain sensitization. *Science*, *304*, 884–887.

Harvey, R. J., Schmieden, V., Von Holst, A., Laube, B., Rohrer, H., & Betz, H. (2000). Glycine receptors containing the alpha4 subunit in the embryonic sympathetic nervous system, spinal cord and male genital ridge. *The European Journal of Neuroscience*, *12*, 994–1001.

Harvey, R. J., Topf, M., Harvey, K., & Rees, M. I. (2008). The genetics of hyperekplexia: More than startle!. *Trends in Genetics*, *24*, 439–447.

Hawthorne, R., Cromer, B. A., Ng, H. L., Parker, M. W., & Lynch, J. W. (2006). Molecular determinants of ginkgolide binding in the glycine receptor pore. *Journal of Neurochemistry*, *98*, 395–407.

Hawthorne, R., & Lynch, J. W. (2005). A picrotoxin-specific conformational change in the glycine receptor M2-M3 loop. *The Journal of Biological Chemistry*, *280*, 35836–35843.

Heads, J. A., Hawthorne, R. L., Lynagh, T., & Lynch, J. W. (2008). Structure-activity analysis of ginkgolide binding in the glycine receptor pore. *Journal of Neurochemistry*, *105*, 1418–1427.

Hejazi, N., Zhou, C., Oz, M., Sun, H., Ye, J. H., & Zhang, L. (2006). Delta9-tetrahydrocannabinol and endogenous cannabinoid anandamide directly potentiate the function of glycine receptors. *Molecular Pharmacology*, *69*, 991–997.

Hoon, M., Bauer, G., Fritschy, J. M., Moser, T., Falkenburger, B. H., & Varoqueaux, F. (2009). Neuroligin 2 controls the maturation of GABAergic synapses and information processing in the retina. *The Journal of Neuroscience*, *29*, 8039–8050.

Hoon, M., Soykan, T., Falkenburger, B., Hammer, M., Patrizi, A., Schmidt, K. F., et al. (2011). Neuroligin-4 is localized to glycinergic postsynapses and regulates inhibition in the retina. *Proceedings of the National Academy of Sciences of the United States of America*, *108*, 3053–3058.

Huang, X., Chen, H., Michelsen, K., Schneider, S., & Shaffer, P. L. (2015). Crystal structure of human glycine receptor-alpha3 bound to antagonist strychnine. *Nature, 526*, 277–280.

Huang, X., Shaffer, P. L., Ayube, S., Bregman, H., Chen, H., Lehto, S. G., et al. (2017). Crystal structures of human glycine receptor alpha3 bound to a novel class of analgesic potentiators. *Nature Structural & Molecular Biology, 24*, 108–113.

Islam, R., & Lynch, J. W. (2012). Mechanism of action of the insecticides, lindane and fipronil, on glycine receptor chloride channels. *British Journal of Pharmacology, 165*, 2707–2720.

James, V. M., Bode, A., Chung, S. K., Gill, J. L., Nielsen, M., Cowan, F. M., et al. (2013). Novel missense mutations in the glycine receptor beta subunit gene (GLRB) in startle disease. *Neurobiology of Disease, 52*, 137–149.

Jensen, A. A., Bergmann, M. L., Sander, T., & Balle, T. (2010). Ginkgolide X is a potent antagonist of anionic cys-loop receptors with a unique selectivity profile at glycine receptors. *The Journal of Biological Chemistry, 285*, 10141–10153.

Jensen, A. A., & Kristiansen, U. (2004). Functional characterisation of the human alpha1 glycine receptor in a fluorescence-based membrane potential assay. *Biochemical Pharmacology, 67*, 1789–1799.

Jonsson, S., Adermark, L., Ericson, M., & Soderpalm, B. (2014). The involvement of accumbal glycine receptors in the dopamine-elevating effects of addictive drugs. *Neuropharmacology, 82*, 69–75.

Kim, E. Y., Schrader, N., Smolinsky, B., Bedet, C., Vannier, C., Schwarz, G., et al. (2006). Deciphering the structural framework of glycine receptor anchoring by gephyrin. *The EMBO Journal, 25*, 1385–1395.

Kirson, D., Cornelison, G. L., Philpo, A. E., Todorovic, J., & Mihic, S. J. (2013). Physiological concentrations of zinc reduce taurine-activated GlyR responses to drugs of abuse. *Neuropharmacology, 75*, 286–294.

Kondratskaya, E. L., Betz, H., Krishtal, O. A., & Laube, B. (2005). The beta subunit increases the ginkgolide B sensitivity of inhibitory glycine receptors. *Neuropharmacology, 49*, 945–951.

Krause, R. M., Buisson, B., Bertrand, S., Corringer, P. J., Galzi, J. L., Changeux, J. P., et al. (1998). Ivermectin: A positive allosteric effector of the alpha7 neuronal nicotinic acetylcholine receptor. *Molecular Pharmacology, 53*, 283–294.

Kruger, W., Gilbert, D., Hawthorne, R., Hryciw, D. H., Frings, S., Poronnik, P., et al. (2005). A yellow fluorescent protein-based assay for high-throughput screening of glycine and GABAA receptor chloride channels. *Neuroscience Letters, 380*, 340–345.

Krusek, J., & Zemkova, H. (1994). Effect of ivermectin on gamma-aminobutyric acid-induced chloride currents in mouse hippocampal embryonic neurones. *European Journal of Pharmacology, 259*, 121–128.

Kuhse, J., Kuryatov, A., Maulet, Y., Malosio, M. L., Schmieden, V., & Betz, H. (1991). Alternative splicing generates two isoforms of the alpha 2 subunit of the inhibitory glycine receptor. *FEBS Letters, 283*, 73–77.

Lara, C. O., Murath, P., Munoz, B., Marileo, A. M., Martin, L. S., San Martin, V. P., et al. (2016). Functional modulation of glycine receptors by the alkaloid gelsemine. *British Journal of Pharmacology, 173*, 2263–2277.

Laube, B., Kuhse, J., Rundstrom, N., Kirsch, J., Schmieden, V., & Betz, H. (1995). Modulation by zinc ions of native rat and recombinant human inhibitory glycine receptors. *The Journal of Physiology, 483*(Pt. 3), 613–619.

Legendre, P. (1998). A reluctant gating mode of glycine receptor channels determines the time course of inhibitory miniature synaptic events in zebrafish hindbrain neurons. *Journal of Neuroscience, 18*, 2856–2870.

Legendre, P., Forstera, B., Juttner, R., & Meier, J. C. (2009). Glycine receptors caught between genome and proteome—Functional implications of RNA editing and splicing. *Frontiers in Molecular Neuroscience, 2*, 23.

Lionel, A. C., Vaags, A. K., Sato, D., Gazzellone, M. J., Mitchell, E. B., Chen, H. Y., et al. (2013). Rare exonic deletions implicate the synaptic organizer gephyrin (GPHN) in risk for autism, schizophrenia and seizures. *Human Molecular Genetics*, *22*, 2055–2066.

Liu, J., Wu, D. C., & Wang, Y. T. (2010). Allosteric potentiation of glycine receptor chloride currents by glutamate. *Nature Neuroscience*, *13*, 1225–1232.

Lobo, I. A., & Harris, R. A. (2005). Sites of alcohol and volatile anesthetic action on glycine receptors. *International Review of Neurobiology*, *65*, 53–87.

Lynagh, T., & Lynch, J. W. (2010). An improved ivermectin-activated chloride channel receptor for inhibiting electrical activity in defined neuronal populations. *The Journal of Biological Chemistry*, *285*, 14890–14897.

Lynagh, T., Webb, T. I., Dixon, C. L., Cromer, B. A., & Lynch, J. W. (2011). Molecular determinants of ivermectin sensitivity at the glycine receptor chloride channel. *Journal of Biological Chemistry*, *286*, 43913–43924.

Lynch, J. W. (2004). Molecular structure and function of the glycine receptor chloride channel. *Physiological Reviews*, *84*, 1051–1095.

Lynch, J. W. (2005). High throughput screening of neuronal Cl− channels: Why and how? *Current Neuropharmacology*, *3*, 207–216.

Lynch, J. W. (2009). Native glycine receptor subtypes and their physiological roles. *Neuropharmacology*, *56*, 303–309.

Lynch, J. W., & Callister, R. J. (2006). Glycine receptors: A new therapeutic target in pain pathways. *Current Opinion in Investigational Drugs*, 7, 48–53.

Lynch, J. W., & Chen, X. (2008). Subunit-specific potentiation of recombinant glycine receptors by NV-31, a bilobalide-derived compound. *Neuroscience Letters*, *435*, 147–151.

Lynch, J. W., Jacques, P., Pierce, K. D., & Schofield, P. R. (1998). Zinc potentiation of the glycine receptor chloride channel is mediated by allosteric pathways. *Journal of Neurochemistry*, *71*, 2159–2168.

Mackowiak, M., Mordalska, P., & Wedzony, K. (2014). Neuroligins, synapse balance and neuropsychiatric disorders. *Pharmacological Reports*, *66*, 830–835.

Maksay, G. (1998). Bidirectional allosteric modulation of strychnine-sensitive glycine receptors by tropeines and 5-HT3 serotonin receptor ligands. *Neuropharmacology*, *37*, 1633–1641.

Maksay, G., Laube, B., & Betz, H. (2001). Subunit-specific modulation of glycine receptors by neurosteroids. *Neuropharmacology*, *41*, 369–376.

Maksay, G., Laube, B., Schemm, R., Grudzinska, J., Drwal, M., & Betz, H. (2009). Different binding modes of tropeines mediating inhibition and potentiation of alpha1 glycine receptors. *Journal of Neurochemistry*, *109*, 1725–1732.

Maleeva, G., Buldakova, S., & Bregestovski, P. (2015). Selective potentiation of alpha 1 glycine receptors by ginkgolic acid. *Frontiers in Molecular Neuroscience*, *8*, 64.

Malosio, M. L., Marqueze-Pouey, B., Kuhse, J., & Betz, H. (1991). Widespread expression of glycine receptor subunit mRNAs in the adult and developing rat brain. *The EMBO Journal*, *10*, 2401–2409.

Manzke, T., Niebert, M., Koch, U. R., Caley, A., Vogelgesang, S., Hulsmann, S., et al. (2010). Serotonin receptor 1A-modulated phosphorylation of glycine receptor alpha3 controls breathing in mice. *The Journal of Clinical Investigation*, *120*, 4118–4128.

Markstahler, U., Kremer, E., Kimmina, S., Becker, K., & Richter, D. W. (2002). Effects of functional knock-out of alpha 1 glycine-receptors on breathing movements in oscillator mice. *Respiratory Physiology & Neurobiology*, *130*, 33–42.

McCavera, S., Rogers, A. T., Yates, D. M., Woods, D. J., & Wolstenholme, A. J. (2009). An ivermectin-sensitive glutamate-gated chloride channel from the parasitic nematode Haemonchus contortus. *Molecular Pharmacology*, *75*, 1347–1355.

McCracken, L. M., Trudell, J. R., Goldstein, B. E., Harris, R. A., & Mihic, S. J. (2010). Zinc enhances ethanol modulation of the alpha1 glycine receptor. *Neuropharmacology, 58*, 676–681.

Meier, J. C., Henneberger, C., Melnick, I., Racca, C., Harvey, R. J., Heinemann, U., et al. (2005). RNA editing produces glycine receptor alpha3(P185L), resulting in high agonist potency. *Nature Neuroscience, 8*, 736–744.

Meyer, G., Kirsch, J., Betz, H., & Langosch, D. (1995). Identification of a gephyrin binding motif on the glycine receptor-beta subunit. *Neuron, 15*, 563–572.

Miller, P. S., Beato, M., Harvey, R. J., & Smart, T. G. (2005). Molecular determinants of glycine receptor alphabeta subunit sensitivities to Zn^{2+}-mediated inhibition. *The Journal of Physiology, 566*, 657–670.

Miller, P. S., Da Silva, H. M. A., & Smart, T. G. (2005). Molecular basis for zinc potentiation at strychnine-sensitive glycine receptors. *Journal of Biological Chemistry, 280*, 37877–37884.

Miller, P. S., Topf, M., & Smart, T. G. (2008). Mapping a molecular link between allosteric inhibition and activation of the glycine receptor. *Nature Structural & Molecular Biology, 15*, 1084–1093.

Molander, A., & Soderpalm, B. (2005a). Accumbal strychnine-sensitive glycine receptors: An access point for ethanol to the brain reward system. *Alcoholism, Clinical and Experimental Research, 29*, 27–37.

Molander, A., & Soderpalm, B. (2005b). Glycine receptors regulate dopamine release in the rat nucleus accumbens. *Alcoholism, Clinical and Experimental Research, 29*, 17–26.

Nevin, S. T., Cromer, B. A., Haddrill, J. L., Morton, C. J., Parker, M. W., & Lynch, J. W. (2003). Insights into the structural basis for zinc inhibition of the glycine receptor. *Journal of Biological Chemistry, 278*, 28985–28992.

Obergrussberger, A., Bruggemann, A., Goetze, T. A., Rapedius, M., Haarmann, C., Rinke, I., et al. (2015). Automated patch clamp meets high-throughput screening: 384 cells recorded in parallel on a planar patch clamp module. *Journal of Laboratory Automation, 21*, 779–793.

Olsen, R. W., Li, G. D., Wallner, M., Trudell, J. R., Bertaccini, E. J., Lindahl, E., et al. (2014). Structural models of ligand-gated ion channels: Sites of action for anesthetics and ethanol. *Alcoholism, Clinical and Experimental Research, 38*, 595–603.

Omura, S. (2008). Ivermectin: 25 Years and still going strong. *International Journal of Antimicrobial Agents, 31*, 91–98.

Perkins, D. I., Trudell, J. R., Crawford, D. K., Alkana, R. L., & Davies, D. L. (2010). Molecular targets and mechanisms for ethanol action in glycine receptors. *Pharmacology & Therapeutics, 127*, 53–65.

Pierrefiche, O., Schwarzacher, S. W., Bischoff, A. M., & Richter, D. W. (1998). Blockade of synaptic inhibition within the pre-Bötzinger complex in the cat suppresses respiratory rhythm generation in vivo. *The Journal of Physiology, 509*(Pt. 1), 245–254.

Pilorge, M., Fassier, C., Le Corronc, H., Potey, A., Bai, J., De Gois, S., et al. (2015). Genetic and functional analyses demonstrate a role for abnormal glycinergic signaling in autism. *Molecular Psychiatry, 21*, 936–945.

Piton, A., Gauthier, J., Hamdan, F. F., Lafreniere, R. G., Yang, Y., Henrion, E., et al. (2011). Systematic resequencing of X-chromosome synaptic genes in autism spectrum disorder and schizophrenia. *Molecular Psychiatry, 16*, 867–880.

Poulopoulos, A., Aramuni, G., Meyer, G., Soykan, T., Hoon, M., Papadopoulos, T., et al. (2009). Neuroligin 2 drives postsynaptic assembly at perisomatic inhibitory synapses through gephyrin and collybistin. *Neuron, 63*, 628–642.

Pribilla, I., Takagi, T., Langosch, D., Bormann, J., & Betz, H. (1992). The atypical M2 segment of the beta subunit confers picrotoxinin resistance to inhibitory glycine receptor channels. *The EMBO Journal, 11*, 4305–4311.

Reinold, H., Ahmadi, S., Depner, U. B., Layh, B., Heindl, C., Hamza, M., et al. (2005). Spinal inflammatory hyperalgesia is mediated by prostaglandin E receptors of the EP2 subtype. *The Journal of Clinical Investigation, 115*, 673–679.

Rundstrom, N., Schmieden, V., Betz, H., Bormann, J., & Langosch, D. (1994). Cyanotriphenylborate: Subtype-specific blocker of glycine receptor chloride channels. *Proceedings of the National Academy of Sciences of the United States of America, 91*, 8950–8954.

Sato, K., Kiyama, H., & Tohyama, M. (1992). Regional distribution of cells expressing glycine receptor alpha 2 subunit mRNA in the rat brain. *Brain Research, 590*, 95–108.

Schmid, K., Bohmer, G., & Gebauer, K. (1991). Glycine receptor-mediated fast synaptic inhibition in the brainstem respiratory system. *Respiration Physiology, 84*, 351–361.

Shalaly, N. D., Aneiros, E., Blank, M., Mueller, J., Nyman, E., Blind, M., et al. (2015). Positive modulation of the glycine receptor by means of glycine receptor-binding aptamers. *Journal of Biomolecular Screening, 20*, 1112–1123.

Shan, Q., Haddrill, J. L., & Lynch, J. W. (2001). Ivermectin, an unconventional agonist of the glycine receptor chloride channel. *The Journal of Biological Chemistry, 276*, 12556–12564.

Singer, J. H., Talley, E. M., Bayliss, D. A., & Berger, A. J. (1998). Development of glycinergic synaptic transmission to rat brain stem motoneurons. *Journal of Neurophysiology, 80*, 2608–2620.

Stead, C., Brown, A., Adams, C., Nickolls, S. J., Young, G., Kammonen, J., et al. (2016). Identification of positive allosteric modulators of glycine receptors from a high-throughput screen using a fluorescent membrane potential assay. *Journal of Biomolecular Screening, 21*, 1042–1053.

Supplisson, S., & Chesnoy-Marchais, D. (2000). Glycine receptor beta subunits play a critical role in potentiation of glycine responses by ICS-205,930. *Molecular Pharmacology, 58*, 763–770.

Sztainberg, Y., & Zoghbi, H. Y. (2016). Lessons learned from studying syndromic autism spectrum disorders. *Nature Neuroscience, 19*, 1408–1417.

Talwar, S., Lynch, J. W., & Gilbert, D. F. (2013). Fluorescence-based high-throughput functional profiling of ligand-gated ion channels at the level of single cells. *PLoS One, 8*, e58479.

Thomas, R. H., Chung, S. K., Wood, S. E., Cushion, T. D., Drew, C. J., Hammond, C. L., et al. (2013). Genotype-phenotype correlations in hyperekplexia: Apnoeas, learning difficulties and speech delay. *Brain, 136*, 3085–3095.

Vanegas, H., & Schaible, H. G. (2001). Prostaglandins and cyclooxygenases [correction of cycloxygenases] in the spinal cord. *Progress in Neurobiology, 64*, 327–363.

Vengeliene, V., Bilbao, A., Molander, A., & Spanagel, R. (2008). Neuropharmacology of alcohol addiction. *British Journal of Pharmacology, 154*, 299–315.

Webb, T. I., & Lynch, J. W. (2007). Molecular pharmacology of the glycine receptor chloride channel. *Current Pharmaceutical Design, 13*, 2350–2367.

Wells, M. M., Tillman, T. S., Mowrey, D. D., Sun, T., Xu, Y., & Tang, P. (2015). Ensemble-based virtual screening for cannabinoid-like potentiators of the human glycine receptor alpha1 for the treatment of pain. *Journal of Medicinal Chemistry, 58*, 2958–2966.

Williams, K. L., Ferko, A. P., Barbieri, E. J., & DiGregorio, G. J. (1995). Glycine enhances the central depressant properties of ethanol in mice. *Pharmacology, Biochemistry, and Behavior, 50*, 199–205.

Woolf, C. J. (2010). What is this thing called pain? *The Journal of Clinical Investigation, 120*, 3742–3744.

Xiong, W., Cheng, K., Cui, T., Godlewski, G., Rice, K. C., Xu, Y., et al. (2011). Cannabinoid potentiation of glycine receptors contributes to cannabis-induced analgesia. *Nature Chemical Biology, 7*, 296–303.

Xiong, W., Cui, T., Cheng, K., Yang, F., Chen, S. R., Willenbring, D., et al. (2012). Cannabinoids suppress inflammatory and neuropathic pain by targeting alpha3 glycine receptors. *The Journal of Experimental Medicine, 209*, 1121–1134.

Xiong, W., Wu, X., Li, F., Cheng, K., Rice, K. C., Lovinger, D. M., et al. (2012). A common molecular basis for exogenous and endogenous cannabinoid potentiation of glycine receptors. *The Journal of Neuroscience, 32*, 5200–5208.

Yang, Z., Aubrey, K. R., Alroy, I., Harvey, R. J., Vandenberg, R. J., & Lynch, J. W. (2008). Subunit-specific modulation of glycine receptors by cannabinoids and N-arachidonyl-glycine. *Biochemical Pharmacology, 76*, 1014–1023.

Yang, Z., Cromer, B. A., Harvey, R. J., Parker, M. W., & Lynch, J. W. (2007). A proposed structural basis for picrotoxinin and picrotin binding in the glycine receptor pore. *Journal of Neurochemistry, 103*, 580–589.

Yang, Z., Ney, A., Cromer, B. A., Ng, H. L., Parker, M. W., & Lynch, J. W. (2007). Tropisetron modulation of the glycine receptor: Femtomolar potentiation and a molecular determinant of inhibition. *Journal of Neurochemistry, 100*, 758–769.

Yang, Z., Taran, E., Webb, T. I., & Lynch, J. W. (2012). Stoichiometry and subunit arrangement of alpha1beta glycine receptors as determined by atomic force microscopy. *Biochemistry, 51*, 5229–5231.

Yevenes, G. E., & Zeilhofer, H. U. (2011a). Allosteric modulation of glycine receptors. *British Journal of Pharmacology, 164*, 224–236.

Yevenes, G. E., & Zeilhofer, H. U. (2011b). Molecular sites for the positive allosteric modulation of glycine receptors by endocannabinoids. *PLoS One, 6*, e23886.

Zeilhofer, H. U. (2005). The glycinergic control of spinal pain processing. *Cellular and Molecular Life Sciences, 62*, 2027–2035.

Zeilhofer, H. U., Wildner, H., & Yevenes, G. E. (2012). Fast synaptic inhibition in spinal sensory processing and pain control. *Physiological Reviews, 92*, 193–235.

Zhang, Y., Bode, A., Nguyen, B., Keramidas, A., & Lynch, J. W. (2016). Investigating the mechanism by which gain-of-function mutations to the alpha1 glycine receptor cause hyperekplexia. *The Journal of Biological Chemistry, 291*, 15332–15341.

Zhang, Y., Dixon, C. L., Keramidas, A., & Lynch, J. W. (2015). Functional reconstitution of glycinergic synapses incorporating defined glycine receptor subunit combinations. *Neuropharmacology, 89*, 391–397.

Zhang, Y., Keramidas, A., & Lynch, J. W. (2016). The free zinc concentration in the synaptic cleft of artificial glycinergic synapses rises to at least 1 μM. *Frontiers in Molecular Neuroscience, 9*, 88.

CHAPTER NINE

Voltage-Gated Sodium Channel Pharmacology: Insights From Molecular Dynamics Simulations

Rong Chen, Amanda Buyan, Ben Corry[1]
Research School of Biology, Australian National University, Canberra, ACT, Australia
[1]Corresponding author: e-mail address: ben.corry@anu.edu.au

Contents

Abstract

Voltage-gated ion channels are the target of a range of naturally occurring toxins and therapeutic drugs. There is a great interest in better understanding how these diverse compounds alter channel function in order to design the next generation of therapeutics that can selectively target one of the channel subtypes found in the body. Since the publication of a number of bacterial sodium channel structures, molecular dynamics simulations have been invaluable in gaining a high resolution understanding where many of these small molecules and toxins bind to the channels, how they find their binding site, and how they can selectively bind to one channel subtype over another. This chapter summarizes these recent studies to highlight what has been learnt about channel pharmacology using computer simulations and to draw out shared conclusions, focusing separately on toxin–channel interactions and small molecule–channel interactions.

Advances in Pharmacology, Volume 79
ISSN 1054-3589
http://dx.doi.org/10.1016/bs.apha.2017.02.002

NONSTANDARD ABBREVIATIONS

MD molecular dynamics
PMF potential of mean force
TTX tetrodotoxin

1. INTRODUCTION

Voltage-gated sodium channels are responsible for rapidly depolarizing cells as required for generating action potentials in nerve and muscle. Malfunctions in sodium channels caused by inherited mutations are responsible for a range of debilitating cardiovascular, muscular, and nerve disorders including cardiac arrhythmias, epilepsy, and chronic pain (Meisler & Kearney, 2005; Roden & George, 1996; Ruan, Liu, & Priori, 2009; Waxman, Dib-Hajj, Cummins, & Black, 1999; Waxman & Hains, 2006). These channels are also targets of a wide range of naturally occurring toxins, which may generate a lethal response when altering channel function (Al-Sabi, McArthur, Ostroumov, & French, 2006; Catterall et al., 2007; Knapp, McArthur, & Adams, 2012; Nicholson, 2007), as well as a range of therapeutic drugs (Catterall, 2000; Catterall & Swanson, 2015; Fozzard, Sheets, & Hanck, 2011). Thus, gaining a detailed understanding of how these channels function, how their function is altered by drugs and toxins, where these agents bind to the channel, and how they reach the active site is of great pharmaceutical interest.

The pore-forming component of voltage-gated sodium channels in eukaryotes is shaped by large protein chains that fold into a pseudo-tetrameric complex surrounding the central, ion-selective pore. At rest, this pore is closed. But, by opening a sodium selective pore in response to small changes in membrane potential, they allow sodium to rush inside, rapidly depolarizing the cell. After a short time in the open or "activated" state, these channels are also known to inactivate. That is, sodium conductance becomes blocked even though the initial activating signal remains. Finally, after the cell repolarises, the channels return to the resting state, ready to contribute to the next electrical signal. Humans express nine different types of sodium channel, termed $Na_v1.1$–$Na_v1.9$, localized in different tissue and cell types around the body (Catterall, Goldin, & Waxman, 2005; Goldin et al., 2000). Modification of each subtype yields a different biological response, and so there is great interest in developing more targeted therapeutic compounds for treating specific conditions. Although most of our current sodium channel targeting drugs are nonselective, many toxins affect only one or a few of the channel subtypes. So, understanding how this selectivity arises is of great use in designing the next generation of targeted therapeutic compounds.

Although we do not have any atomic resolution structures of eukaryotic sodium channels, a number of bacterial channel structures have been published in the last five years (Ahuja et al., 2015; Bagneris et al., 2013, 2014; McCusker et al., 2012; Naylor et al., 2016; Payandeh, Gamal El-Din, Scheuer, Zheng, & Catterall, 2012; Payandeh, Scheuer, Zheng, & Catterall, 2011; Shaya et al., 2014; Tsai et al., 2013; Zhang et al., 2012). Although these bacterial channels are formed by four identical protein subunits, rather than a single long protein chain, they are believed to be a good first model of the structure of their eukaryotic counterparts. This is because of evidence that they share similar structural folds, despite the overall sequence similarity between them being low. Small segments of the channels contain areas with higher similarity (from 15% to 77%), although there are great differences in other areas such as the P-loop turret region which is ~100 residues longer in mammalian channels than bacterial sodium channels. In these channels, each subunit contains six α-helices. The first four helices (named S1–S4) form the voltage-sensing domains, which surround the central pore-forming domains created by the last two helices (S5 & S6) and a reentrant extracellular loop. This loop makes up the narrowest part of the pore known as the selectivity filter, which is responsible for sodium selection. The cytoplasmic half of the pore is shaped by the S6 helices, which come together to form the activation gate at the bottom of the channel. Schematic depictions of eukaryotic and bacterial sodium channels are given in Fig. 1.

The publication of the bacterial sodium channel structures has enabled a number of molecular dynamics (MD) simulation studies to be conducted to help understand how these channels are affected by drugs and toxins. These studies aim to address questions such as where different drugs and toxins bind to the channel, how they reach this site, why some toxins selectively bind to specific channel subtypes, and how we can make more selective channel inhibitors. This chapter aims to summarize these studies and shed light on what they have contributed to our understanding of sodium channel pharmacology. We start by briefly discussing the simulation methodology itself so that the specific examples given can be more easily interpreted. We then look at studies examining channel–toxin interactions before moving to those looking at the interaction of small molecules with sodium channel proteins.

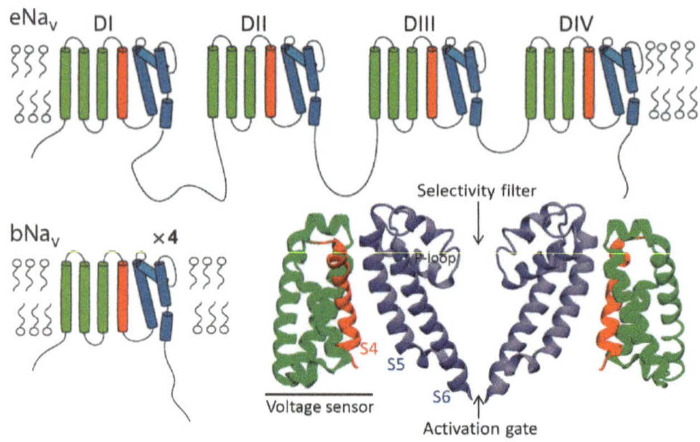

Fig. 1 Schematic depictions of eukaryotic Na$_V$ (eNa$_V$) and bacterial Na$_V$ (bNa$_V$) channels showing the predicted topologies and the X-ray structure of a bacterial channel. Topologies are adapted from Corry, Lee, and Ahern (2014), while the structure depicts two out of four subunits of each of the voltage sensors and pore domains of the bacterial channel Na$_V$Ab (PDB accession code 3RVY Payandeh et al., 2011).

2. MOLECULAR DYNAMICS SIMULATION APPROACHES

The idea of molecular dynamics simulations is to monitor how all the atoms in a system of interest move over time. If this is done carefully, it can be used to follow the dynamics and structural changes of proteins as well as to examine the interaction of the proteins with ions, water, small molecules, lipids, peptides, and other proteins. As such, it has the potential to gain information about the interactions of sodium channels with pharmacological agents at a high level of spatial and time resolution that is difficult to obtain with any other technique.

Conducting molecular dynamics simulations on sodium channels requires first having an atomic resolution structure or model of the channel protein and its environment, including the lipid bilayer, water, ions, etc. Next, a method for determining the forces acting on each atom is needed, including all the covalent bonds between atoms, electrostatic, van der Waals interactions, and any external electric fields. In classical molecular dynamics, this is done using a so-called force field, which describes these interactions by representing each atom as a charged ball with bonds represented by springs. These force fields are carefully parameterized to be able to reproduce a number of microscopic and macroscopic properties. With these in hand, Newton's equations of motion can be used to determine how all of the atoms move over a large number of short discrete time steps (for more information, see Corry, 2015; van Gunsteren et al., 2006).

There are a number of challenges in extracting useful information from MD simulations. First, because of the large number of atoms involved in a sodium channel simulation system, a large amount of computer power is required to calculate the interatomic forces. In addition, these forces must be recalculated every time step (typically 1–2 fs) to accurately reproduce the motion of the atoms. This limits the duration over which simulations can be run. Although computer hardware and algorithm improvements have now extended simulations into the μs (and in exceptional cases ms range; Jensen et al., 2012), this is often much shorter than the timescales of drug binding or the functional consequences of binding to be apparent in the channel. Methods are also required to extract statistically significant data out of the complex output information about the positions of all the atoms. This not only requires repetition of experiments, but also careful statistical analysis of the simulation data.

A number of approaches are often applied on top of the basic simulation method to overcome the challenges described earlier. These can speed up slow events, improve the conformational sampling of the protein and drugs, and aid in extracting significant conclusions from a simulation. Because these extra methods are used in almost all the studies described later, we briefly introduce them here, with examples of how they can be employed to study protein–drug/toxin interactions.

Unbiased or equilibrium simulations are the simple implementation of the molecular dynamics method. As the system evolves, it often moves toward low energy conformations. Drugs, for example, may move into a binding site which can be evidenced by them remaining in a stable position for a long time. However, unless the drug starts near the site, binding is likely to take longer than can be simulated. Also, the drug may dwell in a low-affinity site rather than moving toward a high-affinity position. Thus, replication of results with different starting coordinates is generally necessary to prove significance.

"Flooding" is a simple extension of unbiased simulations in which a very high concentration of the drug or toxin is used in the simulation to speed up binding events and to aid in the drug sampling all possible positions in the system (Vemparala, Domene, & Klein, 2008). Even at high concentrations, very long simulations are generally required and slow processes can be missed. There is also the possibility that results may be influenced by interaction between drug molecules that may not be relevant at lower concentrations.

But, if adequate sampling of drug positions is achieved, it is possible to determine the free energy landscape (more correctly a "potential of mean force" (PMF)) of the drug in the system, which can pinpoint likely binding locations and barriers to movement.

Umbrella sampling is a method aiming to improve the sampling of the system along selected coordinates of interest, specifically forcing the system into conformations that are poorly sampled in unbiased simulations (Torrie & Valleau, 1977). In the context of interactions of a protein with a pharmacological agent, typically the agent will be forced to move to a series of positions of interest—such as steps along a proposed access route to the binding site—and the rest of the system allowed to evolve accordingly. The data from these simulations can be used to generate an energy landscape indicating location and size of energetic barriers and the location and affinity of binding sites (Deng & Roux, 2009). However, the method requires the coordinates of interest to be predefined.

Metadynamics is another approach to speed up slow processes, forcing a system to sample all available conformations and generate a complete free energy landscape for chosen characteristics of a system (Laio & Gervasio, 2008; Laio & Parrinello, 2002). In the studies described in this chapter, metadynamics is used to make it harder for a drug to return to positions it has already been, by gently pushing it away from previously visited locations. Not only does this speed up how quickly it moves about the system, but by keeping track of the forces used to do so, this allows the "unbiased" behavior of the system (such as the free energy surface and binding locations) to be reconstructed. As for umbrella sampling, this method also requires certain coordinates of interest to be preselected prior to starting the simulation.

Steered Molecular Dynamics is a method where an external force is applied to a molecule to pull it along a chosen reaction coordinate (Park & Schulten, 2004). This is often used to determine the amount of work a biological process takes, such as protein unfolding experiments, but can also be used to compare the energies required for drugs to access a site by different routes.

Alchemical transformations allow parts of a system to be chemically transformed during a simulation and the energetics of the process to be determined (Deng & Roux, 2009). Typically, this is used to find the free energy change involved in mutating an amino acid, to add or remove a drug (or other small molecule) from the system, or to move a side chain from one configuration to another. Combining such transformations, such as the removal of a drug from the protein and insertion of the drug into aqueous solution, is one of the most accurate ways to predict binding free energies and dissociation constants in simulations if a binding pose is known (Gumbart, Roux, & Chipot, 2013).

3. SODIUM CHANNEL–TOXIN INTERACTIONS

Various toxins isolated from animal venoms, ranging from small molecules to large polypeptides, modulate the conduction and gating properties of Na_V channels. For example, tetrodotoxin (TTX) and saxitoxin are small compounds isolated from the puffer fish. Both compounds are comparable to two amino acids in size, but they can potently inhibit certain Na_V channels with nanomolar affinities. On the other hand, scorpion α- and β-toxins are polypeptides consisting of 60–80 amino acids. They interfere with the gating mechanisms of Na_V channels by binding to the voltage sensor domain. Since Na_V channels are important drug targets, the toxins are potential scaffolds for drug discovery.

The structures of Na_V channels from several different bacterial species have been solved (Payandeh et al., 2012; Zhang et al., 2012), providing excellent templates for computational studies of mammalian Na_V channels. A number of computational studies have focused on the binding of toxins to bacterial and mammalian Na_V channels. We will briefly discuss how these studies have helped to gain a structural understanding of toxin action.

3.1 Tetrodotoxin

TTX (molecular formula $C_{11}H_{17}N_3O_8$) is a guanidinium compound synthesized by bacteria in animals, such as puffer fish (Noguchi et al., 1987), octopus (Hwang et al., 1989), and chaetognatha (Thuesen & Kogure, 1989). It has a cage-like rigid structure and carries one positive charge at neutral pH (Fig. 2A).

TTX selectively inhibits several mammalian Na_V channel isoforms such as $Na_V1.4$, which is predominantly expressed in the skeletal muscle cells, with IC_{50} values in the nanomolar range (Catterall et al., 2007; French, Yoshikami, Sheets, & Olivera, 2010; Kao & Nishiyama, 1965). However, it is much less effective for certain isoforms such as $Na_V1.5$, $Na_V1.8$, $Na_V1.9$, with much higher IC_{50} values in the micromolar range (Lee & Ruben, 2008). TTX does not inhibit bacterial Na_V channels even at micromolar toxin concentrations (Ren et al., 2001), which may yield insights into TTX binding and selectivity, but also generates difficulties in using bacterial Na_V structures as models for understanding TTX binding.

A

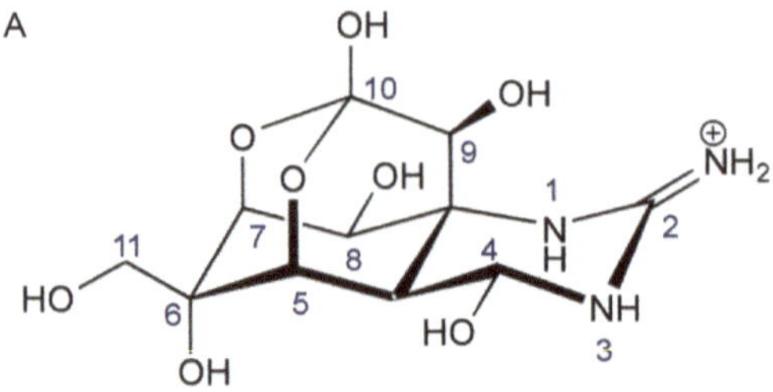

B

	160	177	192	
Na_VAb	FGTLGESFYTLFQVM	TLESW	SMGIVRPLMEVYP	
I	YDTFSWAFLALFRLM	TQDYW	ENLFQLTLRAAGK	421
II	MHDFFHSFLIVFRIL	CGEWI	ETMWDCMEVAAMC	778
III	YDNVGLGYLSLLQVA	TFKGW	MDIMYAAVDSREK	1259
IV	FETFGNSIICLFEIT	TSAGW	DGLLNPILNSGPP	1551

Fig. 2 (A) Structure of tetrodotoxin. (B) Sequence alignment of Na_VAb and human Na_V1.4 in the pore region. The selectivity filter is highlighted in *shadow* and the Tyr407 residue of the domain I filter with an *underscore*. Basic residues are colored in *blue* and acidic residues in *red*. *Adapted with permission from Chen, R., & Chung, S. H. (2014). Mechanism of tetrodotoxin block and resistance in sodium channels.* Biochemical and Biophysical Research Communications, 446, *370–374. Copyright Elsevier.*

Experimental studies suggest that the tyrosine residue in the filter of domain I (Tyr401 of rat and Tyr407 of human Na_V1.4) is crucial for TTX sensitivity and the lack of this tyrosine in Na_V1.5, Na_V1.8, Na_V1.9 may be responsible for their resistance to TTX (Santarelli, Eastwood, Dougherty, Horn, & Ahern, 2007). Earlier models proposed that the guanidinium group of TTX protrudes into the pore and interacts intimately with the tyrosine, thereby blocking the channel (Fozzard & Lipkind, 2010).

Fig. 2B shows a sequence alignment of the bacterial channel Na_VAb and the human Na_V1.4 in the pore region. In contrast to Na_VAb, which is a homotetramer, Na_V1.4 is an integral protein consisted of four homologous domains (I–IV). The selectivity filter of Na_VAb carries four negative charges (EEEE ring at position 177), while that of Na_V1.4 carries two negative charges and one positive charge (DEKA ring). The difference in the filter charges may account for the sensitivity and resistance of the two channels to TTX (Chen & Chung, 2014). Another key difference between the two channels is that there is a second charge ring EEDD just outside the filter in Na_V1.4, at a position corresponding to Ser180 or Met181 of Na_VAb (Fig. 2B).

Molecular dynamics studies have revealed that at least two Na^+ ions would occupy the filter of Na_VAb in a nonconducting state (Carnevale, Treptow, & Klein, 2011; Chakrabarti et al., 2013; Corry & Thomas, 2012). Simulations of Na_VAb and TTX revealed that TTX is able to form strong interactions with the EEEE ring in the presence of one filter ion (Fig. 3A). However, in the presence of two filter ions, the second ion weakens the interaction between TTX and the charged EEEE ring (Fig. 3B), resulting in the binding affinity to reduce by five orders of magnitude (Chen & Chung, 2014).

In the case of $Na_V1.4$, only one Na^+ ion is stably bound to the filter, possibly due to fewer negative charges in the DEKA ring than that in the EEEE ring of Na_VAb (Chen & Chung, 2014). The fewer charges would also mean weaker electrostatic interactions with TTX. Molecular dynamics simulations suggest that TTX forms a hydrogen-bond network with the outer charge ring of $Na_V1.4$, rather than the DEKA ring (Chen & Chung, 2014). The hydrogen-bond network collectively stabilizes the binding of TTX to $Na_V1.4$. The guanidine group of TTX adopts a lateral orientation relative to the filter of $Na_V1.4$, thereby fully blocking the outer entrance of the channel (Fig. 3C). The binding of TTX is stabilized by six H-bonds formed with the

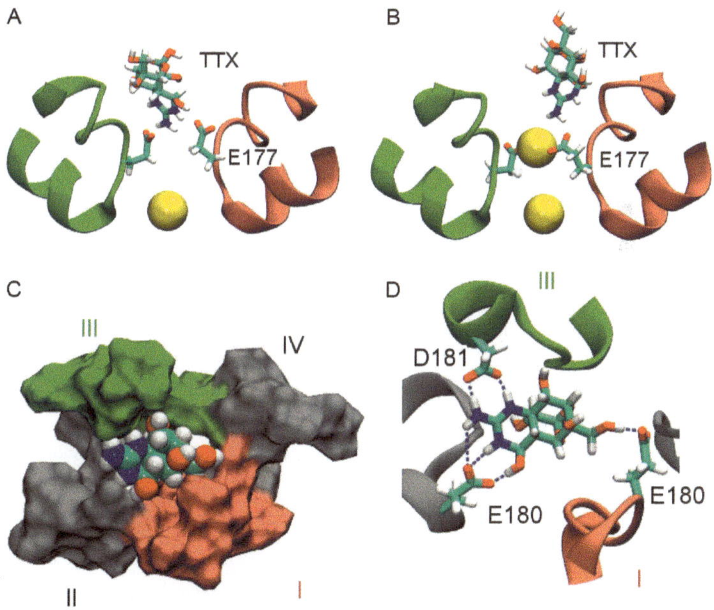

Fig. 3 Tetrodotoxin (TTX) bound to the selectivity filter of Na_VAb (A, B) and $Na_V1.4$ (C, D) as predicted from molecular dynamics. The Na^+ ions in the filter of Na_VAb are shown as *yellow spheres*. In (C) and (D), residue numbering is that of Na_VAb. *Adapted with permission from Chen, R., & Chung, S. H. (2014). Mechanism of tetrodotoxin block and resistance in sodium channels.* Biochemical and Biophysical Research Communications, 446, *370–374. Copyright Elsevier.*

outer charge ring (Fig. 3D). TTX is also in close proximity to Tyr407 of $Na_V1.4$, which has been proposed to be important for TTX sensitivity (Santarelli et al., 2007).

Computational mutagenesis results suggest that the formation of a stable hydrogen-bond network is crucial for the high-affinity binding of TTX, and the weakening of this hydrogen bonding interactions accounts for the resistance of several mutant $Na_V1.4$ channels to TTX (Chen & Chung, 2014). When the key tyrosine residue at the extracellular end of the filter in domain I is replaced by a cysteine or aspartate, the total number of hydrogen bonds between TTX and $Na_V1.4$ is reduced from six to four or five, thus reducing the binding affinity of TTX–$Na_V1.4$ by more than two orders of magnitude (Chen & Chung, 2014).

3.2 Pore-Blocking Toxins

A family of short polypeptides isolated from the venom of cone snails, known as μ-conotoxins, inhibit Na_V channels potently with a pore-blocking mechanism. The μ-conotoxins that have been characterized typically comprise 15–25 amino acids, with six cysteine residues forming three disulfide bridges arranged in a class III framework (Terlau & Olivera, 2004). The primary structures of four example μ-conotoxins are given in Fig. 4A, and the secondary and atomic structures of PIIIA in Fig. 4B.

Many μ-conotoxins with distinct potency and selectivity to mammalian Na_V channels have been characterized. Two of the most widely studied are

A

```
μ-PIIIA    ZRLCCGFOKS-CRSRQCKOHR-CC*
μ-SxIIIA     RCCTGKKGSCSGRACKNLK-CCA*
μ-GIIIA     RDCCTOOKK-CKDRQCKOQR-CCA*
μ-KIIIA       CC-N----CSSKWCRDHSRCC*
```

B

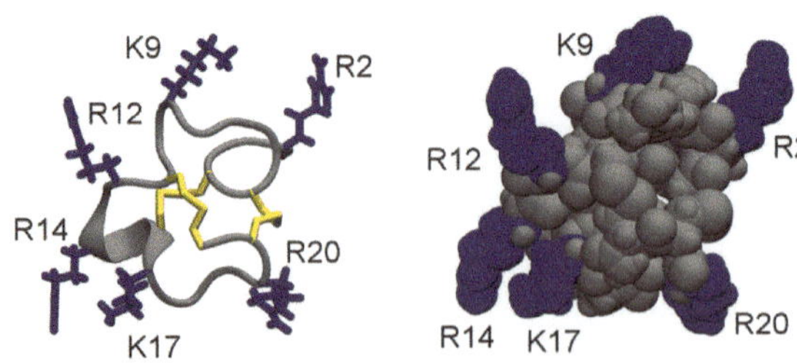

Fig. 4 Structure of μ-conotoxins. (A) Primary structures of four example μ-conotoxins. (B) NMR solution structure of PIIIA (PDB ID 1R9I), highlighting the six basic residues it carries in either *blue licorice or spheres*. The three disulfide bonds are shown in *yellow*.

GIIIA and PIIIA (Al-Sabi et al., 2006). GIIIA isolated from *Conus geographus* is selective for the skeletal muscle channel, $Na_V1.4$ (Safo et al., 2000). On the other hand, PIIIA from *Conus purpurascens* blocks both skeletal muscle and neuronal Na_V channels with IC_{50} values in the nanomolar range (Safo et al., 2000). Experimental studies, in which the alanine mutation of a basic residue caused drastic reduction in toxin inhibition, suggested that μ-conotoxins act via a pore-blocking mechanism (Al-Sabi et al., 2006; Catterall et al., 2007; Dutertre & Lewis, 2010).

Several molecular dynamics studies have focused on the binding modes of PIIIA and GIIIA to the pore domain of bacterial and mammalian Na_V channels (Chen & Chung, 2012b; Chen, Robinson, & Chung, 2014; Mahdavi & Kuyucak, 2014a, 2014b). The simulations, for the first time, predicted that PIIIA should be an extremely potent blocker of Na_VAb, with a predicted K_d value of 10–30 pM (Chen & Chung, 2012b). The picomolar affinity was unexpected as it is substantially lower than the values of between 36 nM and 3.2 μM for the block of mammalian Na_V channels by PIIIA determined experimentally (Wilson et al., 2011). However, subsequent experiments showed that PIIIA indeed inhibits NaChBac, which is a bacterial sodium channel highly related to Na_VAb, with a K_d of 5 pM (Finol-Urdaneta, Glavica, McArthur, & French, 2013), in very good agreement with the computational predictions, indicating the binding affinity of a peptide toxin to a channel can be calculated fairly accurately. The simulations also showed that PIIIA blocks Na_VAb with alternative pore-blocking basic residues such as Arg2 and Lys9 (Chen & Chung, 2012b), as opposed to a single dominant residue. Two example binding modes predicted from the simulations are shown in Fig. 5A. In both binding modes, three salt bridges between the channel and the toxin are formed. While Arg2 or Lys9 of the toxin protrudes into the selectivity filter, two other basic residues from the toxin form salt bridges with acidic residues from the outer vestibular wall of the channel, thereby stabilizing the binding (Fig. 5A). The PMF profiles derived from the two binding modes are comparable in depth and shape (Fig. 5B), indicating that they are of similar energetics.

Simulations of PIIIA and the mammalian $Na_V1.4$ channel showed that the toxin also forms three salt bridges with the channel when one of its basic residues protrudes into the channel filter (Chen et al., 2014; Mahdavi & Kuyucak, 2014b). The diverse models of PIIIA–$Na_V1.4$ complex proposed by Mahdavi and Kuyucak (Mahdavi & Kuyucak, 2014b) and Chen and Chung (Chen et al., 2014) are consistent with the multiple-binding-mode mechanism proposed previously for PIIIA–Na_VAb (Chen & Chung, 2012b).

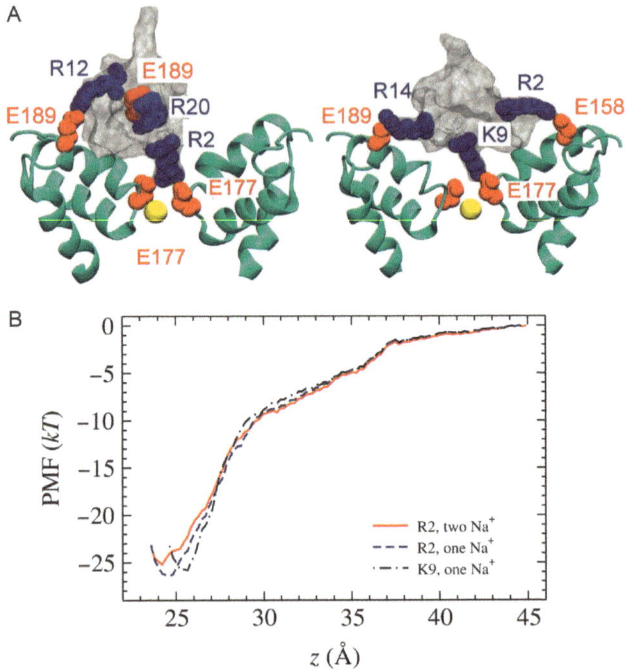

Fig. 5 Binding modes and PMF profiles for the binding of μ-conotoxin PIIIA to Na_VAb. (A) Two binding modes in which Arg2 or Lys9 protrudes into the selectivity filter of the channel are shown. The *yellow sphere* denotes the Na^+ ion in the filter. (B) PMF profiles of the two binding modes in the presence of one or two Na^+ ions in the filter. The reaction coordinate is the center of mass distance between the toxin and channel backbones along the channel axis. *Adapted with permission from Chen, R., & Chung, S. H. (2012b). Binding modes of μ-conotoxin to the bacterial sodium channel (Na_VAb).* Biophysical Journal, 102, *483–488. Copyright Elsevier.*

The exceptionally high affinities of PIIIA for bacterial Na_V channels could be due to the four negative charges in the channel filter (EEEE ring), which are absent in mammalian Na_V channels (DEKA ring). In conclusion, computational studies provided insights into the molecular mechanisms of toxin action that were otherwise difficult to obtain from physical experiments.

3.3 Voltage-Sensing Toxins

Many peptide toxins isolated from spiders, cone snails, and scorpions that have been characterized regulate the gating mechanisms of Na_V channels by binding to the voltage sensor domain of the channel (Bosmans & Swartz, 2010; Heinemann & Leipold, 2007; Possani, Becerril, Delepierre, & Tytgat, 1999). Some toxins show exceptional selectivity for $Na_V1.7$, a target for the treatment of acute and inflammatory pain (Nassar et al., 2004) as well as neuropathic pain (Minett et al., 2012). For example, ProTx-II from *Thrixopelma pruriens* is 100-fold selective for $Na_V1.7$ over six other Na_V channel isoforms (Schmalhofer et al., 2008). Similarly, scorpion α- and β-toxins are also selective for certain Na_V channels. Due to the lack of high-resolution structures, relatively few studies focusing on Na_V channel voltage-sensing toxins have been reported.

Scorpion α- and β-toxins are short peptides consisting of 60–80 residues. They share a similar structural fold (Fig. 6), but their mechanisms of action are rather different. Available experimental data suggest that scorpion α-toxins interfere with the fast inactivation by binding to the voltage sensor of domain IV, whereas β-toxins interfere with the activation of the channel by binding to the domain II voltage sensor.

Experimental studies have suggested that the functional surface of both α- and β-toxins consists of two key domains, the NC domain and the core domain. The NC domain consists of a five-residue turn (residues 8–12) and the C-terminal segment (residues 56–64), whereas the core domain is formed by several residues spatially in close proximity to the residue at

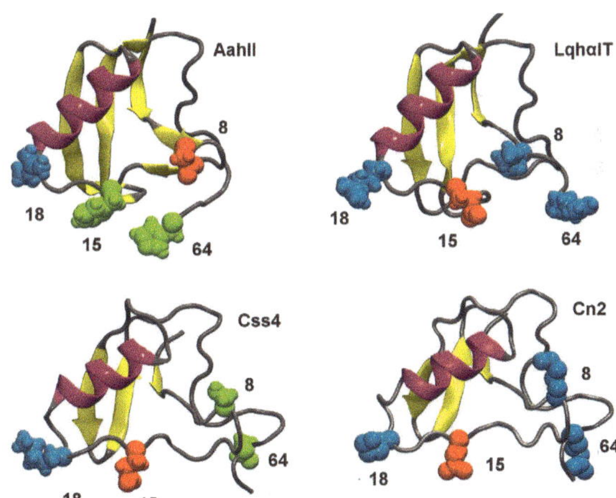

Fig. 6 Structures of two scorpion α-toxins, AahII (PDB ID 1PTX) and LqhαIT (PDB ID 1LQH) and two β-toxins, Cn2 (PDB ID 1CN2) and Css4 (modeled on Cn2). The side chains of residues at positions 8, 18, 15, and 64 are highlighted (*blue*, basic; *red*, acidic; *green*, polar). *Adapted with permission from Chen, R., & Chung, S. H. (2012a). Binding modes and functional surface of anti-mammalian scorpion α-toxins to sodium channels.* Biochemistry, 51, *7775–7782; Chen, R., & Chung, S. H. (2012c). Conserved functional surface of anti-mammalian scorpion β-toxins.* The Journal of Physical Chemistry B, 116, *4796–4800. Copyright American Chemical Society.*

position 18 (Fig. 7A). The NC domain and the core domain are less conserved compared to other regions of the toxins, and several key residues of these two domains have been found to largely determine the selectivity of these toxins (Kahn et al., 2009; Schiavon et al., 2006).

Using molecular dynamics, the critical role of the linker domain, which interconnects the NC domain and the core domain, in the binding of the toxins to mammalian Na_V channels was proposed (Chen & Chung, 2012a, 2012c) (Fig. 7B). Molecular docking was used to predict the possible binding modes between scorpion β-toxin Css4 and domain II voltage sensor of $Na_V1.2$. The most highly ranked conformation in which the NC domain and the core domain the toxin are in close proximity to the voltage sensor was selected for subsequent refinement in a lipid bilayer using molecular dynamics with explicit solvent (Chen & Chung, 2012c). The resulting model shows that the linker domain wedges into the outer crevice of the voltage sensor (Fig. 7B) (Chen & Chung, 2012c). One acidic residue from the toxin forms a salt bridge with an arginine from the extracellular end of the S4 helix of the voltage sensor (Fig. 7C), thereby stabilizing the binding. The salt bridge involving the equivalent S4 arginine is also observed when the conotoxin EVIA binds to the domain IV voltage sensor of $Na_V1.2$. EVIA spontaneously binds to the extracellular end of the voltage sensor over a

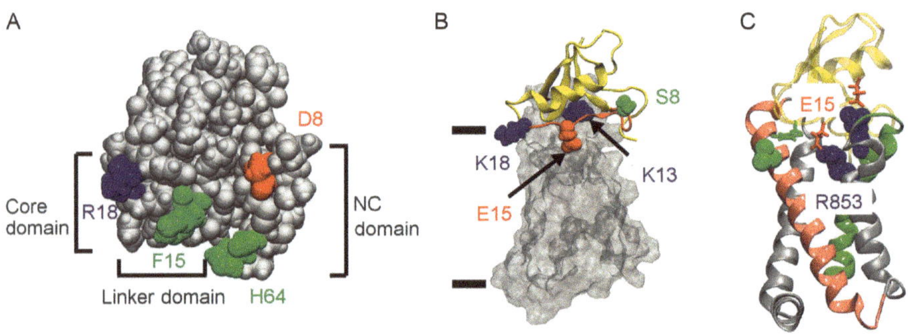

Fig. 7 (A) Structure of AahII with three domains important for Na^+ channel binding indicated. (B) Binding mode of Css4 to the domain II voltage sensor of $Na_V1.2$ predicted from molecular dynamics. The linker domain of the toxin is highlighted in *red*. The *horizontal bars* indicate the approximate position of the membrane surface. (C) Binding of Css4 (*top, yellow ribbons*) to $Na_V1.2$ domain II voltage sensor (*bottom*). *Adapted with permission from Chen, R., & Chung, S. H. (2012a). Binding modes and functional surface of anti-mammalian scorpion α-toxins to sodium channels.* Biochemistry, 51, *7775–7782; Chen, R., & Chung, S. H. (2012c). Conserved functional surface of anti-mammalian scorpion β-toxins.* The Journal of Physical Chemistry B, 116, *4796–4800. Copyright American Chemical Society.*

simulation period of 50 ns, forming a salt bridge between Asp2 of EVIA and the arginine of the S4 helix (Chen & Chung, 2012a). This finding was subsequently reproduced with EVIA and $Na_V1.7$ using docking and molecular dynamics (Tietze et al., 2016). More studies are to be carried out to elucidate the mechanisms of selectivity of these toxins among different species (e.g., mammals vs insects) and channel isoforms (e.g., $Na_V1.1$–$Na_V1.9$).

4. SODIUM CHANNEL–SMALL MOLECULE INTERACTIONS

Voltage-gated sodium channels are known to be key targets of a variety of analgesics, antiepileptic, and antiarrhythmic drugs (Catterall, 2000; Fozzard et al., 2011). Even though these small molecules are known to affect sodium channel function, much about the mechanism of how this happens is still under investigation. These diverse compounds, collectively known as "local anesthetics," block the central ion conducting pore in sodium channels, thereby preventing Na^+ influx and hampering membrane depolarization. Recently, a number of compounds have been discovered that inhibit sodium channels by binding to the voltage sensor domains (Ahuja et al., 2015; McCormack et al., 2013). However, these are not yet used clinically and have not been the subject of simulations at the time of writing, so are not discussed further here.

Many local anesthetics have a pK_a in the neutral range, meaning that they exist in both neutral and charged forms at physiological pH. Parallel to this, these compounds are known to be able to block the pore in at least two distinct ways. Small hydrophobic compounds and neutral species of the drugs are known to be able to enter and block the pore in the resting state, or to leave the pore while the channel remains closed (Hille, 1977). The so-called tonic block of resting channels led to the hypothesis that such compounds might enter the pore using a "hydrophobic route"—directly from the bilayer via gaps in the side of the sodium channel protein (Hille, 1977). Drug binding in tonic block is generally low affinity (high μM to mM) but is effective at completely blocking nerve impulses at high concentration. The presence of a hydrophobic entrance route in the form of lateral fenestrations proposed by Hille in 1977 was confirmed in 2011, upon publication of the first structure of the bacterial sodium channel Na_VAb (Payandeh et al., 2011). This was shown to have four lipid-filled gaps in the protein that extend to the center of the lipid bilayer, which could represent the proposed hydrophobic path taken by tonic blocking compounds. Since then, a number of bacterial sodium channel structures have been solved (Ahuja et al., 2015; Bagneris et al., 2013, 2014; McCusker et al., 2012; Naylor et al., 2016; Payandeh et al., 2012; Shaya et al., 2014; Tsai et al., 2013; Zhang et al., 2012), all of which contain fenestrations. Although the presence of fenestrations in the crystal structures is suggestive of a route for tonic block, there is no direct evidence to show that small molecules can pass through these gaps in the protein. Thus, important questions remain about the process of tonic block: (i) What small molecules will enter the lipid bilayer? (ii) Are the fenestrations seen in the crystal structures large enough to allow small molecules to pass? (iii) Can a compound pass all the way from the aqueous solution to the pore-blocking site via this route? (iv) Can differences in the fenestrations in different channel isoforms generate selective binding? (v) Are there any other routes by which small hydrophobic compounds could enter the pore? As described later, recent simulation studies have assisted in answering all of these questions.

Alternatively, amphiphilic compounds or charged drug species can cause open-channel block, or "use-dependent" block (Hille, 2001), by entering through the cytoplasmic gate when the channel opens. Presumably charged use-dependent blockers must permeate the membrane in the neutral form, before becoming reprotonated in the cytoplasm. Because such compounds bind to open or inactivated channels and have little affinity for resting channels, they are valuable tools for subtly reducing electrical signaling in hyperexcitable cells, which have many channels in these states. In addition, channels can only recover from use-dependent block once the compound has unbound from the blocking site, meaning that they can limit the frequency of sodium channel activation. Use-dependent block is typically of higher affinity (low μM) than tonic block.

Mutagenesis studies show that both tonic and use-dependent inhibitors bind in the central pore, as a number of pore lining residues are implicated in binding. While there are small differences between the sites inferred for each class of compound the approximate similarity has led to this site being termed the "local anesthetic site." This site lies in the central cavity of the pore, toward the cytoplasmic activation gate (Ahern, Eastwood, Dougherty, & Horn, 2008; Gingrich, Beardsley, & Yue, 1993; Kimbrough & Gingrich, 2000; McNulty et al., 2007; Pless, Galpin, Frankel, & Ahern, 2011; Ragsdale, McPhee, Scheuer, & Catterall, 1994, 1996; Zamponi, Doyle, & French, 1993). However, different residues contribute to use-dependent and tonic block (Ragsdale et al., 1994), suggesting that there may be conformational changes in the pore associated with channel opening and/or inactivation. Most of the pharmacological and mutagenesis data comes from studies of eukaryotic channels, and the lack of a corresponding structure makes it difficult to clearly discern the nature and differences between the tonic and use-dependent binding sites. Thus, it is hoped that the bacterial channel structures may provide a template for understanding the location and nature of binding, although there are a number of sequence differences in amino acids lining the pore walls. As discussed later, molecular simulations may provide a way to help determine how well binding to bacterial channels can mimic that in eukaryotic channels and to pinpoint the location and interactions in the binding site.

A final, as yet unexplored, area is to determine which species of the drug enters and binds to the channel in each case. For example, do protonatable tonic blockers reach the site in the neutral form, but revert to the charged form prior to binding in the aqueous interior of the pore? Do use-dependent blockers have to enter through the cytoplasmic gate in the charged form, or can they enter resting channels in the neutral form, but change charge state in the pore and display high-affinity binding once the channel enters the open or inactivated state?

4.1 Bilayer Partitioning

A compound's potency is often positively correlated with its lipophilicity, suggesting that entry into and crossing the cell membrane is essential to a compound's efficacy (Langerman, Bansinath, & Grant, 1994; Štolc, Nemček, & Szöcsová, 1989; Strichartz, Sanchez, Arthur, Chafetz, & Martin, 1990). Indeed, entering or crossing the membrane is a requirement for both use-dependent block through the cytoplasmic gate or tonic entry via the fenestrations. A number of simulations studies have been conducted to examine the interaction of benzocaine (Boiteux et al., 2014; Cascales, Costa, & Porasso, 2011; Martin, Chao, & Corry, 2014; Porasso, Bennett, Oliveira-Costa, & Cascales, 2009), lidocaine (Högberg & Lyubartsev, 2008; Högberg, Maliniak, & Lyubartsev, 2007), articaine (Mojumdar & Lyubartsev, 2010), and phenytoin (Boiteux et al., 2014; Martin et al., 2014) with lipid bilayers. Benzocaine exists only in a neutral form and displays only tonic block, while lidocaine, articaine, and phenytoin can block in both a tonic and use-dependent fashion (Hille, 1977, 2001; Quan, Mok, & Wang, 1996; Schwarz, Palade, & Hille, 1977; Wang, Calderon, Jaw, & Wang, 2009). Interestingly, lidocaine and articaine exist in both neutral and charged states at neutral pH, but phenytoin is almost exclusively in a neutral form.

A variety of simulation techniques, such as flooding and PMF calculations, were used to study the interaction of these compounds with lipid bilayers. All found that, irrespective of the charge state, the drugs preferred to partition into the bilayer and sit just below the lipid head groups, slightly above the position at which the fenestrations appear as seen in Fig. 8. This would suggest the plausibility of the compounds finding the fenestration

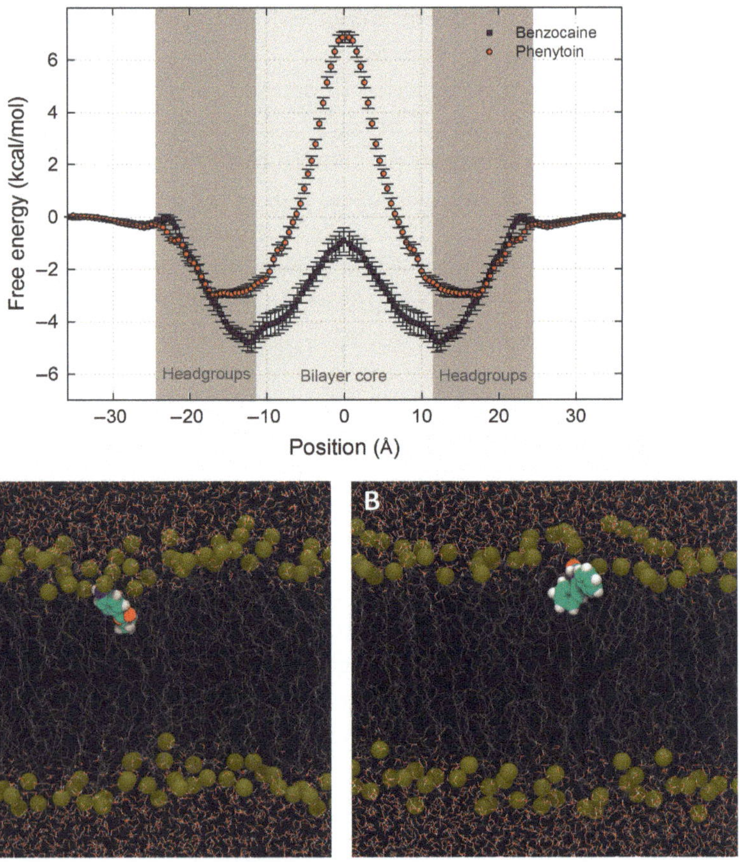

Fig. 8 Simulations of bilayer partitioning. The free energy (PMF) for the tonic blocker benzocaine (*blue*) and the primarily use-dependent blocker phenytoin (*red*) is shown as a function of position in a POPC bilayer. Included are snapshots of benzocaine (A) and phenytoin (B) sitting at their most favorable position near the head groups of the bilayer. *Adapted from Martin, L. J., Chao, R., & Corry, B. (2014). Molecular dynamics simulation of the partitioning of benzocaine and phenytoin into a lipid bilayer.* Biophysical Chemistry, 185, *98–107. Copyright Elsevier.*

entrance as required for tonic block. However, all compounds do face an energy barrier in the center of the bilayer, which is large for phenytoin (as shown in Fig. 8A), which will limit the rate at which they can enter the cytoplasm. It is important that use-dependent blockers do not partition too strongly into the bilayer and that they do not face a large barrier to cross the bilayer, otherwise they will not accumulate in the cytoplasm. The presence of two charge states may be essential to achieving this balance. In contrast, compounds with only a neutral form, such as benzocaine, are generally attracted more strongly to the bilayer, as seen in Fig. 8A. As a consequence, they only display tonic block, as they never reach large concentrations in the cytoplasm.

4.2 Route of Entry of Tonic Blocking Drugs

An obvious question to ask when assessing the route of tonic blocking compounds into the pore is whether the lipid-filled fenestrations seen in the crystal structures are large enough for small molecules to pass. One can start answering this by simply measuring the dimensions in the published structures. A recent analysis of a number of the published bacterial Na_V structures indicates that the radius at the narrowest point in fenestrations is generally a little larger than 2 Å, almost the size required to pass a benzene ring (r=2.4 Å) (Corry et al., 2014). However, the dimensions differ among the published structures. While the "preopen" structures contain four identical fenestrations, the potentially inactivated channels have two narrow fenestrations and two wider ones (Payandeh et al., 2012). In addition, the structure of the potentially open state channel is reported to have wider fenestrations than the preopen states (McCusker et al., 2012). This has led to the hypothesis that there may be differential access to the channel in different channel states. However, the size differences are small (<1 Å) and mostly occur at the external end of the fenestration rather than altering the bottleneck diameter (Corry et al., 2014). In addition, the differences between the preopen and open structures reflect sequence differences rather than state-dependent structural changes (Kaczmarski & Corry, 2014), so it is not clear if such variations can be exploited for pharmacological targeting of functional states.

Before inferring too much from the crystal structures of the bacterial channels, it is important to remember that these are only snapshots, which do not capture the full range of motion possible for each structure. Thus, it is possible that the fenestration sizes may fluctuate with time due to side chain motions or larger scale structural changes. Molecular dynamics can help answer this by simulating the channel and tracking the fenestration size over a long period of time. Two studies have systematically investigated how the fenestration sizes change over time in Na_VAb (Boiteux et al., 2014; Kaczmarski & Corry, 2014). It was found that the fenestration radii is dynamic, and for at least part of the time they are wide enough ($r=2.6$ Å) to get a benzene ring ($r=2.4$ Å) through the fenestration into the pore (Fig. 9). The key residues that are responsible for the dynamic nature of the pore radius are hydrophobic. The dynamic, hydrophobic nature of the fenestrations would allow a number of local anesthetic drugs to pass through the fenestrations. One of these studies also examined differences in the fenestration size among six different bacterial protein structures and a homology model of $Na_v1.4$ (Kaczmarski & Corry, 2014). It suggested

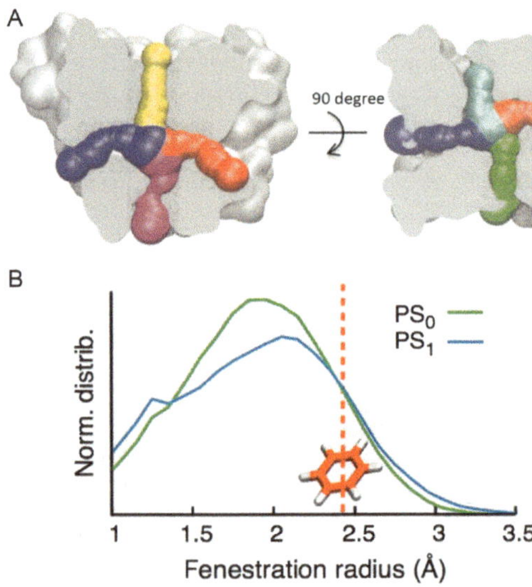

Fig. 9 Fenestration location and size. (A) Representative volumes of individual fenestrations over a simulation shown by colored surfaces, with a *side view* (*left*) and *top view* (*right*) of the fenestrations. The selectivity filter (*yellow*) and cytoplasmic pore (*purple*) are also visible. (B) Distribution of fenestration radii from a long (ca. 2–3 μs) simulation. The radius of a benzene ring is highlighted by a *dashed red line*, along with the structure of benzene. *Panel (A) adapted from Kaczmarski, J. A., & Corry, B. (2014). Investigating the size and dynamics of voltage-gated sodium channel fenestrations: A molecular dynamics study.* Channels, 8*(3), 264–277. Copyright Taylor and Francis. Panel (B) adapted from Boiteux, C., Vorobyov, I., & Allen, T. W. (2014). Ion conduction and conformational flexibility of a bacterial voltage-gated sodium channel.* Proceedings of the National Academy of Sciences of the United States of America, 111*(9), 3454–3459. Copyright National Academy of Sciences.*

that there is no clear evidence that the fenestration size changes in different functional states of the channel, but sequence differences among the proteins could yield differential access for tonic blockers to different proteins. While the eukaryotic model had two very narrow fenestrations, two were large enough to pass small blocking drugs.

Final proof that small molecules can pass through the fenestrations comes from studies that directly simulate this process, with a number of studies showing that small molecules can penetrate the fenestration. For example, when benzocaine was initially placed inside the pore, it was observed to pass outward through the fenestration in a 125 ns unbiased simulation (Martin & Corry, 2014). Conversely, the flooding approach has been used to witness the movement of isoflurane (Raju, Barber, LeBard, Klein, & Carnevale, 2013), benzocaine (Boiteux et al., 2014), and sevoflurane (Barber, Carnevale, Klein, Eckenhoff, & Covarrubias, 2014) from the aqueous solution, into the bilayer, through the fenestration, and into the pore. The fenestrations are often occupied by lipid tails in the absence of any drug molecules. However, in the presence of the small molecules, the lipid tails are displaced from the fenestrations when the drugs enter into the pore via the lateral fenestrations and move to the bottom of the pore, remaining there for much of the simulation.

The energetic barriers for benzocaine and phenytoin entry through the fenestrations have been quantified using the approach of umbrella sampling simulations (Martin & Corry, 2014). These showed that benzocaine faced only very small barriers in the order of 2 kcal/mol to pass from the bilayer into the pore. Phenytoin is bulkier and faces larger barriers (~5 kcal/mol), but these primarily arise from penetrating deep into the bilayer to access the fenestration rather than being impeded in the fenestration itself (Fig. 10A). These barriers are consistent with the tonic blocking on-rates of these compounds. The free energy barriers seen by benzocaine to pass through the fenestrations and bilayer have also be quantified from long flooding simulations (Boiteux et al., 2014), which show similar magnitudes to the umbrella sampling results (Fig. 10B). Phenytoin does enter the fenestration in the flooding simulations so similar data could not be obtained in this case.

Another study (O'Reilly et al., 2012) ran steered molecular dynamics simulations on a homology model of $Na_V1.5$ to determine how Bisphenol-A and mexiletine enter resting channels. This study found that it is more favorable for both compounds to enter the pore via the lateral fenestrations than the selectivity filter, which agrees with previous studies on the bacterial channels.

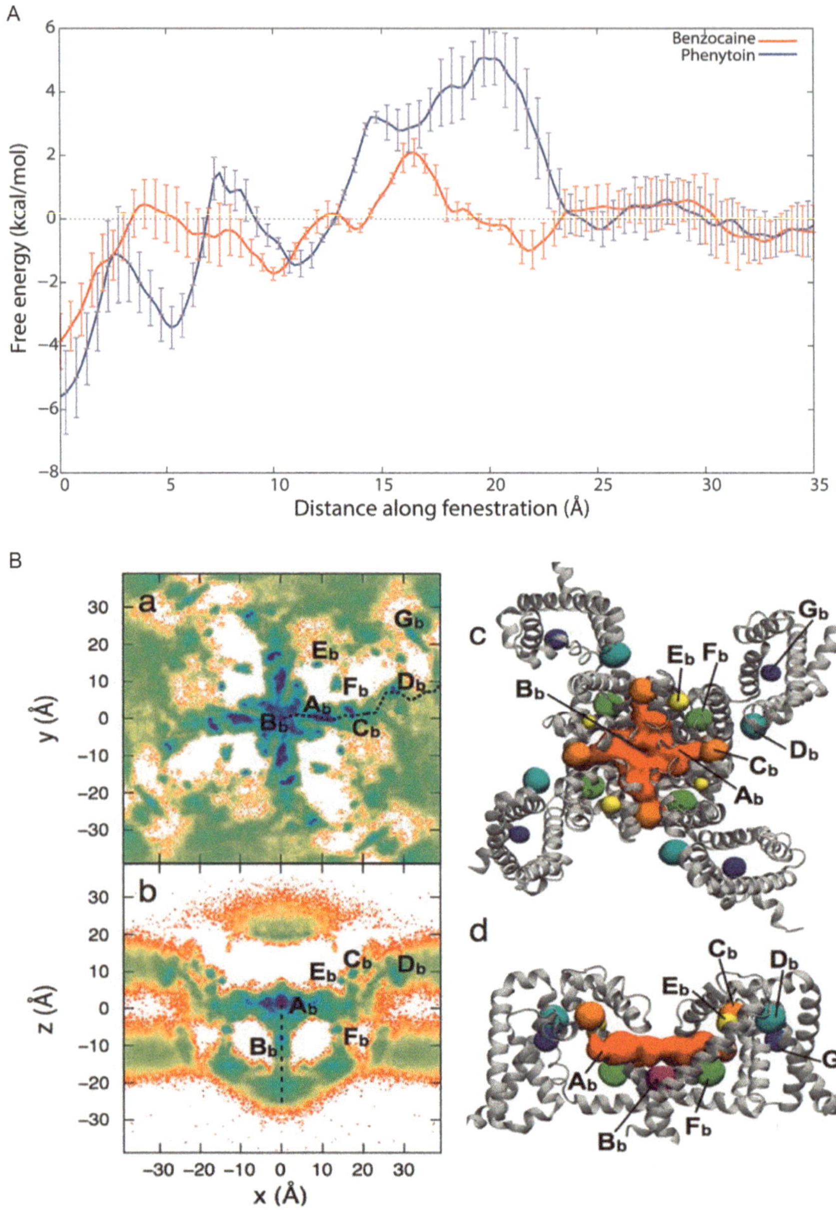

Fig. 10 Passage of drugs through the fenestrations. (A) PMF of benzocaine and phenytoin traveling from the bilayer (*right side* of the graph) through a fenestration into the pore (*left side* of the graph). Benzocaine is represented by the *red line* and Phenytoin by the *blue line*. (B) Energy landscapes of benzocaine and phenytoin from flooding simulations. The location of the low energy regions are represented by capitalized letters in the graphs on the *left side* and are represented by colored surfaces in the structure to the

A surprise finding from the MD simulations has been that small molecules may be able to pass through the closed activation gate (Boiteux et al., 2014; Martin & Corry, 2014; Smith & Corry, 2016). All these studies presented evidence that benzocaine faced only a very small barrier to move from the cytoplasm into the pore in Na_VAb. This aqueous route, could, therefore represent a way for tonic blocking compounds to enter the pore. But, this result needs to be taken with caution. The crystal structure of Na_VAb is truncated just beyond the cytoplasmic gate, and it is possible that additional barriers for entry would exist in the presence of the full C-terminus. In addition, eukaryotic sodium channels contain additional aromatic residues in the pore, and when these are added to Na_VAb, entry of benzocaine through the gate becomes much harder (Smith & Corry, 2016). Finally, due to its strong preference to partition into the bilayer, benzocaine may not reach high enough concentrations in the cytoplasm for this aqueous route to be commonly used.

4.3 Location of Binding Sites

The locations of binding have been examined using molecular dynamics in a number of studies using a variety of methods. Martin et al. (2014) used equilibrium simulations starting with drugs in the pore, metadynamics simulations and umbrella sampling to locate the most likely positions inside the Na_VAb pore. It found two likely sites for benzocaine and phenytoin using each of the methods: (1) near the activation gate and (2) at the internal entrance of the fenestrations (Fig. 11A). Either of these could represent the local anesthetic site. Similar sites were found using flooding simulations of two inhalation anesthetics isoflurane (Raju et al., 2013) and sevoflurane (Barber et al., 2014) with NaChBac, and flooding of benzocaine with Na_VAb (Boiteux et al., 2014). Flooding simulations also found additional binding sites (3), an extracellular site at the top of the selectivity filter between P loops and (4) a linker site at a "corner" formed by the

right (with corresponding labels). *Top* and *side views* are shown. *Panel (A) adapted from Martin, L. J., & Corry, B. (2014). Locating the route of entry and binding sites of benzocaine and phenytoin in a bacterial voltage gated sodium channel.* PLoS Computational Biology, 10*(7). Panel (B) adapted from Boiteux, C., Vorobyov, I., French, R. J., French, C., Yarov-yarovoy, V., & Allen, T. W. (2014). Local anesthetic and antiepileptic drug access and binding to a bacterial voltage-gated sodium channel.* Proceedings of the National Academy of Sciences of the United States of America, 111*(36), 13057–13062.*

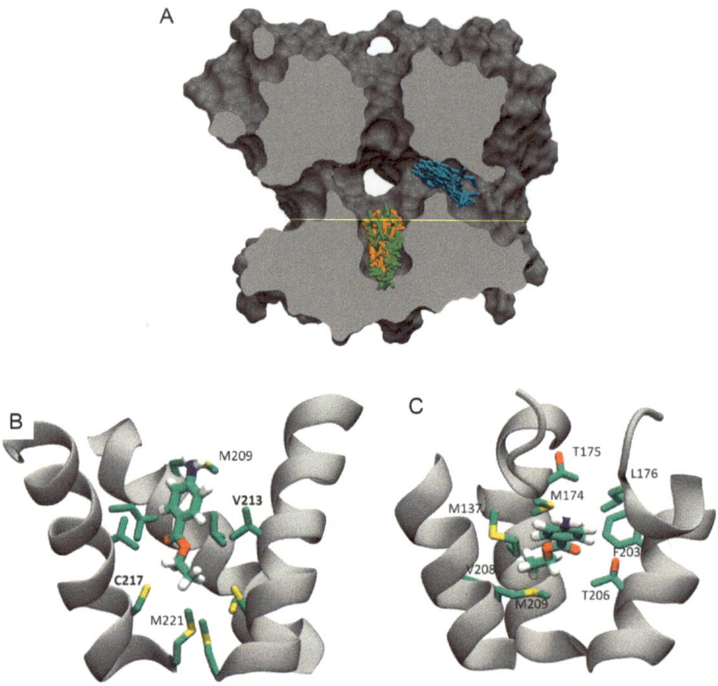

Fig. 11 Binding sites of small molecules in Na_VAb. (A) A cut-through *side view* of Na_VAb, highlighting benzocaine clusters binding to the activation gate site (*green* and *orange*) and fenestration site (*blue*). (B) Binding site of benzocaine in the activation gate region, with relevant residues highlighted. (C) Binding site of benzocaine in the fenestrations, with relevant residues highlighted. Note that strong interactions of benzocaine with F203 are common but not obvious in this picture. Numbering corresponds with associated residue numbers in the Na_VAb sequence. *Adapted from Martin, L. J., & Corry, B. (2014). Locating the route of entry and binding sites of benzocaine and phenytoin in a bacterial voltage gated sodium channel.* PLoS Computational Biology, 10*(7), e1003688.*

N-terminus of one S6 helix, and the C-terminus of the helix that links the S4–S5 helices together.

The simulations allow a number of observations about the binding sites to be made, and we focus here on those for the sites in the pore, which most closely resemble the typical local anesthetic site. First, multiple drug molecules are able to occupy the pore in flooding simulations (Barber et al., 2014; Boiteux et al., 2014; Raju et al., 2013), something that may be physiologically relevant or may be caused by the very high drug concentrations used. Second, both these pore sites involve hydrophobic interactions rather than the formation of specific hydrogen bonds. The activation gate site is a nonpolar pocket formed by the S6 helices, which is probably only present in the resting channel (Fig. 11B). The fenestration site involves interacting with the aromatic phenylalanine F203 in Na_VAb, although there is no equivalent aromatic residue in NachBac, and a number of methionine and hydrophobic residues (Fig. 11C). It is perhaps not surprising that there are not specific polar interactions with these bacterial channels given the low affinity of tonic block and the large number of compounds that are known to block the pore.

The relative binding affinity of the different sites can be determined if the sampling of positions is good in the flooding simulations, or directly from the metadynamics and umbrella sampling simulations. While the flooding simulations for benzocaine show a slight preference for the fenestration site (Fig. 10B) (Boiteux et al., 2014), the umbrella sampling and metadynamics suggest a stronger affinity at the activation gate site than at the fenestrations (Martin & Corry, 2014). This is reinforced by alchemical free energy perturbations which also indicate that phenytoin binds at higher affinity than benzocaine (Martin & Corry, 2014). That the activation gate site is preferred over the fenestration site is slightly surprising, as the latter is more compatible with mutagenesis data in eukaryotic channels. One hypothesis put forward is that the activation gate could represent the site for tonic block, but as this disappears upon channel activation the fenestration site would represent the use-dependent site (Martin & Corry, 2014). However, the absolute binding affinity for benzocaine at the fenestration site found from FEP (80 ± 30 μM) and flooding (140 ± 30 μM) is also more consistent with experimental measurements of tonic block in eukaryotic channels (300–1200 μM) (Neguliaev & Nosyreva, 1979; Wang, Mitchell, Moczydlowski, & Wang, 2004), than is the higher affinity binding at the activation gate.

This uncertainty has been largely clarified in a more recent simulation in which mutations were introduced into the Na_VAb pore to make it more closely represent the sequence found in eukaryotic channels (Smith & Corry, 2016). Aromatic residues are known to be important for binding in eukaryotic channels (Ahern et al., 2008; Kimbrough & Gingrich, 2000; McNulty et al., 2007; Pless et al., 2011; Ragsdale et al., 1994, 1996), but these are largely absent in the bacterial pores. Introducing these into Na_VAb altered the location of binding and the predicted dissociation constants. The bulky aromatic groups obscure the activation gate site, and so favor binding at the fenestration. They also alter the interactions with blocking drugs, reducing the affinity for benzocaine but increasing them for phenytoin to be more in line with experimental measurements in eukaryotic channels. It is suggested that such mutant bacterial channels may be a better model of local anesthetic binding to eukaryotic channels than are the wild type proteins.

5. CONCLUSION

In this chapter, we have summarized how computational methods, in particular molecular dynamics, have advanced our understanding of the detailed mechanisms by which short globular toxin peptides and small drug molecules interfere with the conduction and gating of Na^+ channels. With the rapid advancement in structural biology, such as the recent publication of the high-resolution structure of a mammalian Ca^{2+} channel (Wu et al., 2016), which is highly homologous to Na^+ channels, more insights into Na^+ channel gating and modulation will be gleaned from computational methods in the near future.

ACKNOWLEDGMENTS

R.C. is grateful for financial support from the National Health and Medical Research Council of Australia (APP1070030). B.C. gratefully acknowledges financial support from the Australian Research Council (FT-130100781).

Conflict of interest statement: None.

REFERENCES

Ahern, C. A., Eastwood, A. L., Dougherty, D. A., & Horn, R. (2008). Electrostatic contributions of aromatic residues in the local anesthetic receptor of voltage-gated sodium channels. *Circulation Research*, *102*(1), 86–94.

Ahuja, S., Mukund, S., Deng, L., Khakh, K., Chang, E., Ho, H., ... Payandeh, J. (2015). Structural basis of $Na_V1.7$ inhibition by an isoform-selective small-molecule antagonist. *Science*, *350*(6267), aac5464.

Al-Sabi, A., McArthur, J., Ostroumov, V., & French, R. J. (2006). Marine toxins that target voltage-gated sodium channels. *Marine Drugs*, *4*(3), 157–192.

Bagneris, C., Decaen, P. G., Hall, B. A., Naylor, C. E., Clapham, D. E., Kay, C. W. M., & Wallace, B. A. (2013). Role of the C-terminal domain in the structure and function of tetrameric sodium channels. *Nature Communications*, *4*, 2465.

Bagneris, C., DeCaen, P. G., Naylor, C. E., Pryde, D. C., Nobeli, I., Clapham, D. E., ... Bagnéris, C. (2014). Prokaryotic Na_VMs channel as a structural and functional model for eukaryotic sodium channel antagonism. *Proceedings of the National Academy of Sciences of the United States of America*, *111*(23), 8428–8433.

Barber, A. F., Carnevale, V., Klein, M. L., Eckenhoff, R. G., & Covarrubias, M. (2014). Modulation of a voltage-gated Na+ channel by sevoflurane involves multiple sites and distinct mechanisms. *Proceedings of the National Academy of Sciences of the United States of America*, *111*(18), 6726–6731.

Boiteux, C., Vorobyov, I., French, R. J., French, C., Yarov-yarovoy, V., & Allen, T. W. (2014). Local anesthetic and antiepileptic drug access and binding to a bacterial voltage-gated sodium channel. *Proceedings of the National Academy of Sciences of the United States of America*, *111*(36), 13057–13062.

Bosmans, F., & Swartz, K. J. (2010). Targeting voltage sensors in sodium channels with spider toxins. *Trends in Pharmacological Sciences*, *31*(4), 175–182.

Carnevale, V., Treptow, W., & Klein, M. L. (2011). Sodium ion binding sites and hydration in the lumen of a bacterial ion channel from molecular dynamics simulations. *Journal of Physical Chemistry Letters, 2*, 2504–2508.

Cascales, J. J. L., Costa, S. D. O., & Porasso, R. D. (2011). Thermodynamic study of benzocaine insertion into different lipid bilayers. *The Journal of Chemical Physics, 135*(13), 135103.

Catterall, W. A. (2000). From ionic currents to molecular mechanisms: The structure and function of voltage-gated sodium channels. *Neuron, 26*, 13–25.

Catterall, W. A., Cestele, S., Yarov-Yarovoy, V., Yu, F. H., Konoki, K., & Scheuer, T. (2007). Voltage-gated ion channels and gating modifier toxins. *Toxicon, 49*(2), 124–141.

Catterall, W. A., Goldin, A. L., & Waxman, S. G. (2005). International Union of Pharmacology. XLVII. Nomenclature and structure-function relationships of voltage-gated sodium channels. *Pharmacological Reviews, 57*(4), 397–409.

Catterall, W. A., & Swanson, T. M. (2015). Structural basis for pharmacology of voltage-gated sodium and calcium channels. *Molecular Pharmacology, 88*(1), 141–150.

Chakrabarti, N., Ing, C., Payandeh, J., Zheng, N., Catterall, W. A., & Pomès, R. (2013). Catalysis of Na^+ permeation in the bacterial sodium channel Na_VAb. *Proceedings of the National Academy of Sciences of the United States of America, 110*, 11331–11336.

Chen, R., & Chung, S. H. (2012a). Binding modes and functional surface of anti-mammalian scorpion α-toxins to sodium channels. *Biochemistry, 51*, 7775–7782.

Chen, R., & Chung, S. H. (2012b). Binding modes of μ-conotoxin to the bacterial sodium channel (Na_VAb). *Biophysical Journal, 102*, 483–488.

Chen, R., & Chung, S. H. (2012c). Conserved functional surface of anti-mammalian scorpion β-toxins. *The Journal of Physical Chemistry. B, 116*, 4796–4800.

Chen, R., & Chung, S. H. (2014). Mechanism of tetrodotoxin block and resistance in sodium channels. *Biochemical and Biophysical Research Communications, 446*, 370–374.

Chen, R., Robinson, A., & Chung, S. H. (2014). Mechanism of μ-conotoxin PIIIA binding to the voltage-gated Na^+ channel $Na_V1.4$. *PLoS One, 9*, e93267.

Corry, B. (2015). Long timescale molecular simulations for understanding ion channel function. In R. J. Clarke & M. A. A. Khalid (Eds.), *Pumps, channels and transporters: Methods of functional analysis* (pp. 411–441). Hoboken, New Jersey: Wiley.

Corry, B., Lee, S., & Ahern, C. A. (2014). Pharmacological insights and quirks of bacterial sodium channels. *Handbook of Experimental Pharmacology, 221*, 251–267.

Corry, B., & Thomas, M. (2012). Mechanism of ion permeation and selectivity in a voltage gated sodium channel. *Journal of the American Chemical Society, 134*(3), 1840–1846.

Deng, Y., & Roux, B. (2009). Computations of standard binding free energies with molecular dynamics simulations. *The Journal of Physical Chemistry. B*, 2234–2246.

Dutertre, S., & Lewis, R. J. (2010). Use of venom peptides to probe ion channel structure and function. *The Journal of Biological Chemistry, 285*(18), 13315–13320.

Finol-Urdaneta, R. K., Glavica, R., McArthur, J. R., & French, R. J. (2013). Polymodal, high affinity actions of μ-conotoxins on a bacterial voltage-gated sodium channel. *Biophysical Journal, 104*, 136a–137a.

Fozzard, H. A., & Lipkind, G. M. (2010). The tetrodotoxin binding site is within the outer vestibule of the sodium channel. *Marine Drugs, 8*(2), 219–234.

Fozzard, H. A., Sheets, M. F., & Hanck, D. A. (2011). The sodium channel as a target for local anesthetic drugs. *Frontiers in Pharmacology, 2*, 68.

French, R. J., Yoshikami, D., Sheets, M. F., & Olivera, B. M. (2010). The tetrodotoxin receptor of voltage-gated sodium channels—Perspectives from interactions with μ-conotoxins. *Marine Drugs, 8*(7), 2153–2161.

Gingrich, K. J., Beardsley, D., & Yue, D. T. (1993). Ultra-deep blockade of Na + channels by a quaternary ammonium ion: Catalysis by a transition-intermediate state? *The Journal of Physiology, 471*, 319–341.

Goldin, A. L., Barchi, R. L., Caldwell, J. H., Hofmann, F., Howe, J. R., Hunter, J. C., … Catterall, W. A. (2000). Nomenclature of voltage-gated sodium channels. *Neuron*, *28*(2), 365–368.

Gumbart, J. C., Roux, B., & Chipot, C. (2013). Standard binding free energies from computer simulations: What is the best strategy? *Journal of Chemical Theory and Computation*, *9*(1), 794–802.

Heinemann, S. H., & Leipold, E. (2007). Conotoxins of the O-superfamily affecting voltage-gated sodium channels. *Cellular and Molecular Life Sciences*, *64*(11), 1329–1340.

Hille, B. (1977). Local anesthetics: Hydrophilic and hydrophobic pathways for the drug-receptor reaction. *The Journal of General Physiology*, *69*(4), 497–515.

Hille, B. (2001). *Ion channels of excitable membranes* (3rd ed.). Sunderland, Mass: Sinauer.

Högberg, C.-J., & Lyubartsev, A. P. (2008). Effect of local anesthetic lidocaine on electrostatic properties of a lipid bilayer. *Biophysical Journal*, *94*(2), 525–531. http://dx.doi.org/10.1529/biophysj.107.104208.

Högberg, C. J., Maliniak, A., & Lyubartsev, A. P. (2007). Dynamical and structural properties of charged and uncharged lidocaine in a lipid bilayer. *Biophysical Chemistry*, *125*(2–3), 416–424.

Hwang, D. F., Arakawa, O., Saito, T., Noguchi, T., Simidu, U., Tsukamoto, K., … Hashimoto, K. (1989). Tetrodotoxin-producing bacteria from the blue-ringed octopus *Octopus maculosus*. *Marine Biology*, *100*, 327–332.

Jensen, M. Ø., Jogini, V., Borhani, D. W., Leffler, A. E., Dror, R. O., & Shaw, D. E. (2012). Mechanism of voltage gating in potassium channels. *Science*, *336*(6078), 229–233.

Kaczmarski, J. A., & Corry, B. (2014). Investigating the size and dynamics of voltage-gated sodium channel fenestrations: A molecular dynamics study. *Channels*, *8*(3), 264–277.

Kahn, R., Karbat, I., Ilan, N., Cohen, L., Sokolov, S., Catterall, W. A., … Gurevitz, M. (2009). Molecular requirements for recognition of brain voltage-gated sodium channels by scorpion α-toxins. *The Journal of Biological Chemistry*, *284*(31), 20684–20691.

Kao, C. Y., & Nishiyama, A. (1965). Actions of saxitoxin on peripheral neuromuscular systems. *The Journal of Physiology*, *180*(1), 50–66.

Kimbrough, J. T., & Gingrich, K. J. (2000). Quaternary ammonium block of mutant Na+ channels lacking inactivation: Features of a transition-intermediate mechanism. *The Journal of Physiology*, *529*, 93–106.

Knapp, O., McArthur, J. R., & Adams, D. J. (2012). Conotoxins targeting neuronal voltage-gated sodium channel subtypes: Potential analgesics? *Toxins*, *4*(11), 1236–1260.

Laio, A., & Gervasio, F. L. (2008). Metadynamics: A method to simulate rare events and reconstruct the free energy in biophysics, chemistry and material science. *Reports on Progress in Physics*, *71*(12), 126601.

Laio, A., & Parrinello, M. (2002). Escaping free-energy minima. *Proceedings of the National Academy of Sciences of the United States of America*, *99*, 12562–12566.

Langerman, L., Bansinath, M., & Grant, G. J. (1994). The partition coefficient as a predictor of local anesthetic potency for spinal anesthesia: Evaluation of five local anesthetics in a mouse model. *Anesthésie et Analgésie*, *79*, 490–494.

Lee, C. H., & Ruben, P. C. (2008). Interaction between voltage-gated sodium channels and the neurotoxin, tetrodotoxin. *Channels*, *2*(6), 407–412.

Mahdavi, S., & Kuyucak, S. (2014a). Molecular dynamics study of binding of μ-conotoxin GIIIA to the voltage-gated sodium channel $Na_V1.4$. *PLoS One*, *9*(8), e105300.

Mahdavi, S., & Kuyucak, S. (2014b). Systematic study of binding of mu-conotoxins to the sodium channel $Na_V1.4$. *Toxins*, *6*(12), 3454–3470.

Martin, L. J., Chao, R., & Corry, B. (2014). Molecular dynamics simulation of the partitioning of benzocaine and phenytoin into a lipid bilayer. *Biophysical Chemistry*, *185*, 98–107.

Martin, L. J., & Corry, B. (2014). Locating the route of entry and binding sites of benzocaine and phenytoin in a bacterial voltage gated sodium channel. *PLoS Computational Biology, 10*(7), e1003688.
McCormack, K., Santos, S., Chapman, M. L., Krafte, D. S., Marron, B. E., West, C. W., ... Castle, N. A. (2013). Voltage sensor interaction site for selective small molecule inhibitors of voltage-gated sodium channels. *Proceedings of the National Academy of Sciences of the United States of America, 110*(29), E2724–E2732.
McCusker, E. C., Bagnéris, C., Naylor, C. E., Cole, A. R., D'Avanzo, N., Nichols, C. G., & Wallace, B. A. (2012). Structure of a bacterial voltage-gated sodium channel pore reveals mechanisms of opening and closing. *Nature Communications, 3*, 1102.
McNulty, M. M., Edgerton, G. B., Shah, R. D., Hanck, D. A., Fozzard, H. A., & Lipkind, G. M. (2007). Charge at the lidocaine binding site residue Phe-1759 affects permeation in human cardiac voltage-gated sodium channels. *The Journal of Physiology, 5812*, 741–755.
Meisler, M. H., & Kearney, J. A. (2005). Sodium channel mutations in epilepsy and other neurological disorders. *The Journal of Clinical Investigation, 115*(8), 2010–2017.
Minett, M. S., Nassar, M. A., Clark, A. K., Passmore, G., Dickenson, A. H., Wang, F., ... Wood, J. N. (2012). Distinct Na_V1.7-dependent pain sensations require different sets of sensory and sympathetic neurons. *Nature Communications, 3*, 791.
Mojumdar, E. H., & Lyubartsev, A. P. (2010). Molecular dynamics simulations of local anesthetic articaine in a lipid bilayer. *Biophysical Chemistry, 153*(1), 27–35.
Nassar, M. A., Stirling, L. C., Forlani, G., Baker, M. D., Matthews, E. A., Dickenson, A. H., & Wood, J. N. (2004). Nociceptor-specific gene deletion reveals a major role for Na_V1.7 (PN1) in acute and inflammatory pain. *Proceedings of the National Academy of Sciences of the United States of America, 101*(34), 12706–12711.
Naylor, C. E., Bagnéris, C., DeCaen, P. G., Sula, A., Scaglione, A., Clapham, D. E., & Wallace, B. A. (2016). Molecular basis of ion permeability in a voltage-gated sodium channel. *The EMBO Journal, 35*(8), 820–830.
Neguliaev, A., & Nosyreva, E. D. (1979). Comparative study of the action of procaine and benzocaine on normal and aconitine-modified sodium channels. *Tsitologiia, 21*(6), 697–702.
Nicholson, G. M. (2007). Insect-selective spider toxins targeting voltage-gated sodium channels. *Toxicon, 49*(4), 490–512.
Noguchi, T., Hwang, D. F., Arakawa, O., Sugita, H., Deguchi, Y., Shida, Y., & Hashimoto, K. (1987). *Vibrio alginolyticus*, a tetrodotoxin-producing bacterium, in the intestines of the fish *Fugu vermicularis vermicularis*. *Marine Biology, 94*, 625–630.
O'Reilly, A. O., Eberhardt, E., Weidner, C., Alzheimer, C., Wallace, B. A., & Lampert, A. (2012). Bisphenol A binds to the local anesthetic receptor site to block the human cardiac sodium channel. *PLoS One*, 7(7), e41667.
Park, S., & Schulten, K. (2004). Calculating potentials of mean force from steered molecular dynamics simulations. *The Journal of Chemical Physics, 120*(13), 5946–5961.
Payandeh, J., Gamal El-Din, T. M., Scheuer, T., Zheng, N., & Catterall, W. A. (2012). Crystal structure of a voltage-gated sodium channel in two potentially inactivated states. *Nature, 486*(7401), 135–139.
Payandeh, J., Scheuer, T., Zheng, N., & Catterall, W. A. (2011). The crystal structure of a voltage-gated sodium channel. *Nature, 475*(7356), 353–358.
Pless, S. A., Galpin, J. D., Frankel, A., & Ahern, C. A. (2011). Molecular basis for class Ib anti-arrhythmic inhibition of cardiac sodium channels. *Nature Communications, 2*, 351.
Porasso, R. D., Bennett, W. F. D., Oliveira-Costa, S. D., & Cascales, J. J. L. (2009). Study of the benzocaine transfer from aqueous solution to the interior of a biological membrane. *The Journal of Physical Chemistry. B, 113*(29), 9988–9994.

Possani, L. D., Becerril, B., Delepierre, M., & Tytgat, J. (1999). Scorpion toxins specific for Na^+-channels. *European Journal of Biochemistry*, *264*(2), 287–300.
Quan, C., Mok, W. M., & Wang, G. K. (1996). Use-dependent inhibition of Na+ currents by benzocaine homologs. *Biophysical Journal*, *70*(1), 194–201.
Ragsdale, D. S., McPhee, J. C., Scheuer, T., & Catterall, W. A. (1994). Molecular determinants of state-dependent block of Na+ channels by local anesthetics. *Science*, *265*(5179), 1724–1728.
Ragsdale, D. S., McPhee, J. C., Scheuer, T., & Catterall, W. A. (1996). Common molecular determinants of local anesthetic, antiarrhythmic, and anticonvulsant block of voltage-gated Na+ channels. *Proceedings of the National Academy of Sciences of the United States of America*, *93*, 9270–9275.
Raju, S. G., Barber, A. F., LeBard, D. N., Klein, M. L., & Carnevale, V. (2013). Exploring volatile general anesthetic binding to a closed membrane-bound bacterial voltage-gated sodium channel via computation. *PLoS Computational Biology*, *9*(6), 1–10.
Ren, D., Navarro, B., Xu, H., Yue, L., Shi, Q., & Clapham, D. E. (2001). A prokaryotic voltage-gated sodium channel. *Science*, *294*(5550), 2372–2375.
Roden, D. M., & George, A. L. (1996). The cardiac ion channels: Relevance to management of arrhythmias. *Annual Review of Medicine*, *47*, 135–148.
Ruan, Y., Liu, N., & Priori, S. G. (2009). Sodium channel mutations and arrhythmias. *Nature Reviews Cardiology*, *6*(5), 337–348.
Safo, P., Rosenbaum, T., Shcherbatko, A., Choi, D. Y., Han, E., Toledo-Aral, J. J., … Mandel, G. (2000). Distinction among neuronal subtypes of voltage-activated sodium channels by μ-conotoxin PIIIA. *The Journal of Neuroscience*, *20*(1), 76–80.
Santarelli, V. P., Eastwood, A. L., Dougherty, D. A., Horn, R., & Ahern, C. A. (2007). A cation-π interaction discriminates among sodium channels that are either sensitive or resistant to tetrodotoxin block. *The Journal of Biological Chemistry*, *282*(11), 8044–8051.
Schiavon, E., Sacco, T., Cassulini, R. R., Gurrola, G., Tempia, F., Possani, L. D., & Wanke, E. (2006). Resurgent current and voltage sensor trapping enhanced activation by a β-scorpion toxin solely in $Na_V1.6$ channel. Significance in mice Purkinje neurons. *The Journal of Biological Chemistry*, *281*(29), 20326–20337.
Schmalhofer, W. A., Calhoun, J., Burrows, R., Bailey, T., Kohler, M. G., Weinglass, A. B., … Priest, B. T. (2008). ProTx-II, a selective inhibitor of $Na_V1.7$ sodium channels, blocks action potential propagation in nociceptors. *Molecular Pharmacology*, *74*(5), 1476–1484.
Schwarz, W., Palade, P. T., & Hille, B. (1977). Local anesthetics. Effect of pH on use-dependent block of sodium channels in frog muscle. *Biophysical Journal*, *20*(3), 343–368.
Shaya, D., Findeisen, F., Abderemane-Ali, F., Arrigoni, C., Wong, S., Nurva, S. R., … Minor, D. L. (2014). Structure of a prokaryotic sodium channel pore reveals essential gating elements and an outer ion binding site common to eukaryotic channels. *Journal of Molecular Biology*, *426*(2), 467–483.
Smith, N. E., & Corry, B. (2016). Mutant bacterial sodium channels as models for local anesthetic block of eukaryotic proteins. *Channels*, *10*(3), 225–237.
Štolc, S., Nemček, V., & Szöcsová, H. (1989). Local anesthetics: Lipophilicity, charge, diffusion and site of action in isolated neuron. *European Journal of Pharmacology*, *164*(2), 249–256.
Strichartz, G. R., Sanchez, V., Arthur, G. R., Chafetz, R., & Martin, D. (1990). Fundamental properties of local anesthetics. II. Measured octanol: Buffer partition coefficients and pK_a values of clinically used drugs. *Anesthesia and Analgesia*, *71*(2), 158–170.
Terlau, H., & Olivera, B. M. (2004). *Conus* venoms: A rich source of novel ion channel-targeted peptides. *Physiological Reviews*, *84*(1), 41–68.
Thuesen, E. V., & Kogure, K. (1989). Bacterial production of tetrodotoxin in four species of chaetognatha. *The Biological Bulletin*, *176*, 191–194.

Tietze, D., Leipold, E., Heimer, P., Bohm, M., Winschel, W., Imhof, D., ... Tietze, A. A. (2016). Molecular interaction of δ-conopeptide EVIA with voltage-gated Na^+ channels. *Biochimica et Biophysica Acta*, *1860*(9), 2053–2063.

Torrie, G. M., & Valleau, J. P. (1977). Nonphysical sampling distributions in Monte Carlo free-energy estimation: Umbrella sampling. *Journal of Computational Physics*, *23*(2), 187–199.

Tsai, C. J., Tani, K., Irie, K., Hiroaki, Y., Shimomura, T., McMillan, D. G., ... Li, X. D. (2013). Two alternative conformations of a voltage-gated sodium channel. *Journal of Molecular Biology*, *425*(22), 4074–4088.

van Gunsteren, W. F., Bakowies, D., Baron, R., Chandrasekhar, I., Christen, M., Daura, X., ... Yu, H. B. (2006). Biomolecular modeling: Goals, problems, perspectives. *Angewandte Chemie, International Edition*, *45*(25), 4064–4092.

Vemparala, S., Domene, C., & Klein, M. L. (2008). Interaction of anesthetics with open and closed conformations of a potassium channel studied via molecular dynamics and normal mode analysis. *Biophysical Journal*, *94*(11), 4260–4269.

Wang, G. K., Calderon, J., Jaw, S. J., & Wang, S. Y. (2009). State-dependent block of Na+ channels by articaine via the local anesthetic receptor. *The Journal of Membrane Biology*, *229*(1), 1–9.

Wang, S.-Y., Mitchell, J., Moczydlowski, E., & Wang, G. K. (2004). Block of inactivation-deficient Na+ channels by local anesthetics in stably transfected mammalian cells: Evidence for drug binding along the activation pathway. *The Journal of General Physiology*, *124*(6), 691–701.

Waxman, S. G., Dib-Hajj, S., Cummins, T. R., & Black, J. A. (1999). Sodium channels and pain. *Proceedings of the National Academy of Sciences of the United States of America*, *96*, 7635–7639.

Waxman, S. G., & Hains, B. C. (2006). Fire and phantoms after spinal cord injury: Na+ channels and central pain. *Trends in Neurosciences*, *29*(4), 207–215.

Wilson, M. J., Yoshikami, D., Azam, L., Gajewiak, J., Olivera, B. M., Bulaj, G., & Zhang, M. M. (2011). μ-Conotoxins that differentially block sodium channels $Na_V1.1$ through 1.8 identify those responsible for action potentials in sciatic nerve. *Proceedings of the National Academy of Sciences of the United States of America*, *108*(25), 10302–10307.

Wu, J., Yan, Z., Li, Z., Qian, X., Lu, S., Dong, M., ... Yan, N. (2016). Structure of the voltage-gated calcium channel Cav1.1 at 3.6 Å resolution. *Nature*, *537*, 191–196.

Zamponi, G. W., Doyle, D. D., & French, R. J. (1993). Fast lidocaine block of cardiac and skeletal muscle sodium channels: One site with two routes of access. *Biophysical Journal*, *65*(1), 80–90.

Zhang, X., Ren, W., DeCaen, P., Yan, C., Tao, X., Tang, L., ... Yan, N. (2012). Crystal structure of an orthologue of the NaChBac voltage-gated sodium channel. *Nature*, *486*(7401), 130–134.

CHAPTER TEN

Physiology and Pharmacology of Ryanodine Receptor Calcium Release Channels

Angela F. Dulhunty*,[1], Philip G. Board*, Nicole A. Beard*,†, Marco G. Casarotto*

*John Curtin School of Medical Research, Australian National University, Canberra, ACT, Australia
†Health Research Institute, Faculty of Education Science Technology and Mathematics, University of Canberra, Bruce, ACT, Australia
[1]Corresponding author: e-mail address: angela.dulhunty@anu.edu.au

Contents

Abstract

Ryanodine receptor (RyR) ion channels are essential for skeletal and cardiac muscle function. Their knockout leads to perinatal death from respiratory and cardiac failure. Acquired changes or mutations in the protein cause debilitating skeletal myopathy and cardiac arrhythmia which can be deadly. Knowledge of the pharmacology of RyR channels is central to developing effective and specific treatments of these myopathies. The ion channel is a >2.2 MDa homotetamer with distinct structural and functional characteristics giving rise to a myriad of regulatory sites that are potential therapeutic targets. Australian researchers have been intimately involved in the exploration of the proteins since their identification in the mid-1980s. We discuss major

Advances in Pharmacology, Volume 79
ISSN 1054-3589
http://dx.doi.org/10.1016/bs.apha.2016.12.001

aspects of RyR physiology and pharmacology that have been tackled in Australian laboratories. Specific areas of interest include ultrastructural aspects and mechanisms of RyR activation in excitation–contraction (EC) coupling and related pharmacological developments, regulation of RyRs by divalent cations, by associated proteins including the FK506-binding proteins, by redox factors and phosphorylation. We consider adverse effects of anthracycline chemotherapeutic drugs on cardiac RyRs. Phenotypes associated with RyR mutations are discussed with current and developing therapeutic approaches for treating the underlying RyR dysfunction.

ABBREVIATIONS

CaM calmodulin
CaMKII calmodulin kinase 2
CaV1.1 α_{1S} alpha subunit of the skeletal DHPR
CaV1.2 α_{1C} subunit of the cardiac DHPR
CCD central core disease
CICR calcium-induced calcium release
CLIC2 chloride intracellular channel type 2
CPVT catecholaminergic polymorphic ventricular tachycardia
CSQ1 type 1 calsequestrin
CSQ2 type 2 calsequestrin
DHPR dihydropyridine receptor
DR3 divergent region 3
EC coupling excitation–contraction coupling
FKBP FK506-binding protein
GSH reduced glutathione
GSSG oxidized glutathione
GST glutathione transferase
GSTM2 muscle-specific GST
GSTM2C C-terminal helical bundle of GSTM2
II–III loop cytoplasmic loop linking the second and third transmembrane repeats of the DHPR
MH malignant hyperthermia
NADH nicotinamide adenine dinucleotide
NADPH oxidase nicotinamide adenine dinucleotide phosphate-oxidase
NCX sodium calcium exchanger
NO nitric oxide
PKA protein kinase A
ROS reactive oxygen species
RyR1 skeletal ryanodine receptor type 1
RyR2 cardiac ryanodine receptor type 2
SERCA sarcoplasmic endoplasmic reticulum Ca^{2+} ATPase
SR sarcoplasmic reticulum
t-tubule transverse tubule
$\boldsymbol{\alpha_{1C}}$ alpha subunit of the cardiac DHPR
$\boldsymbol{\alpha_{1S}}$ alpha subunit of the skeletal DHPR
$\boldsymbol{\beta_{1a}}$ beta subunit of the skeletal DHPR

1. INTRODUCTION

Ryanodine receptor (RyR) ion channels embedded in the internal sarcoplasmic reticulum (SR) Ca^{2+} store membrane are fundamental to striated muscle contraction. Recently described as "allosteric ion channel giants" (Van Petegem, 2015), RyRs are essential for excitation–contraction (EC) coupling, releasing the Ca^{2+} ions required to activate the contractile proteins in response to surface action potentials (Dulhunty, Casarotto, & Beard, 2011). Knockout of the proteins results in perinatal death with respiratory and circulatory failure, while mutations can cause skeletal myopathies, arrhythmia, and cardiac arrest. Acquired changes in the proteins contribute to muscle weakness and heart failure (Dulhunty, Casarotto, et al., 2011). Skeletal ryanodine receptor type 1 (RyR1) is the major isoform expressed in skeletal muscle and cardiac ryanodine receptor type 2 (RyR2) in cardiac myocytes. RyR1 and RyR2 are expressed along with a third isoform (RyR3) in many other tissues. Mutations causing striated muscle disorders also have significant neurological consequences (e.g., Lehnart et al., 2008). Knowledge of RyR pharmacology is of utmost importance for developing therapeutic strategies for these conditions, but to date there are remarkably few RyR-specific drugs and fewer drugs that target specific RyR isoforms.

The RyR was characterized later than many other ion channels. Its internal location precluded whole cell recording that allowed characterization of many ion currents before the proteins were cloned and techniques developed for single channel recording. Australian physiologists were among the first to examine RyR channels in the early 1990s (Dulhunty, Junankar, & Stanhope, 1992; Lewis, Dulhunty, Junankar, & Stanhope, 1992) and have continued a leading role in the field. This contribution to our present knowledge of RyR channels is highlighted in this chapter in the context of the overall development of the field.

2. RyR OVERVIEW

2.1 Ultrastructural Location

The location of the RyR in specialized membrane systems is fundamental to EC coupling. Ca^{2+} release units form where the intracellular SR membrane is closely coupled to the surface membrane or its transverse (t-)tubule invaginations (Franzini-Armstrong, Protasi, & Ramesh, 1999). The ultrastructural characteristics of the t-tubules and Ca^{2+} release units were described in early studies (Block, Imagawa, Campbell, & Franzini-Armstrong, 1988; Dulhunty, 1984, 1989; Dulhunty & Franzini-Armstrong, 1975; Franzini-Armstrong, 1970) and ultrastructure remains an essential tool for investigating EC coupling (Dayal, Bhat, Franzini-Armstrong, & Grabner, 2013; Eltit, Franzini-Armstrong, & Perez, 2014; Schredelseker, Dayal, Schwerte, Franzini-Armstrong, & Grabner, 2009). In skeletal muscle, Ca^{2+} release units are arranged in triads, which are composed of three elements: two terminal expansions of the SR forming junctions on either side of a t-tubule (Fig. 1). Within each junction, RyRs form a double row of 10–60 or more channels and form "couplons" with dihydropyridine receptors (DHPRs) in the t-tubule membrane (Block et al., 1988). t-Tubules enter muscle fibers via caveolae (Dulhunty & Franzini-Armstrong, 1975) and in mammals are aligned with the A/I band overlap on either side of the Z-line, forming a double band in each sarcomere, repeating at ~2 μM intervals along the length of the fiber. *In cardiac myocytes*, Ca^{2+} release units are arranged in dyads, which contain only two elements, a single terminal SR expansion forming a junction with the surface/t-tubule membrane

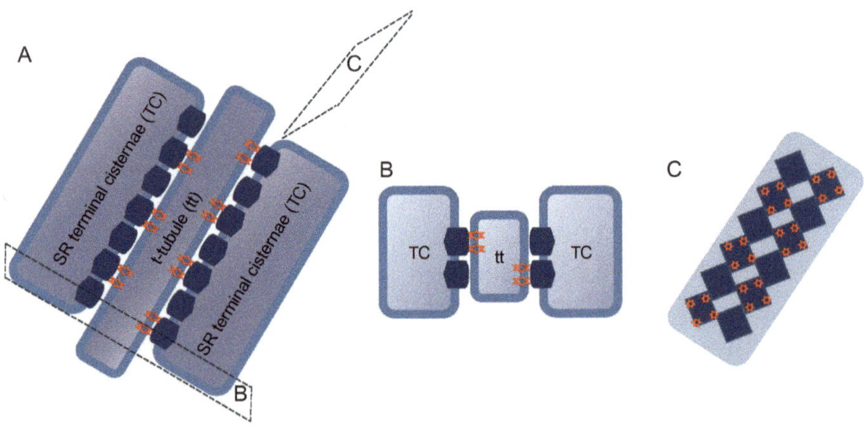

Fig. 1 DHPR and RyR1 in skeletal muscle triad junctions. The crystalline-like array of RyRs (*dark blue*) in the SR membrane and junctional gap is seen in thin section and freeze-fracture electron microscopy. DHPRs (*red stars*) are arranged in tetrads in the t-tubule membrane, with a one tetrad overlying every second RyR1 (Block et al., 1988). (A) A longitudinal section through a triad junction showing terminal cisternae (TC) on either side of a t-tubule (tt). The *rectangle* (B) shows the plane of the transversely sectioned junction in (B) and the *rhombus* (C) shows the plane of the section in (C). Only two of the four DHPRs in each tetrad are seen in the sections in (A) and (B). The full tetrad with four DHPRs are shown overlying RyRs in the junctional SR membrane in (C).

(Franzini-Armstrong et al., 1999). The cardiac SR expansions are relatively narrow and the t-tubules and dyads are aligned with Z-line forming a single band in each sarcomere.

The dimension of the junctional gap is similar to the width of the boundary membranes, and the gap largely occupied by the cytoplasmic domain of the RyR (Fig. 1). These dimensions are important when considering the movement of ions within the gap. The width of the gap is often represented as being much larger in order to include the many interactions that occur within the confined region, however, this gives a false impression of the space. Anchoring of the surface/t-tubules and SR membranes is strong within Ca^{2+} release units and maintained by several proteins including junctophilin (Murphy et al., 2013), triadin (Fourest-Lieuvin et al., 2012), and possibly STAC3 (Horstick et al., 2013). Experimental or pathological separation of the membranes results in degradation of EC coupling, muscle weakness, and paralysis (Lamb, Junankar, & Stephenson, 1995; Verburg, Dutka, & Lamb, 2006).

2.2 Protein Structure

The functional RyR ion channel is formed by four monomers each having >5000 residues, with a total mass of >2 MDa, forming the largest ion channel protein so far identified. One of several major challenges in unravelling RyR function has been the lack of a high-resolution structure. Pioneering cryoelectron microscopy revealed a mushroom-like structure with a fourfold symmetry, a huge cytoplasmic domain, and a small transmembrane/luminal domain (<10% of the protein) (Fig. 7). Until recently, the cryoelectron microscopy resolution has been ~10–30 Å (Peralvarez-Marin et al., 2011; Radermacher et al., 1994; Zhong et al., 2013). In a landmark issue of Nature, two groups reported RyR1 structures at 3–5 Å resolution, sufficient to resolve tertiary structure within stable domains, particularly the ion pore and transmembrane domains (Fig. 2; Yan et al., 2015; Zalk et al., 2015). Notably, the luminal domain is formed only by short loops linking the transmembrane helices and contains <1.5% of the protein. These higher resolution structures allow identification of core elements that could transmit binding signals from the cytoplasmic periphery the pore (Bai, Yan, Wu, Li, & Yan, 2016; des Georges et al., 2016). Protein/protein interaction sites can now be defined (Wium, Dulhunty, & Beard, 2016) and more sophisticated docking of drugs into known binding domains undertaken.

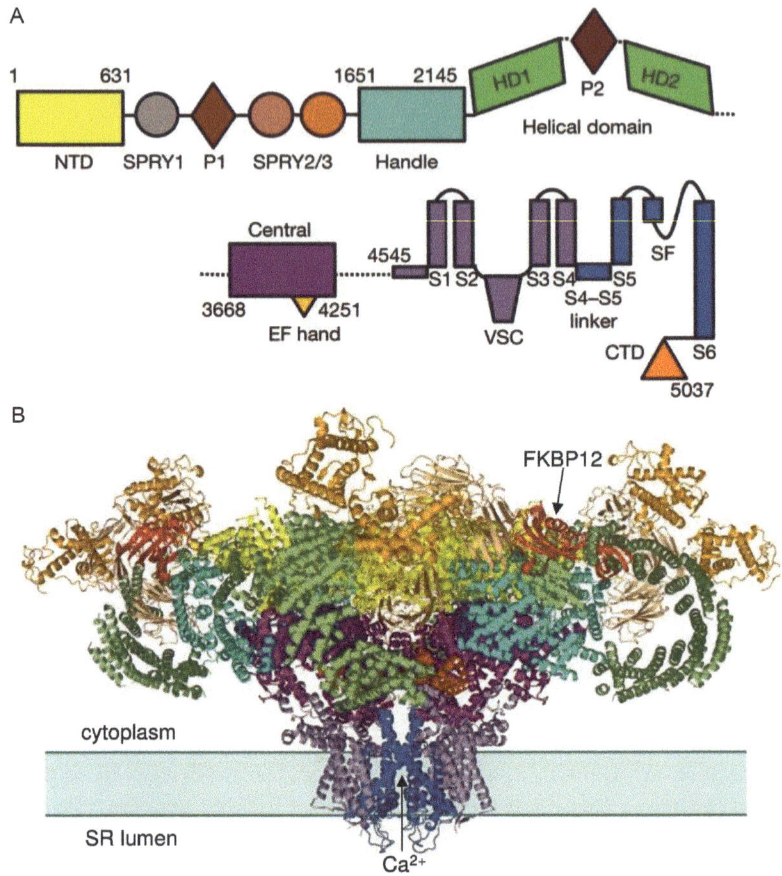

Fig. 2 The near atomic resolution structure of RyR1 (Yan et al., 2015). The structure was obtained using high-resolution cryoelectron microscopy. (A) The linear sequence of RyR1 domains, starting at the N-terminal domain is shown. (B) "Side" view of the structure of two RyR1 protomers with FKBP12 bound is shown, with the cytoplasmic domain uppermost. Domains are color matched to those in (A). The luminal domain is formed by short linkers between membrane spanning helices. *Modified from figure 1 of Yan, Z., Bai, X. C., Yan, C., Wu, J., Li, Z., Xie, T., et al. (2015). Structure of the rabbit ryanodine receptor RyR1 at near-atomic resolution.* Nature, *517, 50–55.*

3. ION CHANNEL RECORDING

Most ion channel studies of RyRs have been performed using artificial lipid bilayer techniques, introduced into Australia and modified for this purpose shortly after identification of the protein (Ahern, Junankar, &

Dulhunty, 1994). Surface membrane patch clamp is not applicable to intracellular ion channels or to SR vesicles with diameters of 20–100 nm that are smaller than the tip of patch electrodes. Patch clamp of fused intracellular membranes on the surface of skinned fibers "sarcoballs" (Hals, Stein, & Palade, 1989; Lewis et al., 1992) proved impractical as did electrode tip–dip bilayer methods (Coronado & Latorre, 1983). Population responses of RyRs are obtained with [^{3}H]ryanodine binding (Lu, Xu, & Meissner, 1995), Ca^{2+} release from SR vesicles (Casarotto et al., 2000), skinned fiber techniques—largely developed in Australia (Fink & Stephenson, 1987), or intracellular Ca^{2+} transients in intact fibers (Dainese et al., 2009; Rebbeck et al., 2015). While yielding significant information, population responses do not reveal molecular events within individual ion channel molecules.

In the lipid bilayer method, single purified RyR protein or RyRs in SR vesicles, incorporate into an artificial lipid bilayer painted across an ~100 μm aperture in a partition separating two chambers. The outside-out SR vesicle is added to the *cis* solution and the cytoplasmic surface remains on *cis* side of the bilayer after fusion, with the luminal surface on the opposite (*trans*) side. When purified RyR is added to the *cis* solution it seems thermodynamically preferable for the small hydrophobic transmembrane domain to penetrate the bilayer, leaving the cytoplasmic domain on the *cis* side. The orientation of the channel can be confirmed with side-specific actions of drugs or ions, so that the cytoplasmic or luminal solutions can be experimentally manipulated (Laver, Baynes, & Dulhunty, 1997).

4. EC COUPLING

EC coupling encompasses the many complex processes linking surface membrane action potentials to shortening of the muscle fiber, but the term has evolved within the field to encompass only the mechanism linking the depolarization-dependent response of the DHPR α_1 voltage sensor with the release of the Ca^{2+} from the SR. Within this definition, EC coupling in the heart is relatively straight forward, while defining the mechanism of EC coupling in skeletal muscle has provided a major and continuing challenge (Rebbeck et al., 2014). *In Cardiac EC coupling* Ca^{2+} ions enter the diadic junction through the DHPR α_{1C} (CaV1.2) and activate RyR2 via calcium-induced calcium release (CICR). The DHPR Ca^{2+} influx is sufficient to activate several RyR2 channels and there is one DHPR for every 4–10 RyR2 tetramers (Bers & Stiffel, 1993). Cardiac-type EC coupling is defined as voltage-activated SR Ca^{2+} release that depends on an influx of extracellular Ca^{2+}. *Skeletal EC coupling* does not depend on CICR as it is maintained in the absence of an extracellular Ca^{2+} influx. Since no other transmitter has been identified, skeletal EC coupling is thought to depend on conformational coupling through protein/protein interactions that link DHPR α_{1S} subunit (CaV1.1) to RyR1 (Rebbeck et al., 2014). The voltage sensor response to depolarization is measured as a "charge movement" across the surface/t-tubule membrane (Schneider & Chandler, 1973). Australians were among the first to record this current in mammalian muscle (Dulhunty & Gage, 1983, 1985; Gage & Dulhunty, 1981) and identify its origin in the DHPR (Dulhunty & Gage, 1988; Lamb, 1986). This was confirmed when charge movement and EC coupling were abolished by knock-out of the α_{1S} subunit (Adams, Tanabe, Mikami, Numa, & Beam, 1990). Similarly, RyR1 was confirmed as the Ca^{2+} release channel when skeletal EC coupling was abolished by RyR1 knock out and rescued with RyR1, but not RyR2, expression (Nakai et al., 1997). The possibility of structural coupling between the DHPR α_{1S} subunit and RyR1 is elegantly revealed in freeze-fracture replicas which show DHPR α_{1S} clusters in groups of four (tetrads) arranged to match the spacing of the four RyR1 subunits of every second RyR1, i.e., two DHPRs per RyR tetramer (Fig. 1 earlier) (Block et al., 1988). The tetrad arrangement is essential for skeletal EC coupling (Schredelseker et al., 2009).

4.1 Transmission of Skeletal EC Coupling Signals

The skeletal EC coupling field has been dominated by the search for protein/protein interactions that allow conformational coupling. The α_{1S} cytoplasmic loop linking the second and third transmembrane repeats of the DHPR (II–III loop) and it's central "C" region are essential (Nakai, Tanabe, Konno, Adams, & Beam, 1998; Tanabe, Beam, Adams, Niidome, & Numa, 1990). The recombinant II–III loop and peptides corresponding to its "A" and "C" regions interact with isolated RyRs (Dulhunty, Karunasekara, et al., 2005; Dulhunty et al., 1999; Dulhunty, Wei-LaPierre, Casarotto, & Beard, 2017; el-Hayek, Antoniu, Wang, Hamilton, & Ikemoto, 1995; Haarmann, Dulhunty, & Laver, 2005; Lu et al., 1995). The II–III loop and peptide C are intrinsically unstructured, with the flexibility for a rapid conformational change during EC coupling (Cui et al., 2009; Dulhunty, Karunasekara, et al., 2005; Haarmann et al., 2005; Haarmann, Green, Casarotto, Laver, & Dulhunty, 2003). The "A" region is α-helical (Casarotto et al., 2000) and, although of pharmacological interest, it is not required for EC coupling (Bannister, 2016; Proenza, Wilkens, & Beam, 2000). As neither direct binding of α_{1S} to RyR1 or specific binding residues in RyR1 have been found, it is likely that another protein or proteins link the II–III loop to RyR1 to enable EC coupling (Bannister, 2016; Rebbeck et al., 2014).

Skeletal DHPR β subunit (β_{1a}) is a likely candidate for a role in conformational coupling as it binds to α_{1S} and RyR1 and is essential for skeletal EC coupling, charge movement and tetrad structures (Dayal et al., 2013; Schredelseker et al., 2005). The final 35–36 residues of the C-terminal tail of β_{1a} bind to RyR1 and are required for skeletal EC coupling (Beurg et al., 1999; Dulhunty et al., 2017; Eltit et al., 2014; Rebbeck et al., 2011). An interaction site on β_{1a} for RyR1 has been identified (Karunasekara et al., 2012), and a binding site on RyR1 for β_{1a} partially identified (Cheng, Altafaj, Ronjat, & Coronado, 2005; Rebbeck et al., 2015). A mutation in β_{1a} was recently reported in a patient with malignant hyperthermia (MH) (Bjorksten, Gillies, Hockey, & du Start, 2016). MH is characterized by uncontrollable Ca^{2+} release and muscle contracture in the presence of volatile anesthetics and neuromuscular blockers. It has been linked to mutations in RyR1, the DHPR α_{1S} subunit, and the Ca^{2+}-binding protein, calsequestrin (CSQ) (Laver et al., 1997; Protasi, Paolini, & Dainese, 2009). A mutation in β_{1a} also causing MH indicates an intimate involvement of β_{1a} with α_{1S} and RyR1 in the regulation of SR Ca^{2+} release. β_{1a} is spatially close to the α_{1S} II–III loop in the DHPR complex (Wu et al., 2016, 2015) and β_{1a} binding to α_{1S} alters II–III loop conformation (Mahalingam, Perez, & Fessenden, 2016). While these observations suggest that β_{1a} is a part of the EC coupling pathway, they are also consistent with an alternative proposal that β_{1a} simply maintains the α_{1S}/RyR1 complex in a conformation that allows EC coupling (Dayal et al., 2013).

5. PHARMACOLOGY ARISING FROM EC COUPLING STUDIES

Australian researchers made a major contribution to defining RyR1 activation by the recombinant II–III loop, its "C" region (peptide C) and "A" region (peptide A) (Casarotto et al., 2000; Casarotto, Green, Pace, Curtis, & Dulhunty, 2001; Casarotto, Green, Pace, Young, & Dulhunty, 2004; Tae, Casarotto, & Dulhunty, 2009; Tae et al., 2011). The activation is explained in terms of a "domain switching" hypothesis which assumes that several central and cytoplasmic domains are in close contact, in a zipped conformation that stabilizes the closed state of the channel. Channel opening occurs when the interactions are weakened by activating signals (e.g., EC coupling, activating peptides, MH or central core disease (CCD) mutations) which "unzip" the domains and switch the channel from a closed to an open state (Bannister & Ikemoto, 2006; Kimlicka, Lau, Tung, & Van Petegem, 2013; Kimura et al., 2009; Yamamoto & Ikemoto, 2002). Signals that originate in different regions of RyR1 can converge on interdomain interfaces through identifiable intramolecular structures (Yan et al., 2015).

Peptide A provides a template for potential RyR-specific pharmacological agents because of a strong structure/function correlation. The peptide activates RyR1 and RyR2, induces Ca^{2+} release from cardiac and skeletal SR and potentiates contraction in skinned muscle fibers (Dulhunty, Curtis, Cengia, Sakowska, & Casarotto, 2004; Lamb, El-Hayek, Ikemoto, & Stephenson, 2000). RyR activation depends on basic residues which stabilize the peptide's α-helical structure: activity and helical structure are enhanced by replacing Asp at position 18 with Arg (peptide A1(D-R18)) (Fig. 3A and B) (Casarotto et al., 2000, 2001; Green et al., 2003). An activating peptide with a sequence of the variably spliced ASI region of RyR1 also contains a strong α-helical structure with aligned basic residues (Fig. 3C; Kimura et al., 2009). The A peptides are not membrane permeable, but penetrate muscle fibers following lipo-amino acid conjugation, with fortuitously enhanced RyR-activating action (Dulhunty, Cengia, et al., 2005).

The A and ASI peptides are functionally similar to the scorpion toxins, Imperatoxin A, maurocalcine, and U1-liotoxin-Lw1a (Green et al., 2003; Mosbah et al., 2000; Smith, Vetter, et al., 2013). The structural alignment of the positively charged residues is similar to the peptides despite the toxins having a disulfide-stabilized β-sheet Inhibitor Cystine Knot (Fig. 3D and E) or a "disulfide-directed" hairpin (Fig. 3F) structures that contrast with the α-helical peptides. Imperatoxin A increases transient full conductance gating in competition with peptide A (Dulhunty, Curtis, Watson, Cengia, & Casarotto, 2004). High concentrations of Imperatoxin A and peptide A inhibit RyRs and induce substate activity (Dulhunty, Curtis, Watson, et al., 2004; Tripathy, Resch, Xu, Valdivia, & Meissner, 1998). U1-liotoxin-Lw1a has similar action to Imperatoxin A and peptides A1, A1(DR-18), but activates with fM affinity (Smith, Vetter, et al., 2013). Although not fully explored, it is likely that the positive charge on U1-liotoxin-Lw1a is again involved (Smith, Vetter, et al., 2013).

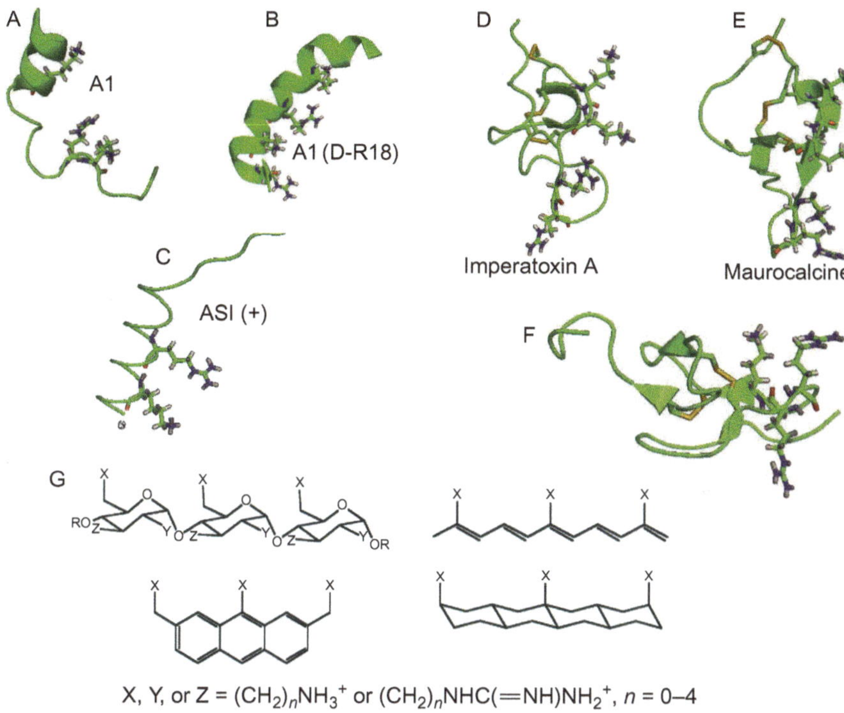

Fig. 3 Nuclear magnetic resonance structures of DHPR α1S II–III loop peptides, the ASI/polybasic RyR1 region and scorpion toxins. Although structurally diverse, the peptides and toxins present a compact positively charged surface available to interact with RyRs, which provides a template for a peptidomimetic. (A) A1 peptide (PDB 1DU1) (Casarotto et al., 2000). (B) The more active and more structured A1 analogue, A1(D-R18) (PDB 1JZP) (Green et al., 2003). (C) The ASI/polybasic RyR1 region (Kimura et al., 2009). (D, E) Inhibitor cysteine knot toxins, imperatoxin A (PDB 1IE6) and maurocalcine (PDB 1C6W) (Green et al., 2003). (F) U1-liotoxin-Lw1a, LITX (PDB LW1A) (Smith et al., 2013). (G) Potential peptidomimetic scaffolds: X, Y, and Z denote amine or guandino head groups from lysine and arginine side chains, *n* denotes the alkyl chain number.

The next step is to develop peptidomimetics as pharmacological tools and lead molecules for treatment of RyR-based diseases. The common structural trait in the activating peptides and toxins is the alignment of positively charged residues along one surface of the molecule (Fig. 3A–F). We can replace the peptide backbone with a nonpeptidic framework, while maintaining a positively charged surface as in Fig. 3G, to circumvent the many issues encountered when using peptides as therapeutic agents and to open the door for the development of small-molecule drugs.

Although maurocalcine binds to RyR1 and RyR2, it does not modify RyR2 activity (Altafaj et al., 2007) and thus has potential as a rare RyR1-specific pharmacological agent. In a separate therapeutic strategy, its cell penetrating ability and lack of toxicity, has enabled maurocalcine to transport therapeutic cargo into cells (Ronjat et al., 2016) and to overcome doxorubicin resistance in cancer cells (Aroui et al., 2009).

6. REGULATION BY DIVALENT CATIONS AND CSQ

This section highlights the major Australian contribution to biophysical characterization of regulatory sites for Ca^{2+} activation and Ca^{2+} inhibition of RyRs and interactions with Mg^{2+} and ATP. [Ca^{2+}] in the cytoplasm and SR lumen changes rhythmically during each contraction/relaxation cycle, with significant effects on RyRs that underlie dynamic activation and deactivation of Ca^{2+} release during each heartbeat, breath, and daily activity.

Cytoplasmic Ca^{2+} and Mg^{2+}. Cytoplasmic Ca^{2+} activation is a basic to RyR1 and RyR2. Both RyR1 and RyR2 demonstrate a bell-shaped cytoplasmic [Ca^{2+}] dependence, being activated when cytoplasmic [Ca^{2+}] increases above resting levels (~100 nM) to a maximum ~10–30 μM (Meissner, 1994; Xu, Mann, & Meissner, 1996). RyR1 activity declines with increases to >100 μM Ca^{2+} (Laver et al., 1995), levels seldom reached physiologically without cell damage and EC coupling loss as junctophilin is cleaved (Murphy et al., 2013). In contrast to RyR1, maximum Ca^{2+}-activated activity of RyR2 declines only when [Ca^{2+}] is increased to supraphysiological levels of ≥500 μM (Laver et al., 1995; Xu et al., 1996). Cytoplasmic Ca^{2+} inhibition sites in RyR1 are functionally significant in a cellular context as they can be occupied by Mg^{2+}, which is present in the cytoplasm at ~1 mM and reduces RyR1 activity at rest to desirably low levels (Laver, Baynes, et al., 1997). Mg^{2+} inhibition must be relieved to allow Ca^{2+} release from SR during skeletal EC coupling (Lamb & Stephenson, 1994). RyR1 from MH pigs are "leaky" at rest due to defective Mg^{2+} inhibition (Laver, O'Neill, & Lamb, 2004; Laver, Owen, et al., 1997). Cytoplasmic Mg^{2+} inhibition of RyR2 is an essential in regulating CICR and is likely compromised in ischemia (Gusev & Niggli, 2008). Cytoplasmic Ca^{2+}-activation of RyR1 provides a backup for muscle activation when conformational EC coupling fails in myopathies or sarcopenia (Weisleder et al., 2006). It may also allow activation of the 50% of RyRs not linked to DHPR tetrads that may be activated by Ca^{2+} released through linked RyRs (Meissner & Lu, 1995). In the latter case, Mg^{2+} inhibition of the unlinked RyRs would have to be relieved, perhaps by allosteric transmission of the EC coupling signal from DHPR-linked RyRs though regions of contact between adjacent RyRs (Fig. 1).

RyR regulation by luminal [Ca^{2+}] and [Mg^{2+}] is important in resting muscle. Whole cell and SR vesicle studies show that RyR activity increases as luminal [Ca^{2+}] increases (Chen et al., 2014; Donoso, Prieto, & Hidalgo, 1995; Wei, Varsanyi, Dulhunty, & Beard, 2006). RyR activity in bilayers also increases in many instances as luminal [Ca^{2+}] increases within cellular levels between 0.1 and 1.5 mM (Dulhunty et al., 2012; Hanna, Lam, Thekkedam, et al., 2014; Walweel et al., 2014; Wei et al., 2006). The dynamic range of free [Ca^{2+}] in skeletal SR is ~20 to ~400 μM (Ziman, Ward, Rodney, Lederer, & Bloch, 2010) and in the heart is 400 to ~1500 μM (Guo, Ai, Shannon, Pogwizd, & Bers, 2007; Shannon, Wang, & Bers, 2005). RyR1 and RyR2 differ in their regulation by luminal [Ca^{2+}].

The luminal Ca^{2+} sensitivity of RyR2 in the cell depends on the summation of several mechanisms. Luminal Ca^{2+} can pass through the RyR2 pore and bind to cytoplasmic Ca^{2+} activation sites, while luminal Ca^{2+} activation sites are engaged when the cytoplasmic Ca^{2+} sites are occupied (Dulhunty et al., 2012; Hanna, Lam, Thekkedam, et al., 2014; Laver, 2007). One intrinsic luminal Ca^{2+} sensor in RyR2 is E4872 (Chen et al., 2014). A second luminal sensor is type 2 calsequestrin (CSQ2) which communicates with RyR2 via triadin and junctin (Dulhunty et al., 2012; Gyorke, Hester, Jones, & Gyorke, 2004; Wei, Hanna, Beard, & Dulhunty, 2009). CSQ2 binding to triadin/junctin increases RyR2 activity (Wei, Hanna, et al., 2009), but reduces the relative increase in activity as luminal [Ca^{2+}] increases from 0.1 to 1.0 mM (Dulhunty et al., 2012). In the presence of CSQ2, RyR2 activity increases with luminal [Ca^{2+}] when the cytoplasmic redox potential is oxidising, but decreases at more reducing potentials (Hanna, Lam, Thekkedam, et al., 2014). This suggests the RyR2 environment in intact cell is more oxidizing than the bulk cytoplasm, as increasing luminal Ca^{2+} in the cell induces spontaneous Ca^{2+} release, e.g., (Jiang et al., 2010). Luminal Ca^{2+} regulation of RyR2 also depends on cytoplasmic [Ca^{2+}], [Mg^{2+}], [ATP], bilayer potential, and luminal [Mg^{2+}] (Laver, 2007; Laver & Honen, 2008; Walweel et al., 2014).

RyR2 responses to luminal Ca^{2+} are altered in catecholaminergic polymorphic ventricular tachycardia (CPVT) and arrhythmogenic right ventricular cardiomyopathy. In these severe albeit rare genetic disorders, sudden cardiac death occurs when arrhythmia is triggered by stress, in the absence of any structural heart disease. The phenotype is associated with RyR2, CSQ2, or calmodulin (CaM) mutations (Hwang et al., 2014; Jiang et al., 2005; Terentyev et al., 2008) in which RyR2 activity increases to higher than normal levels as the SR refills during diastole, a time when healthy RyR2 activity is very low. The resulting diastolic SR "Ca^{2+} leak" leads to spontaneous Ca^{2+} release and high diastolic cytoplasmic [Ca^{2+}] (Jiang et al., 2005; Koop, Goldmann, Chen, Thieleczek, & Varsanyi, 2008; Fig. 4). The surface Na^{+}/Ca^{2+} exchanger (NCX) removes Ca^{2+} from the cell and depolarizes the membrane as 3 Na^{+} ions are imported for 1 Ca^{2+} extruded. This delayed after depolarization in individual myocytes triggers unsynchronized action potentials and arrhythmia.

The effect of the RyR2, CSQ2, and CaM mutations is to alter the relation between RyR activity and luminal [Ca^{2+}] so that activity exceeds the threshold for spontaneous Ca^{2+} release (Jiang et al., 2008; Jones et al., 2008; Koop et al., 2008; Terentyev et al., 2008). Fig. 4 suggests that activity

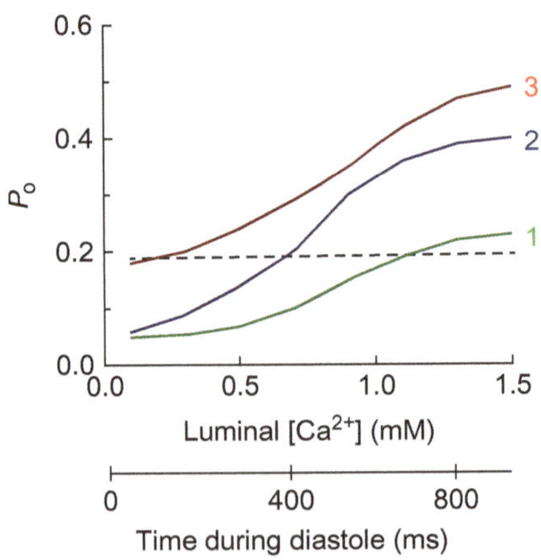

Fig. 4 Hypothetical luminal Ca^{2+}-sensitivity profiles. RyR2 open probability (P_o) vs luminal [Ca^{2+}] over the range experienced during diastole. [Ca^{2+}] increases with time during diastole, so the *x* axis can be approximated as time (lower *x* axis). The horizontal line is a hypothetical threshold P_o for spontaneous Ca^{2+} release. Curve 1 (*green*): a "healthy" increase in P_o remains below spontaneous release threshold until the SR SR is overloaded as [Ca^{2+}] exceeds ~1.0 mM. Curve 2 (*blue*): P_o exceeds spontaneous release threshold with partial SR loading. In curve 3 (*red*): P_o is above threshold for spontaneous release at all [Ca^{2+}]s.

exceeds this threshold if the slope of the curve increases (curve 2) as with CSQ2 dissociation (Dulhunty et al., 2012), or if open probability is higher than normal at all luminal [Ca^{2+}] (curve 3) as in many CPVT mutations (Jiang et al., 2005). Carvedilol and its analogues bind to RyR2, reducing its activity and reducing spontaneous Ca^{2+} release (Smith, Wang, et al., 2013; Zhou et al., 2011). Other drugs that reduce diastolic RyR activity (e.-g., dantrolene, S107, flecainide, or C-terminal helical bundle of GSTM2 (GSTM2C)), irrespective of mechanism, could keep RyR2 activity below threshold for spontaneous Ca^{2+} release.

As an aside, the greatest increase in RyR2 activity occurs when luminal [Ca^{2+}] is increased through nonphysiological Ca^{2+} levels of $\leq 10^{-5}$ to >0.01 mM (Chen et al., 2014; Laver, 2007; Walweel et al., 2014). The relationship is bell shaped over a wide range of luminal [Ca^{2+}] *($\leq 10^{-5}$ to 20 mM), with the [Ca^{2+}] for maximum activity varying greatly under different experimental conditions (Chen et al., 2014; Laver, 2007; Walweel et al., 2014). Thus, in the relatively narrow physiological range (0.1–1.0 mM), the slope can be positive, negative, or flat, depending on the profile of the overall curve. As a result, the reported relationship between RyR2 activity and luminal [Ca^{2+}] varies substantially between laboratories.

The RyR1 activity vs luminal [Ca^{2+}] curve reflects changes in Ca^{2+} efflux from intact vesicles (Donoso et al., 1995) only in the presence of type 1 calsequestrin (CSQ1) (Wei et al., 2006), which inhibits RyR1 through binding to junctin (Beard, Sakowska, Dulhunty, & Laver, 2002; Beard et al., 2008; Wei, Gallant, Dulhunty, & Beard, 2009). The curve relating RyR1 activity to luminal [Ca^{2+}] is not bell shaped, but is flat between 10^{-7} and 10^{-4}M Ca^{2+}, increases slightly between 10^{-4} and 10^{-3}M and steeply as Ca^{2+} is increased beyond 10^{-3}M (Wei et al., 2006). The curve is steeper in MH pig muscle and in a mouse model of Duchenne Muscular Dystrophy (Cully & Launikonis, 2016; Jiang et al., 2008). A mutation in CSQ1 is linked to MH in one Australian family, a significant finding as human MH has previously been associated only with RyR1 and CaV1.1 mutations (Bjorksten et al., 2016). CSQ1 knockout in mice, like RyR1 MH mutations, increases RyR1 leak (Dainese et al., 2009; Protasi et al., 2009) and reduces tetanic force in fast twitch, but not in slow-twitch fibers which also express CSQ2 (Paolini, Quarta, D'Onofrio, Reggiani, & Protasi, 2011). The "leaky" RyR1 with CSQ1 knockout is consistent with removal of the inhibitory influence of CSQ1 on RyR1 (Beard et al., 2002) and likely alters luminal Ca^{2+} sensitivity of RyR1 (Wei et al., 2006). MH-like episodes in CSQ1 knockout mice are alleviated by dantrolene, a drug that is effective against MH episodes in humans (Dainese et al., 2009), and may act by dampening the enhanced luminal Ca^{2+} sensitivity.

7. THE FK506-BINDING PROTEINS

FK506 (tacrolimas), is a common immunosuppressant used with organ and bone marrow transplants. It binds to FK506-binding proteins (FKBPs) which range in size from 12 to 135 kDa (Galat, 2008; Gothel & Marahiel, 1999). The 12 kDa FKBP12 and 12.6 kDa FKBP12.6 associate with RyRs. Skeletal muscle expresses only FKBP12, while cardiac muscle expresses both FKBP12 and 12.6 in a variable species-dependent ratio (Zissimopoulos, Seifan, Maxwell, Williams, & Lai, 2012). FKBP12.6 binds to RyR2 with a Kd of ~0.7 nM, while FKBP12 has a lower affinity with a K_d of ~206 nM (Guo et al., 2010), although [FKBP]s reported to modulate RyR activity range from pM to μM concentrations (Brillantes et al., 1994; Galfre et al., 2012; Mei et al., 2013; Venturi et al., 2014; Wehrens et al., 2003). FKBP regulation of RyRs is mechanistically important as their dissociation increases substate activity (Ahern et al., 1994; Ahern, Junankar, & Dulhunty, 1997; Brillantes et al., 1994). Substate levels (Fig. 5) are contrary to the concept that channel opening is an all-or-none event, but have long been recognized as a characteristic of RyR gating (Ahern et al., 1994; Liu, Lai, Rousseau, Jones, & Meissner, 1989), although the underlying molecular events remain a fascinating mystery.

FKBP regulation of RyRs has clinical significance as FKBP dissociation and the "leaky" RyR phenotype are implicated in skeletal myopathies, cardiac arrhythmia, heart failure, and seizures linked to RyR2 mutations (Chelu, Danila, Gilman, & Hamilton, 2004; Lehnart et al., 2008; Marks, 2013; Wehrens et al., 2003). JTV519 (a 1,4-benzothiazepine) and 2,3,4,5,-tetrahydro-7-methoxy-4-methyl-1,4-benzothiazepine (S107), stabilize the RyR/FKBP complex, improve muscle function and reduce seizures (Bellinger et al., 2009; Lehnart et al., 2008; Mei et al., 2013; Wehrens et al., 2004). Therefore, S107 has significant potential for treatment of these FKBP dissociation-related conditions (Matecki et al., 2016).

8. CaM, DANTROLENE, AND S100A1

CaM is a 17-kDa cytoplasmic Ca^{2+}-binding protein involved in Ca^{2+} signaling in most tissues. In muscle, CaM binding to RyR1 and RyR2 regulates channel activity and is required for RyR phosphorylation by

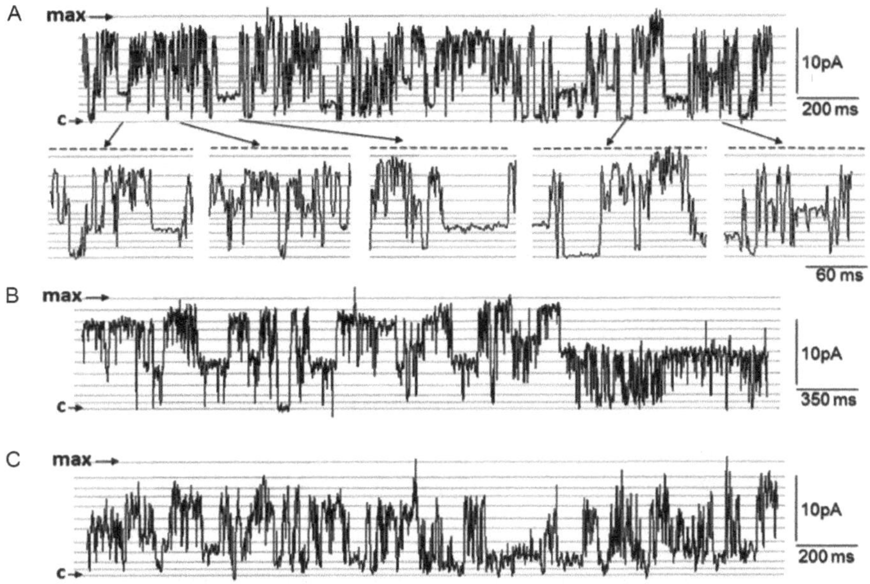

Fig. 5 Substate levels in purified RyR1 activity. (A)–(C) Current recordings from three different purified RyR1 channels obtained at +40 mV with symmetrical 250 mM Cs^{+}, 1.0 μM *cis* Ca^{2+}, and 1 mM *trans* Ca^{2+} (Beard et al., 2002; Casarotto et al., 2000). Openings to levels less than maximum are maintained for tens of milliseconds and therefore their amplitude are limited by the 200 Hz filter used to display the data. Lines are drawn through some of the more obvious levels. "c" indicates the closed level and "max" the maximum open level. In (A), lower records are shown on an expanded time base to reveal dwell times; *arrows* indicate the origin of the segment in the full record above (E. Wium, A.F. Dulhunty, N.A. Beard, unpublished).

calmodulin kinase 2 (CaMKII) (Balshaw, Xu, Yamaguchi, Pasek, & Meissner, 2001; Tripathy, Xu, Mann, & Meissner, 1995). Ca^{2+} binding to EF hand Ca^{2+}-binding domains in CaMs N- and C-terminal lobes exposes hydrophobic sites that bind to target proteins (Park et al., 2008). The three CaM genes in humans, CALM1, CALM2, and CALM3, encode identical proteins. The CaM-binding domains in RyRs are potential therapeutic targets (Oo et al., 2015; Walweel, Oo, & Laver, 2017). *In the heart,* Ca–CaM binds to RyR2 with high affinity (K_d 20–100 nM) at high (100 μM) cytoplasmic [Ca^{2+}], inhibiting the channel (Balshaw et al., 2001; Guo et al., 2011; Huang et al., 2013). Ca^{2+}-depleted apoCaM at lower [Ca^{2+}] either weakly inhibits RyR2 (Balshaw et al., 2001) or has no effect (Fruen, Bardy, Byrem, Strasburg, & Louis, 2000). Two missense mutations in CALM1 and one in CALM3 are associated with CPVT (Gomez-Hurtado et al., 2016; Vassilakopoulou et al., 2015) and impact on

RyR2's luminal Ca^{2+} sensitivity (Sondergaard et al., 2015). *In skeletal muscle*, RyR1 is regulated by CaM in a highly cytoplasmic [Ca^{2+}]-dependent manner. With a resting cytoplasmic [Ca^{2+}] of 100 nM, apoCaM activates RyR1 (Tripathy et al., 1995) while at an activating 10 μM Ca^{2+}, Ca–CaM partially inhibits the channel (Tripathy et al., 1995). Three CaM-binding sites are conserved in RyR1, RyR2, and RyR3; ApoCaM and Ca–CaM bind to all three sites in RyR1 and RyR2, with highest affinity to a site which also contains MH and CCD mutations that alter CaM/RyR1 binding (Lau, Chan, & Van Petegem, 2014).

Dantrolene and CaM. Dantrolene inhibits Ca^{2+} release from skeletal muscle SR and is one of the few muscle-specific relaxants. It is recommended for treatment of potentially fatal MH episodes and reduces arrhythmia associated with CPVT mutations and heart failure (Jung et al., 2012; Protasi et al., 2009). Dantrolene-binding sites are located in RyR1 and RyR2 (Kobayashi et al., 2009), but dantrolene has no effect on isolated single channel activity (Szentesi et al., 2001); unless, as discovered in Australia, CaM is added to the RyRs (Oo et al., 2015; Walweel et al., 2017).

S100A1 and CaM. S100 proteins are small 16–26 kDa Ca^{2+}-binding proteins found in most cell types. S100A1 is strongly expressed in striated muscle and exists as a dimer which, like CaM, contains four EF hand Ca^{2+}-binding motifs (Prosser, Hernandez-Ochoa, & Schneider, 2011). Both S100A and CaM contribute to skeletal and cardiac EC coupling (Prosser et al., 2011). *In skeletal muscle*, S100A1 potentiates RyR1 activity, caffeine-evoked force in skinned fibers and Ca^{2+} release and twitch tension in intact fibers (Most et al., 2003; Prosser et al., 2011; Treves et al., 1997). It is suggested that S100A1 and CaM bind to the same site as they compete in activating RyR1 and S100A1 competes with Ca–CaM in inactivation of Ca^{2+} release (Prosser et al., 2011). Also a mutation in the RyR1 S100A1-binding domain interrupts both CaM and S100A1 binding, reduces apoCaM and S100A1 activation and Ca–CaM inhibition (Prosser et al., 2011). However, FRET studies indicate that S100A1 and CaM bind at the same time to RyRs, and that RyR/CaM binding allosterically affects the S100A1/RyR interaction rather than competing for the same binding site (Rebbeck et al., 2016). *In the heart*, the RyR1 S100A1-binding domain is conserved in RyR2, S100A1 expression is decreased in cardiomyopathies, knockout mice are susceptible to heart failure and S100A1 increases the gain of CICR (Prosser et al., 2011). Evaluating CaM and S100A1 role in myocytes is complex as both interact with other Ca^{2+}-signaling proteins including CaV1.2 and SERCA2A (the cardiac sarcoplasmic endoplasmic reticulum Ca^{2+} ATPase (SERCA) isoform)/phospholamban complex (Prosser et al., 2011). However, S100A1 interacts with RyR2, enhancing [^{3}H]-ryanodine binding with μM [Ca^{2+}] or reducing [^{3}H]-ryanodine binding with diastolic nM [Ca^{2+}] and reducing Ca^{2+} leak from SR and Ca^{2+} spark frequency (Prosser et al., 2011). A therapeutic role for S100A1 is indicated by prevention of RyR2-dependent arrhythmia by an S100A1 DNA-based therapy (Ritterhoff et al., 2015).

9. THE GLUTATHIONE TRANSFERASE STRUCTURAL FAMILY

Glutathione transferases (GSTs). GSTs are a large family of cytoplasmic proteins that are best known for their role in phase II detoxification reactions, although many GSTs have additional functions (Board, 2007; Board & Menon, 2013; Mannervik, Board, Hayes, Listowsky, & Pearson, 2005). At the ANU, we discovered an unexpected function of GSTs in strongly inhibiting RyR2 and mildly activating RyR1 (Abdellatif et al., 2007; Dulhunty, Gage, Curtis, Chelvanayagam, & Board, 2001; Dulhunty, Hewawasam, Liu, Casarotto, & Board, 2011). RyR2 inhibition, but not RyR1 activation, requires only the nonenzymatic C-terminal half of GSTM2 (GSTM2C), particularly helices 5–8 (Fig. 6; Dulhunty, Hewawasam, et al., 2011; Hewawasam, Liu, Casarotto, Dulhunty, & Board, 2010; Liu et al., 2009). RyR2-specific inhibition is explained by GSTM2C binding to a unique sequence in divergent region 3 (DR3) of RyR2 (Liu et al., 2012). GSTM2C and its analogues reduce Ca^{2+} transients and contractility in mouse myocytes (Hewawasam, Liu, Casarotto, Board, & Dulhunty, 2016; Samarasinghe et al., 2015). The RyR2-specific inhibition, added to GSTM2Cs endosomal transport into myocytes is therapeutically significant (Hewawasam et al., 2016; Morris, Craig, Sutherland, Board, & Casarotto, 2009; Morris, Liu, Weaver, Board, & Casarotto, 2011; Samarasinghe et al., 2015).

Chloride intracellular channels (CLIC) belong to the GST structural family (Fig. 6), but lack enzyme activity (Dulhunty, Gage, et al., 2001). The proteins are soluble at cellular redox potentials and pH, but embed in membranes and conduct Cl^- ions with acidic pH and oxidizing redox potentials (Cromer et al., 2007; Littler et al., 2010). We discovered that the soluble chloride intracellular channel type 2 (CLIC2) inhibits RyR1 and RyR2 channels (Board, Coggan, Watson, Gage, & Dulhunty, 2004), indicating that they bind to a conserved site in the RyRs, contrasting with the RyR2-specific DR3-binding site for the GSTs. CLIC2 binding to

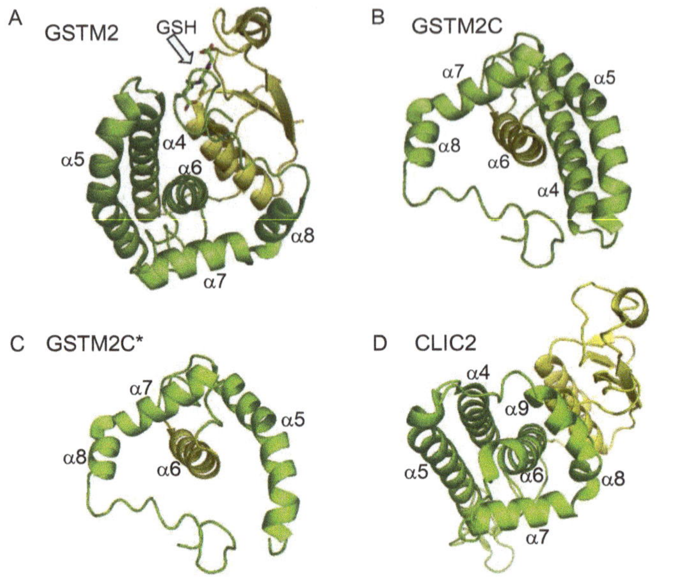

Fig. 6 GST structural family members. (A)–(C) Structures of GSTM2 and deletion constructs that inhibit RyR2. (A) Crystal structure of GSTM2 (PDB 1XW5) (Raghunathan et al., 1994). The N-terminal catalytic domain is in gold and C-terminal α-helical domain in green. Helices α4 to α8 as labeled. GSH is shown in the active site in CPK color code. (B) Structure of GSTM2C predicted from the GSTM2 structure. Helix 6 (in *gold*) maintains an activating conformation. (C) Predicted structure of GSTM2C*, the most active deletion construct contains helices 5, 6, 7, and 8 (Liu et al., 2009). (D) Crystal structure of CLIC2, PDB R5G (Cromer et al., 2007).

domains 5 and 6 in the clamp region of RyR1 dramatically changes RyR conformational, breaking a structural bridge between domains 9 and 10 (Fig. 7; Meng et al., 2009), a significant structural change that is also observed in the RyR1 open conformation (Orlova, Serysheva, van Heel, Hamilton, & Chiu, 1996).

The effect of CLIC2 on RyR activity is complex as it inhibits RyR2 when the redox potential is oxidizing, but activates channels under more reducing conditions (Jalilian, Gallant, Board, & Dulhunty, 2008). CLIC2 potentiates [^{3}H]ryanodine binding, but inhibits RyR channels and Ca^{2+} release from skeletal and cardiac SR, questioning the dogma that [^{3}H] ryanodine-binding simply reflects RyR open probability (Dulhunty, Pouliquin, Coggan, Gage, & Board, 2005; Meng et al., 2009). Finally, CLIC2 enhances substate activity in individual RyRs and increases coupled gating events, where several channels in the bilayer open simultaneously (Dulhunty, Pouliquin, et al., 2005). Coupled gating may allow

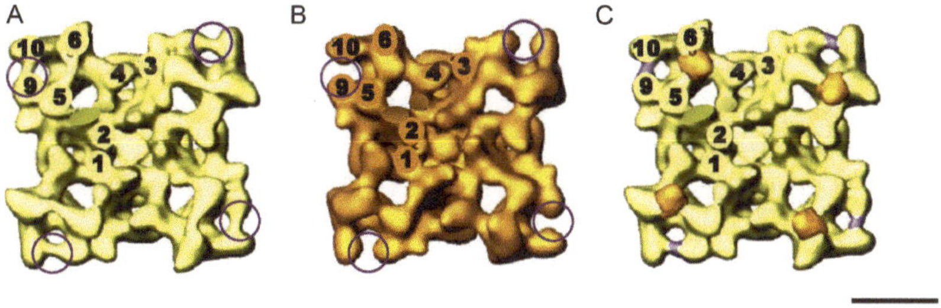

Fig. 7 Structural consequences of CLIC2 binding to RyR1. The t-tubule-facing surface of the RyR1 homotetramer is shown. Domains are numbered according to the convention for cryoelectron microscopy used at the time of publication (Meng et al., 2009). Images in the absence (A) and presence (B) of CLIC2, with the difference image in (C). There is an additional mass of CLIC2 between domains 5 and 6 and separation of domains 9 and 10 (*blue circle* in A–C) and *blue* region in (C). The scale bar is 10 nm. *Modified from Meng, X., Wang, G., Viero, C., Wang, Q., Mi, W., Su, X. D., et al. (2009). CLIC2-RyR1 interaction and structural characterization by cryo-electron microscopy.* Journal of Molecular Biology, 387, *320–334.*

DHPR-linked RyR1 to activate unlinked RyRs during skeletal EC coupling (Porta et al., 2012; Yin, Han, Wei, & Lai, 2005). Therefore, CLIC2 interacts profoundly with the RyR channel and can be used as an experimental tool in unravelling RyR gating (Jalilian et al., 2008).

CLIC2 is associated with cardiac and neurological disorders. It is downregulated in dilated cardiomyopathy (Molina-Navarro et al., 2013) and is implicated in behavioral and cognitive impairment (El-Hattab et al., 2015). An H101Q substitution in a patient with intellectual deficit and cardiac hypertrophy activates RyR channels, reversing the inhibitory action of WT CLIC2 (Takano et al., 2012).

10. OXIDATION, PHOSPHORYLATION, DOXORUBICIN, AND FLECAINIDE

Oxidation. RyRs contain ~80 (RyR2) to ~101 (RyR1) cysteine residues per subunit (320–404 per channel); of these, between 25% and 50% are free and available for *S*-oxidation, *S*-nitrosylation *S*-glutathionylation, or *S*-palmitoylation, reinforcing the notion that the protein is an "allosteric ion channel giant" (Van Petegem, 2015). Mild oxidation increases RyR1 and RyR2 activity and can be reversed by reducing agents, while stronger oxidation produces a mainly irreversible inhibition (Eager & Dulhunty, 1998; Eager, Roden, & Dulhunty, 1997; Favero, Zable, & Abramson, 1995; Green et al., 2000; Haarmann, Fink, & Dulhunty, 1999; Hidalgo, Aracena,

Sanchez, & Donoso, 2002; Liu, Abramson, Zable, & Pessah, 1994). Various oxidizing and reducing agents cause different effects on channel gating, suggesting that different classes of cysteine residues can be modified (Dulhunty, Haarmann, Green, & Hart, 2000). In this context, mild oxidation decreases the number of thiols from ~48 to ~38/subunit, without affecting RyR1 activity (Sun, Xu, Eu, Stamler, & Meissner, 2001). Further oxidation reduces thiol numbers to ~23/subunit and reversibly activates RyR1, while extreme oxidation decreases thiols to ~13/subunit and irreversibly inactivates channels (Sun et al., 2001). *S*-nitrosylation and *S*-glutathionylation reduce apoCaM and Ca–CaM binding to RyR1, while *S*-glutathionylation alone decreases RyR1 affinity for FKBP12 (Aracena, Tang, Hamilton, & Hidalgo, 2005). Stress-related increases in reactive oxygen species (ROS) underlie oxidation of RyRs in many pathologies (Prosser, Khairallah, Ziman, Ward, & Lederer, 2013). (TGF)-β upregulation of NADPH oxidase 4 leads to oxidation and activation of RyR1 causing muscle weakness (Waning et al., 2015). RyRs are also sensitive to transmembrane redox potential, set by redox buffers in the cytoplasm and SR lumen and detected by a redox sensor comprised of six to eight hyperreactive cysteines per subunit (Pessah & Feng, 2000; Voss, Lango, Ernst-Russell, Morin, & Pessah, 2004). The reduced glutathione (GSH)/GSSG ratio and $NADH/NAD^+$ couple may both contribute to redox buffering (Cherednichenko et al., 2004). Changes in redox potential alter the electron distribution within CH_2–SH groups, without covalent cysteine modification (Pessah & Feng, 2000). The redox sensor allows RyRs to respond to small changes in redox potential and alter Ca^{2+} release during oxidative stress (Feng, Liu, Allen, & Pessah, 2000; Hanna, Lam, Thekkedam, et al., 2014).

Phosphorylation. In the heart, although there are numerous potential phosphorylation sites in RyR2, three residues are mainly examined: S2808 and S2030, phosphorylated by protein kinase A (PKA) and S2814, phosphorylated by CaMKII. Debate surrounds the relative importance of these sites and the effects of phosphorylation of each site on RyR2 gating, however it is generally agreed that CaMKII phosphorylation of S2814 increases RyR2 activity (Dobrev & Wehrens, 2014). A synergy between S2808 phosphorylation, RyR2 thiol modification, and FKBP12.6 dissociation in adversely modifying RyR2 activity is suggested by some authors and disputed by others (Dobrev & Wehrens, 2014). An Australian study found that in rat heart, RyR2 S2808 and S2814 are basally phosphorylated to 69% and 15% of maximum respectively and that β-adrenergic stimulation increases the respective levels to 83% and 60% (Li et al., 2013). Increased phosphorylation is correlated with higher diastolic RyR2 activity due to reduced cytoplasmic Mg^{2+} and Ca^{2+} inhibition and increased luminal Ca^{2+} activation. Significant differences between human, sheep, and rat RyR2 in response to changes in [Ca^{2+}] and [Mg^{2+}] may indeed result from different levels of endogenous phosphorylation (Walweel et al., 2014). *In skeletal muscle.* Australians were among the first to show that skeletal muscle SR Ca^{2+} release and contraction are enhanced by β-adrenergic stimulation and PKA phosphorylation (Cairns & Dulhunty, 1993a, 1993b; Cairns, Westerblad, & Allen, 1993), possibly due to RyR1-S2844 phosphorylation leading to FKBP12 depletion (Andersson et al., 2012; Gehlert et al., 2012). Skeletal muscle weakness in heart failure is attributed to PKA hyper-phosphorylation of RyR1, with *S*-nitrosylation, *S*-oxidation, and FKBP12 depletion (Rullman et al., 2013).

It is likely that a synergy between oxidation of RyRs, *S*-nitrosylation, phosphorylation, and FKBP association alters RyR responses to changes in cytoplasmic and luminal [Ca^{2+}] and [Mg^{2+}] leading to the "leaky" RyR phenotype in cardiac and skeletal myopathies (Belevych et al., 2011; Kyrychenko et al., 2013; Marx & Marks, 2013; Walweel et al., 2017). It is notable that stabilization of FKBP binding to RyRs by S107 prevents Ca^{2+} leak through RyRs and overcomes effects of excess *S*-oxidation, S-nitrosylation, and phosphorylation (Matecki et al., 2016).

Doxorubicin. Anthracyclines are some of the most successful chemotherapeutic agents, but their use is limited by cardiotoxicity. Chronic changes cardiac myocytes are due to ROS generation, impaired mitochondrial function and targeting to topoisomerase 2, DNA replication, transcription, recombination, and chromatin remodeling (Damiani et al., 2016). ANU researchers found that anthracycline interactions with RyR2 and SERCA2A contribute to acute drug effects. RyR2 is activated by low clinical concentrations of the drugs binding to RyR2, while higher clinical concentrations lead to RyR2 oxidation and irreversible inhibition (Hanna, Janczura, Cho, Dulhunty, & Beard, 2011; Hanna, Lam, Tham, Dulhunty, & Beard, 2014). There are also redox-dependent and -independent actions as SERCA2A oxidation leading to reduced SR Ca^{2+} uptake, although Ca^{2+} uptake is enhanced if oxidation is prevented by DTT (Hanna, Lam, Tham, et al., 2014). In addition, anthracycline binding to CSQ2 prevents its polymerization and Ca^{2+}-binding capacity (Beard, Laver, & Dulhunty, 2004). Therefore, RyR2, SERCA2A, and CSQ2 are all potential targets for therapeutic reduction of acute cardiotoxic effects of anthracyclines.

Flecainide is a class 1c antiarrhythmic Na^+ channel blocker. It reduces arrhythmia in patients with CPVT, and in mice with CSQ2 or RyR2 mutations, that are resistant to β-blocker therapy (Lieve, Wilde, & van der Werf, 2016; Watanabe et al., 2009). Australian researchers first examined the effects of flecainide on RyR2 gating, finding that it inhibits the channels and suppresses SR Ca^{2+} release and spontaneous Ca^{2+} release in myocytes (Mehra, Imtiaz, van Helden, Knollmann, & Laver, 2014; Watanabe et al., 2009). The mechanism of flecainide's antiarrhythmic action in CPVT requires further investigation. The clinical effects on CPVT may be independent of RyR2 as a high affinity action on RyR2 is seen only when the cations flow into the SR (Bannister et al., 2015; Mehra et al., 2014). Cellular studies suggest that flecainide increases the action potential threshold without altering Ca^{2+} signaling (Liu et al., 2011). In addition, NCX Ca^{2+} efflux is stimulated by flecainide and would reduce the cytoplasmic $[Ca^{2+}]$ and thus reduce RyR2 activity (Sikkel et al., 2013).

11. CONCLUSION

Understanding the regulation of RyR ion channels by many diverse factors, commensurate with the size of the protein and its multiple regulatory sites, has progressed rapidly given the late discovery of the protein in the mid- to late 1980s. Indeed, a PubMed search for "ryanodine receptor" yields ~6000 hits, increasing from only two in 1985 to several hundred every year from 1998 to the present time. Australian researchers have a proud history of contribution to some of the major aspects of RyR physiology and pharmacology as outlined in this chapter. As the emphasis has been on the Australian contribution, we apologize for the many excellent publications that have not been cited, although many of these are covered in reviews that have been cited.

CONFLICT OF INTEREST

None of the authors have a conflict of interest to declare.

REFERENCES

Abdellatif, Y., Liu, D., Gallant, E. M., Gage, P. W., Board, P. G., & Dulhunty, A. F. (2007). The Mu class glutathione transferase is abundant in striated muscle and is an isoform-specific regulator of ryanodine receptor calcium channels. *Cell Calcium*, *41*, 429–440.

Adams, B. A., Tanabe, T., Mikami, A., Numa, S., & Beam, K. G. (1990). Intramembrane charge movement restored in dysgenic skeletal muscle by injection of dihydropyridine receptor cDNAs. *Nature*, *346*, 569–572.

Ahern, G. P., Junankar, P. R., & Dulhunty, A. F. (1994). Single channel activity of the ryanodine receptor calcium release channel is modulated by FK-506. *FEBS Letters*, *352*, 369–374.

Ahern, G. P., Junankar, P. R., & Dulhunty, A. F. (1997). Subconductance states in single-channel activity of skeletal muscle ryanodine receptors after removal of FKBP12. *Biophysical Journal*, *72*, 146–162.

Altafaj, X., France, J., Almassy, J., Jona, I., Rossi, D., Sorrentino, V., et al. (2007). Maurocalcine interacts with the cardiac ryanodine receptor without inducing channel modification. *The Biochemical Journal*, *406*, 309–315.

Andersson, D. C., Betzenhauser, M. J., Reiken, S., Umanskaya, A., Shiomi, T., & Marks, A. R. (2012). Stress-induced increase in skeletal muscle force requires protein kinase A phosphorylation of the ryanodine receptor. *The Journal of Physiology*, *590*, 6381–6387.

Aracena, P., Tang, W., Hamilton, S. L., & Hidalgo, C. (2005). Effects of S-glutathionylation and S-nitrosylation on calmodulin binding to triads and FKBP12 binding to type 1 calcium release channels. *Antioxidants & Redox Signaling*, 7, 870–881.

Aroui, S., Ram, N., Appaix, F., Ronjat, M., Kenani, A., Pirollet, F., et al. (2009). Maurocalcine as a non toxic drug carrier overcomes doxorubicin resistance in the cancer cell line MDA-MB 231. *Pharmaceutical Research*, *26*, 836–845.

Bai, X. C., Yan, Z., Wu, J., Li, Z., & Yan, N. (2016). The central domain of RyR1 is the transducer for long-range allosteric gating of channel opening. *Cell Research*, *26*, 995–1006.

Balshaw, D. M., Xu, L., Yamaguchi, N., Pasek, D. A., & Meissner, G. (2001). Calmodulin binding and inhibition of cardiac muscle calcium release channel (ryanodine receptor). *The Journal of Biological Chemistry*, *276*, 20144–20153.

Bannister, R. A. (2016). Bridging the myoplasmic gap II: More recent advances in skeletal muscle excitation-contraction coupling. *The Journal of Experimental Biology*, *219*, 175–182.

Bannister, M. L., & Ikemoto, N. (2006). Effects of peptide C corresponding to the Glu724-Pro760 region of the II-III loop of the DHP (dihydropyridine) receptor alpha1 subunit on the domain- switch-mediated activation of RyR1 (ryanodine receptor 1) Ca^{2+} channels. *The Biochemical Journal*, *394*, 145–152.

Bannister, M. L., Thomas, N. L., Sikkel, M. B., Mukherjee, S., Maxwell, C., MacLeod, K. T., et al. (2015). The mechanism of flecainide action in CPVT does not involve a direct effect on RyR2. *Circulation Research*, *116*, 1324–1335.

Beard, N. A., Laver, D. R., & Dulhunty, A. F. (2004). Calsequestrin and the calcium release channel of skeletal and cardiac muscle. *Progress in Biophysics and Molecular Biology*, *85*, 33–69.

Beard, N. A., Sakowska, M. M., Dulhunty, A. F., & Laver, D. R. (2002). Calsequestrin is an inhibitor of skeletal muscle ryanodine receptor calcium release channels. *Biophysical Journal*, *82*, 310–320.

Beard, N. A., Wei, L., Cheung, S. N., Kimura, T., Varsanyi, M., & Dulhunty, A. F. (2008). Phosphorylation of skeletal muscle calsequestrin enhances its Ca^{2+} binding capacity and promotes its association with junctin. *Cell Calcium*, *44*, 363–373.

Belevych, A. E., Terentyev, D., Terentyeva, R., Nishijima, Y., Sridhar, A., Hamlin, R. L., et al. (2011). The relationship between arrhythmogenesis and impaired contractility in heart failure: Role of altered ryanodine receptor function. *Cardiovascular Research*, *90*, 493–502.

Bellinger, A. M., Reiken, S., Carlson, C., Mongillo, M., Liu, X., Rothman, L., et al. (2009). Hypernitrosylated ryanodine receptor calcium release channels are leaky in dystrophic muscle. *Nature Medicine*, *15*, 325–330.

Bers, D. M., & Stiffel, V. M. (1993). Ratio of ryanodine to dihydropyridine receptors in cardiac and skeletal muscle and implications for E-C coupling. *The American Journal of Physiology*, *264*, C1587–C1593.

Beurg, M., Sukhareva, M., Ahern, C. A., Conklin, M. W., Perez-Reyes, E., Powers, P. A., et al. (1999). Differential regulation of skeletal muscle L-type Ca^{2+} current and excitation-contraction coupling by the dihydropyridine receptor beta subunit. *Biophysical Journal, 76*, 1744–1756.

Bjorksten, A. R., Gillies, R. L., Hockey, B., & du Start, D. (2016). Sequencing of genes involved in the movement of calcium across human skeletal muscle sarcoplasmic reticulum: Continuing the search for genes associated with malignant hyperthermia. *Anaesthesia and Intensive Care, 44*, 762–768.

Block, B. A., Imagawa, T., Campbell, K. P., & Franzini-Armstrong, C. (1988). Structural evidence for direct interaction between the molecular components of the transverse tubule/sarcoplasmic reticulum junction in skeletal muscle. *The Journal of Cell Biology, 107*, 2587–2600.

Board, P. G. (2007). The use of glutathione transferase-knockout mice as pharmacological and toxicological models. *Expert Opinion on Drug Metabolism & Toxicology, 3*, 421–433.

Board, P. G., Coggan, M., Watson, S., Gage, P. W., & Dulhunty, A. F. (2004). CLIC-2 modulates cardiac ryanodine receptor Ca^{2+} release channels. *The International Journal of Biochemistry & Cell Biology, 36*(8), 1599–1612.

Board, P. G., & Menon, D. (2013). Glutathione transferases, regulators of cellular metabolism and physiology. *Biochimica et Biophysica Acta, 1830*, 3267–3288.

Brillantes, A. B., Ondrias, K., Scott, A., Kobrinsky, E., Ondriasova, E., Moschella, M. C., et al. (1994). Stabilization of calcium release channel (ryanodine receptor) function by FK506-binding protein. *Cell, 77*, 513–523.

Cairns, S. P., & Dulhunty, A. F. (1993a). Beta-adrenergic potentiation of E-C coupling increases force in rat skeletal muscle. *Muscle & Nerve, 16*, 1317–1325.

Cairns, S. P., & Dulhunty, A. F. (1993b). The effects of beta-adrenoceptor activation on contraction in isolated fast- and slow-twitch skeletal muscle fibres of the rat. *British Journal of Pharmacology, 110*, 1133–1141.

Cairns, S. P., Westerblad, H., & Allen, D. G. (1993). Changes of tension and $[Ca^{2+}]i$ during beta-adrenoceptor activation of single, intact fibres from mouse skeletal muscle. *Pflügers Archiv, 425*, 150–155.

Casarotto, M. G., Gibson, F., Pace, S. M., Curtis, S. M., Mulcair, M., & Dulhunty, A. F. (2000). A structural requirement for activation of skeletal ryanodine receptors by peptides of the dihydropyridine receptor II-III loop. *The Journal of Biological Chemistry, 275*, 11631–11637.

Casarotto, M. G., Green, D., Pace, S. M., Curtis, S. M., & Dulhunty, A. F. (2001). Structural determinants for activation or inhibition of ryanodine receptors by basic residues in the dihydropyridine receptor II-III loop. *Biophysical Journal, 80*, 2715–2726.

Casarotto, M. G., Green, D., Pace, S., Young, J., & Dulhunty, A. F. (2004). Activating the ryanodine receptor with dihydropyridine receptor II-III loop segments: Size and charge do matter. *Frontiers in Bioscience, 9*, 2860–2872.

Chelu, M. G., Danila, C. I., Gilman, C. P., & Hamilton, S. L. (2004). Regulation of ryanodine receptors by FK506 binding proteins. *Trends in Cardiovascular Medicine, 14*, 227–234.

Chen, W., Wang, R., Chen, B., Zhong, X., Kong, H., Bai, Y., et al. (2014). The ryanodine receptor store-sensing gate controls Ca^{2+} waves and Ca^{2+}-triggered arrhythmias. *Nature Medicine, 20*, 184–192.

Cheng, W., Altafaj, X., Ronjat, M., & Coronado, R. (2005). Interaction between the dihydropyridine receptor Ca^{2+} channel beta-subunit and ryanodine receptor type 1 strengthens excitation-contraction coupling. *Proceedings of the National Academy of Sciences of the United States of America, 102*, 19225–19230.

Cherednichenko, G., Zima, A. V., Feng, W., Schaefer, S., Blatter, L. A., & Pessah, I. N. (2004). NADH oxidase activity of rat cardiac sarcoplasmic reticulum regulates calcium-induced calcium release. *Circulation Research, 94*, 478–486.
Coronado, R., & Latorre, R. (1983). Phospholipid bilayers made from monolayers on patch-clamp pipettes. *Biophysical Journal, 43*, 231–236.
Cromer, B. A., Gorman, M. A., Hansen, G., Adams, J. J., Coggan, M., Littler, D. R., et al. (2007). Structure of the Janus protein human CLIC2. *Journal of Molecular Biology, 374*, 719–731.
Cui, Y., Tae, H. S., Norris, N. C., Karunasekara, Y., Pouliquin, P., Board, P. G., et al. (2009). A dihydropyridine receptor alpha1s loop region critical for skeletal muscle contraction is intrinsically unstructured and binds to a SPRY domain of the type 1 ryanodine receptor. *The International Journal of Biochemistry & Cell Biology, 41*, 677–686.
Cully, T. R., & Launikonis, B. S. (2016). Leaky ryanodine receptors delay the activation of store overload-induced Ca^{2+} release, a mechanism underlying malignant hyperthermia-like events in dystrophic muscle. *American Journal of Physiology. Cell Physiology, 310*, C673–C680.
Dainese, M., Quarta, M., Lyfenko, A. D., Paolini, C., Canato, M., Reggiani, C., et al. (2009). Anesthetic- and heat-induced sudden death in calsequestrin-1-knockout mice. *The FASEB Journal, 23*, 1710–1720.
Damiani, R. M., Moura, D. J., Viau, C. M., Caceres, R. A., Henriques, J. A., & Saffi, J. (2016). Pathways of cardiac toxicity: Comparison between chemotherapeutic drugs doxorubicin and mitoxantrone. *Archives of Toxicology, 90*, 2063–2076.
Dayal, A., Bhat, V., Franzini-Armstrong, C., & Grabner, M. (2013). Domain cooperativity in the beta1a subunit is essential for dihydropyridine receptor voltage sensing in skeletal muscle. *Proceedings of the National Academy of Sciences of the United States of America, 110*, 7488–7493.
des Georges, A., Clarke, O. B., Zalk, R., Yuan, Q., Condon, K. J., Grassucci, R. A., et al. (2016). Structural basis for gating and activation of RyR1. *Cell, 167*, 145–157, e117.
Dobrev, D., & Wehrens, X. H. (2014). Role of RyR2 phosphorylation in heart failure and arrhythmias: Controversies around ryanodine receptor phosphorylation in cardiac disease. *Circulation Research, 114*, 1311–1319. discussion 1319.
Donoso, P., Prieto, H., & Hidalgo, C. (1995). Luminal calcium regulates calcium release in triads isolated from frog and rabbit skeletal muscle. *Biophysical Journal, 68*, 507–515.
Dulhunty, A. F. (1984). Heterogeneity of T-tubule geometry in vertebrate skeletal muscle fibres. *Journal of Muscle Research and Cell Motility, 5*, 333–347.
Dulhunty, A. F. (1989). Feet, bridges, and pillars in triad junctions of mammalian skeletal muscle: Their possible relationship to calcium buffers in terminal cisternae and T-tubules and to excitation-contraction coupling. *The Journal of Membrane Biology, 109*, 73–83.
Dulhunty, A. F., Casarotto, M. G., & Beard, N. A. (2011). The ryanodine receptor: A pivotal Ca^{2+} regulatory protein and potential therapeutic drug target. *Current Drug Targets, 12*, 709–723.
Dulhunty, A. F., Cengia, L., Young, J., Pace, S. M., Harvey, P. J., Lamb, G. D., et al. (2005). Functional implications of modifying RyR-activating peptides for membrane permeability. *British Journal of Pharmacology, 144*, 743–754.
Dulhunty, A. F., Curtis, S. M., Cengia, L., Sakowska, M., & Casarotto, M. G. (2004a). Peptide fragments of the dihydropyridine receptor can modulate cardiac ryanodine receptor channel activity and sarcoplasmic reticulum Ca^{2+} release. *The Biochemical Journal, 379*, 161–172.
Dulhunty, A. F., Curtis, S. M., Watson, S., Cengia, L., & Casarotto, M. G. (2004b). Multiple actions of imperatoxin A on ryanodine receptors: Interactions with the II-III loop "A" fragment. *The Journal of Biological Chemistry, 279*, 11853–11862.

Dulhunty, A. F., & Franzini-Armstrong, C. (1975). The relative contributions of the folds and caveolae to the surface membrane of frog skeletal muscle fibres at different sarcomere lengths. *The Journal of Physiology*, *250*, 513–539.
Dulhunty, A. F., & Gage, P. W. (1983). Asymmetrical charge movement in slow- and fast-twitch mammalian muscle fibres in normal and paraplegic rats. *The Journal of Physiology*, *341*, 213–231.
Dulhunty, A. F., & Gage, P. W. (1985). Excitation-contraction coupling and charge movement in denervated rat extensor digitorum longus and soleus muscles. *The Journal of Physiology*, *358*, 75–89.
Dulhunty, A. F., & Gage, P. W. (1988). Effects of extracellular calcium concentration and dihydropyridines on contraction in mammalian skeletal muscle. *The Journal of Physiology*, *399*, 63–80.
Dulhunty, A., Gage, P., Curtis, S., Chelvanayagam, G., & Board, P. (2001). The glutathione transferase structural family includes a nuclear chloride channel and a ryanodine receptor calcium release channel modulator. *The Journal of Biological Chemistry*, *276*, 3319–3323.
Dulhunty, A., Haarmann, C., Green, D., & Hart, J. (2000). How many cysteine residues regulate ryanodine receptor channel activity? *Antioxidants & Redox Signaling*, *2*, 27–34.
Dulhunty, A. F., Hewawasam, R., Liu, D., Casarotto, M. G., & Board, P. G. (2011). Regulation of the cardiac muscle ryanodine receptor by glutathione transferases. *Drug Metabolism Reviews*, *43*, 236–252.
Dulhunty, A. F., Junankar, P. R., & Stanhope, C. (1992). Extra-junctional ryanodine receptors in the terminal cisternae of mammalian skeletal muscle fibres. *Proceedings of the Biological Sciences*, *247*, 69–75.
Dulhunty, A. F., Karunasekara, Y., Curtis, S. M., Harvey, P. J., Board, P. G., & Casarotto, M. G. (2005). The recombinant dihydropyridine receptor II-III loop and partly structured 'C' region peptides modify cardiac ryanodine receptor activity. *The Biochemical Journal*, *385*, 803–813.
Dulhunty, A. F., Laver, D. R., Gallant, E. M., Casarotto, M. G., Pace, S. M., & Curtis, S. (1999). Activation and inhibition of skeletal RyR channels by a part of the skeletal DHPR II-III loop: Effects of DHPR Ser687 and FKBP12. *Biophysical Journal*, *77*, 189–203.
Dulhunty, A. F., Pouliquin, P., Coggan, M., Gage, P. W., & Board, P. G. (2005). A recently identified member of the glutathione transferase structural family modifies cardiac RyR2 substate activity, coupled gating and activation by Ca^{2+} and ATP. *The Biochemical Journal*, *390*, 333–343.
Dulhunty, A. F., Wei-LaPierre, L., Casarotto, M. G., & Beard, N. A. (2017). The core skeletal muscle ryanodine receptor calcium release complex. *Clinical and Experimental Pharmacology & Physiology*, *44*(1), 3–12.
Dulhunty, A. F., Wium, E., Li, L., Hanna, A. D., Mirza, S., Talukder, S., et al. (2012). Proteins within the intracellular calcium store determine cardiac RyR channel activity and cardiac output. *Clinical and Experimental Pharmacology & Physiology*, *39*, 477–484.
Eager, K. R., & Dulhunty, A. F. (1998). Activation of the cardiac ryanodine receptor by sulfhydryl oxidation is modified by Mg^{2+} and ATP. *The Journal of Membrane Biology*, *163*, 9–18.
Eager, K. R., Roden, L. D., & Dulhunty, A. F. (1997). Actions of sulfhydryl reagents on single ryanodine receptor Ca(2+)-release channels from sheep myocardium. *The American Journal of Physiology*, *272*, C1908–C1918.
El-Hattab, A. W., Schaaf, C. P., Fang, P., Roeder, E., Kimonis, V. E., Church, J. A., et al. (2015). Clinical characterization of int22h1/int22h2-mediated Xq28 duplication/deletion: New cases and literature review. *BMC Medical Genetics*, *16*, 12.

el-Hayek, R., Antoniu, B., Wang, J., Hamilton, S. L., & Ikemoto, N. (1995). Identification of calcium release-triggering and blocking regions of the II-III loop of the skeletal muscle dihydropyridine receptor. *The Journal of Biological Chemistry, 270*, 22116–22118.

Eltit, J. M., Franzini-Armstrong, C., & Perez, C. F. (2014). Amino acid residues 489-503 of dihydropyridine receptor (DHPR) beta1a subunit are critical for structural communication between the skeletal muscle DHPR complex and type 1 ryanodine receptor. *The Journal of Biological Chemistry, 289*, 36116–36124.

Favero, T. G., Zable, A. C., & Abramson, J. J. (1995). Hydrogen peroxide stimulates the Ca^{2+} release channel from skeletal muscle sarcoplasmic reticulum. *The Journal of Biological Chemistry, 270*, 25557–25563.

Feng, W., Liu, G., Allen, P. D., & Pessah, I. N. (2000). Transmembrane redox sensor of ryanodine receptor complex. *The Journal of Biological Chemistry, 275*, 35902–35907.

Fink, R. H., & Stephenson, D. G. (1987). Ca^{2+}-movements in muscle modulated by the state of K^{+}-channels in the sarcoplasmic reticulum membranes. *Pflügers Archiv, 409*, 374–380.

Fourest-Lieuvin, A., Rendu, J., Osseni, A., Pernet-Gallay, K., Rossi, D., Oddoux, S., et al. (2012). Role of triadin in the organization of reticulum membrane at the muscle triad. *Journal of Cell Science, 125*, 3443–3453.

Franzini-Armstrong, C. (1970). STUDIES OF THE TRIAD: I. Structure of the junction in frog twitch fibers. *The Journal of Cell Biology, 47*, 488–499.

Franzini-Armstrong, C., Protasi, F., & Ramesh, V. (1999). Shape, size, and distribution of Ca(2+) release units and couplons in skeletal and cardiac muscles. *Biophysical Journal, 77*, 1528–1539.

Fruen, B. R., Bardy, J. M., Byrem, T. M., Strasburg, G. M., & Louis, C. F. (2000). Differential Ca(2+) sensitivity of skeletal and cardiac muscle ryanodine receptors in the presence of calmodulin. *American Journal of Physiology. Cell Physiology, 279*, C724–C733.

Gage, P. W., & Dulhunty, A. F. (1981). Upper motor neuron modulation of charge movement and mechanical activation in rat skeletal muscle fibres. *Neuroscience Letters, 27*, 271–276.

Galat, A. (2008). Functional drift of sequence attributes in the FK506-binding proteins (FKBPs). *Journal of Chemical Information and Modeling, 48*, 1118–1130.

Galfre, E., Pitt, S. J., Venturi, E., Sitsapesan, M., Zaccai, N. R., Tsaneva-Atanasova, K., et al. (2012). FKBP12 activates the cardiac ryanodine receptor Ca^{2+}-release channel and is antagonised by FKBP12.6. *PloS One, 7*, e31956.

Gehlert, S., Bungartz, G., Willkomm, L., Korkmaz, Y., Pfannkuche, K., Schiffer, T., et al. (2012). Intense resistance exercise induces early and transient increases in ryanodine receptor 1 phosphorylation in human skeletal muscle. *PloS One, 7*, e49326.

Gomez-Hurtado, N., Boczek, N. J., Kryshtal, D. O., Johnson, C. N., Sun, J., Nitu, F. R., et al. (2016). Novel CPVT-associated calmodulin mutation in CALM3 (CALM3-A103V) activates arrhythmogenic Ca waves and sparks. *Circulation. Arrhythmia and Electrophysiology, 9*(8). http://dx.doi.org/10.1161/CIRCEP.116.004161. pii: e004161.

Gothel, S. F., & Marahiel, M. A. (1999). Peptidyl-prolyl cis-trans isomerases, a superfamily of ubiquitous folding catalysts. *Cellular and Molecular Life Sciences, 55*, 423–436.

Green, D., Pace, S., Curtis, S. M., Sakowska, M., Lamb, G. D., Dulhunty, A. F., et al. (2003). The three-dimensional structural surface of two beta-sheet scorpion toxins mimics that of an alpha-helical dihydropyridine receptor segment. *The Biochemical Journal, 370*, 517–527.

Green, D., Pace, S. M., Hurne, A. M., Waring, P., Hart, J. D., & Dulhunty, A. F. (2000). Skeletal muscle ryanodine receptor channels are activated by the fungal metabolite, gliotoxin. *The Journal of Membrane Biology, 175*, 223–233.

Guo, T., Ai, X., Shannon, T. R., Pogwizd, S. M., & Bers, D. M. (2007). Intra-sarcoplasmic reticulum free Ca^{2+} and buffering in arrhythmogenic failing rabbit heart. *Circulation Research*, *101*, 802–810.

Guo, T., Cornea, R. L., Huke, S., Camors, E., Yang, Y., Picht, E., et al. (2010). Kinetics of FKBP12.6 binding to ryanodine receptors in permeabilized cardiac myocytes and effects on Ca sparks. *Circulation Research*, *106*, 1743–1752.

Guo, T., Fruen, B. R., Nitu, F. R., Nguyen, T. D., Yang, Y., Cornea, R. L., et al. (2011). FRET detection of calmodulin binding to the cardiac RyR2 calcium release channel. *Biophysical Journal*, *101*, 2170–2177.

Gusev, K., & Niggli, E. (2008). Modulation of the local SR Ca^{2+} release by intracellular Mg^{2+} in cardiac myocytes. *The Journal of General Physiology*, *132*, 721–730.

Gyorke, I., Hester, N., Jones, L. R., & Gyorke, S. (2004). The role of calsequestrin, triadin, and junctin in conferring cardiac ryanodine receptor responsiveness to luminal calcium. *Biophysical Journal*, *86*, 2121–2128.

Haarmann, C. S., Dulhunty, A. F., & Laver, D. R. (2005). Regulation of skeletal ryanodine receptors by dihydropyridine receptor II-III loop C-region peptides: Relief of Mg2+ inhibition. *The Biochemical Journal*, *387*, 429–436.

Haarmann, C. S., Fink, R. H., & Dulhunty, A. F. (1999). Oxidation and reduction of pig skeletal muscle ryanodine receptors. *Biophysical Journal*, *77*, 3010–3022.

Haarmann, C. S., Green, D., Casarotto, M. G., Laver, D. R., & Dulhunty, A. F. (2003). The random-coil 'C' fragment of the dihydropyridine receptor II-III loop can activate or inhibit native skeletal ryanodine receptors. *The Biochemical Journal*, *372*, 305–316.

Hals, G. D., Stein, P. G., & Palade, P. T. (1989). Single channel characteristics of a high conductance anion channel in "sarcoballs" *The Journal of General Physiology*, *93*, 385–410.

Hanna, A. D., Janczura, M., Cho, E., Dulhunty, A. F., & Beard, N. A. (2011). Multiple actions of the anthracycline daunorubicin on cardiac ryanodine receptors. *Molecular Pharmacology*, *80*, 538–549.

Hanna, A. D., Lam, A., Tham, S., Dulhunty, A. F., & Beard, N. A. (2014a). Adverse effects of doxorubicin and its metabolic product on cardiac RyR2 and SERCA2A. *Molecular Pharmacology*, *86*, 438–449.

Hanna, A. D., Lam, A., Thekkedam, C., Gallant, E. M., Beard, N. A., & Dulhunty, A. F. (2014b). Cardiac ryanodine receptor activation by a high Ca(2)(+) store load is reversed in a reducing cytoplasmic redox environment. *Journal of Cell Science*, *127*, 4531–4541.

Hewawasam, R. P., Liu, D., Casarotto, M. G., Board, P. G., & Dulhunty, A. F. (2016). The GSTM2 C-terminal domain depresses contractility and Ca2+ transients in neonatal rat ventricular cardiomyocytes. *PloS One*, *11*(9), e0162415. http://dx.doi.org/10.1371/journal.pone.0162415.

Hewawasam, R., Liu, D., Casarotto, M. G., Dulhunty, A. F., & Board, P. G. (2010). The structure of the C-terminal helical bundle in glutathione transferase M2-2 determines its ability to inhibit the cardiac ryanodine receptor. *Biochemical Pharmacology*, *80*, 381–388.

Hidalgo, C., Aracena, P., Sanchez, G., & Donoso, P. (2002). Redox regulation of calcium release in skeletal and cardiac muscle. *Biological Research*, *35*, 183–193.

Horstick, E. J., Linsley, J. W., Dowling, J. J., Hauser, M. A., McDonald, K. K., Ashley-Koch, A., et al. (2013). Stac3 is a component of the excitation-contraction coupling machinery and mutated in Native American myopathy. *Nature Communications*, *4*, 1952.

Huang, X., Liu, Y., Wang, R., Zhong, X., Liu, Y., Koop, A., et al. (2013). Two potential calmodulin-binding sequences in the ryanodine receptor contribute to a mobile, intra-subunit calmodulin-binding domain. *Journal of Cell Science*, *126*, 4527–4535.

Hwang, H. S., Nitu, F. R., Yang, Y., Walweel, K., Pereira, L., Johnson, C. N., et al. (2014). Divergent regulation of ryanodine receptor 2 calcium release channels by arrhythmogenic human calmodulin missense mutants. *Circulation Research, 114*, 1114–1124.

Jalilian, C., Gallant, E. M., Board, P. G., & Dulhunty, A. F. (2008). Redox potential and the response of cardiac ryanodine receptors to CLIC-2, a member of the glutathione S-transferase structural family. *Antioxidants & Redox Signaling, 10*, 1675–1686.

Jiang, D., Chen, W., Xiao, J., Wang, R., Kong, H., Jones, P. P., et al. (2008). Reduced threshold for luminal Ca^{2+} activation of RyR1 underlies a causal mechanism of porcine malignant hyperthermia. *The Journal of Biological Chemistry, 283*, 20813–20820.

Jiang, D., Jones, P. P., Davis, D. R., Gow, R., Green, M. S., Birnie, D. H., et al. (2010). Characterization of a novel mutation in the cardiac ryanodine receptor that results in catecholaminergic polymorphic ventricular tachycardia. *Channels (Austin, Tex.), 4*, 302–310.

Jiang, D., Wang, R., Xiao, B., Kong, H., Hunt, D. J., Choi, P., et al. (2005). Enhanced store overload-induced Ca^{2+} release and channel sensitivity to luminal Ca^{2+} activation are common defects of RyR2 mutations linked to ventricular tachycardia and sudden death. *Circulation Research, 97*, 1173–1181.

Jones, P. P., Jiang, D., Bolstad, J., Hunt, D. J., Zhang, L., Demaurex, N., et al. (2008). Endoplasmic reticulum Ca^{2+} measurements reveal that the cardiac ryanodine receptor mutations linked to cardiac arrhythmia and sudden death alter the threshold for store-overload-induced Ca^{2+} release. *The Biochemical Journal, 412*, 171–178.

Jung, C. B., Moretti, A., Mederos y Schnitzler, M., Iop, L., Storch, U., Bellin, M., et al. (2012). Dantrolene rescues arrhythmogenic RYR2 defect in a patient-specific stem cell model of catecholaminergic polymorphic ventricular tachycardia. *EMBO Molecular Medicine, 4*, 180–191.

Karunasekara, Y., Rebbeck, R. T., Weaver, L. M., Board, P. G., Dulhunty, A. F., & Casarotto, M. G. (2012). An alpha-helical C-terminal tail segment of the skeletal L-type Ca^{2+} channel beta1a subunit activates ryanodine receptor type 1 via a hydrophobic surface. *The FASEB Journal, 26*, 5049–5059.

Kimlicka, L., Lau, K., Tung, C. C., & Van Petegem, F. (2013). Disease mutations in the ryanodine receptor N-terminal region couple to a mobile intersubunit interface. *Nature Communications, 4*, 1506.

Kimura, T., Lueck, J. D., Harvey, P. J., Pace, S. M., Ikemoto, N., Casarotto, M. G., et al. (2009). Alternative splicing of RyR1 alters the efficacy of skeletal EC coupling. *Cell Calcium, 45*, 264–274.

Kobayashi, S., Yano, M., Suetomi, T., Ono, M., Tateishi, H., Mochizuki, M., et al. (2009). Dantrolene, a therapeutic agent for malignant hyperthermia, markedly improves the function of failing cardiomyocytes by stabilizing interdomain interactions within the ryanodine receptor. *Journal of the American College of Cardiology, 53*, 1993–2005.

Koop, A., Goldmann, P., Chen, S. R., Thieleczek, R., & Varsanyi, M. (2008). ARVC-related mutations in divergent region 3 alter functional properties of the cardiac ryanodine receptor. *Biophysical Journal, 94*, 4668–4677.

Kyrychenko, S., Polakova, E., Kang, C., Pocsai, K., Ullrich, N. D., Niggli, E., et al. (2013). Hierarchical accumulation of RyR post-translational modifications drives disease progression in dystrophic cardiomyopathy. *Cardiovascular Research, 97*, 666–675.

Lamb, G. D. (1986). Components of charge movement in rabbit skeletal muscle: The effect of tetracaine and nifedipine. *The Journal of Physiology, 376*, 85–100.

Lamb, G. D., El-Hayek, R., Ikemoto, N., & Stephenson, D. G. (2000). Effects of dihydropyridine receptor II-III loop peptides on Ca(2+) release in skinned skeletal muscle fibers. *American Journal of Physiology. Cell Physiology, 279*, C891–C905.

Lamb, G. D., Junankar, P. R., & Stephenson, D. G. (1995). Raised intracellular Ca^{2+} abolishes excitation-contraction coupling in skeletal muscle fibres of rat and toad. *The Journal of Physiology, 489*(Pt. 2), 349–362.

Lamb, G. D., & Stephenson, D. G. (1994). Effects of intracellular pH and [Mg2+] on excitation-contraction coupling in skeletal muscle fibres of the rat. *The Journal of Physiology*, *478*(Pt. 2), 331–339.
Lau, K., Chan, M. M., & Van Petegem, F. (2014). Lobe-specific calmodulin binding to different ryanodine receptor isoforms. *Biochemistry*, *53*, 932–946.
Laver, D. R. (2007). Ca^{2+} stores regulate ryanodine receptor Ca^{2+} release channels via luminal and cytosolic Ca^{2+} sites. *Biophysical Journal*, *92*, 3541–3555.
Laver, D. R., Baynes, T. M., & Dulhunty, A. F. (1997). Magnesium inhibition of ryanodine-receptor calcium channels: Evidence for two independent mechanisms. *The Journal of Membrane Biology*, *156*, 213–229.
Laver, D. R., & Honen, B. N. (2008). Luminal Mg^{2+}, a key factor controlling RYR2-mediated Ca^{2+} release: Cytoplasmic and luminal regulation modeled in a tetrameric channel. *The Journal of General Physiology*, *132*, 429–446.
Laver, D. R., O'Neill, E. R., & Lamb, G. D. (2004). Luminal Ca^{2+}-regulated Mg^{2+} inhibition of skeletal RyRs reconstituted as isolated channels or coupled clusters. *The Journal of General Physiology*, *124*, 741–758.
Laver, D. R., Owen, V. J., Junankar, P. R., Taske, N. L., Dulhunty, A. F., & Lamb, G. D. (1997). Reduced inhibitory effect of Mg^{2+} on ryanodine receptor Ca^{2+} release channels in malignant hyperthermia. *Biophysical Journal*, *73*, 1913–1924.
Laver, D. R., Roden, L. D., Ahern, G. P., Eager, K. R., Junankar, P. R., & Dulhunty, A. F. (1995). Cytoplasmic Ca^{2+} inhibits the ryanodine receptor from cardiac muscle. *The Journal of Membrane Biology*, *147*, 7–22.
Lehnart, S. E., Mongillo, M., Bellinger, A., Lindegger, N., Chen, B. X., Hsueh, W., et al. (2008). Leaky Ca^{2+} release channel/ryanodine receptor 2 causes seizures and sudden cardiac death in mice. *The Journal of Clinical Investigation*, *118*, 2230–2245.
Lewis, T. M., Dulhunty, A. F., Junankar, P. R., & Stanhope, C. (1992). Ultrastructure of sarcoballs on the surface of skinned amphibian skeletal muscle fibres. *Journal of Muscle Research and Cell Motility*, *13*, 640–653.
Li, J., Imtiaz, M. S., Beard, N. A., Dulhunty, A. F., Thorne, R., vanHelden, D. F., et al. (2013). Beta-adrenergic stimulation increases RyR2 activity via intracellular Ca^{2+} and Mg^{2+} regulation. *PloS One*, *8*, e58334.
Lieve, K. V., Wilde, A. A., & van der Werf, C. (2016). The role of flecainide in the management of catecholaminergic polymorphic ventricular tachycardia. *Arrhythmia & Electrophysiology Review*, *5*, 45–49.
Littler, D. R., Harrop, S. J., Goodchild, S. C., Phang, J. M., Mynott, A. V., Jiang, L., et al. (2010). The enigma of the CLIC proteins: Ion channels, redox proteins, enzymes, scaffolding proteins? *FEBS Letters*, *584*, 2093–2101.
Liu, G., Abramson, J. J., Zable, A. C., & Pessah, I. N. (1994). Direct evidence for the existence and functional role of hyperreactive sulfhydryls on the ryanodine receptor-triadin complex selectively labeled by the coumarin maleimide 7-diethylamino-3-(4'-maleimidylphenyl)-4-methylcoumarin. *Molecular Pharmacology*, *45*, 189–200.
Liu, N., Denegri, M., Ruan, Y., Avelino-Cruz, J. E., Perissi, A., Negri, S., et al. (2011). Short communication: Flecainide exerts an antiarrhythmic effect in a mouse model of catecholaminergic polymorphic ventricular tachycardia by increasing the threshold for triggered activity. *Circulation Research*, *109*, 291–295.
Liu, D., Hewawasam, R., Karunasekara, Y., Casarotto, M. G., Dulhunty, A. F., & Board, P. G. (2012). The inhibitory glutathione transferase M2-2 binding site is located in divergent region 3 of the cardiac ryanodine receptor. *Biochemical Pharmacology*, *83*, 1523–1529.
Liu, D., Hewawasam, R., Pace, S. M., Gallant, E. M., Casarotto, M. G., Dulhunty, A. F., et al. (2009). Dissection of the inhibition of cardiac ryanodine receptors by human glutathione transferase GSTM2-2. *Biochemical Pharmacology*, *77*, 1181–1193.

Liu, Q. Y., Lai, F. A., Rousseau, E., Jones, R. V., & Meissner, G. (1989). Multiple conductance states of the purified calcium release channel complex from skeletal sarcoplasmic reticulum. *Biophysical Journal, 55*, 415–424.

Lu, X., Xu, L., & Meissner, G. (1995). Phosphorylation of dihydropyridine receptor II-III loop peptide regulates skeletal muscle calcium release channel function. Evidence for an essential role of the beta-OH group of Ser687. *The Journal of Biological Chemistry, 270*, 18459–18464.

Mahalingam, M., Perez, C. F., & Fessenden, J. D. (2016). Fluorescence resonance energy transfer-based structural analysis of the dihydropyridine receptor alpha1S subunit reveals conformational differences induced by binding of the beta1a subunit. *The Journal of Biological Chemistry, 291*, 13762–13770.

Mannervik, B., Board, P. G., Hayes, J. D., Listowsky, I., & Pearson, W. R. (2005). Nomenclature for mammalian soluble glutathione transferases. *Methods in Enzymology, 401*, 1–8.

Marks, A. R. (2013). Calcium cycling proteins and heart failure: Mechanisms and therapeutics. *The Journal of Clinical Investigation, 123*, 46–52.

Marx, S. O., & Marks, A. R. (2013). Dysfunctional ryanodine receptors in the heart: New insights into complex cardiovascular diseases. *Journal of Molecular and Cellular Cardiology, 58*, 225–231.

Matecki, S., Dridi, H., Jung, B., Saint, N., Reiken, S. R., Scheuermann, V., et al. (2016). Leaky ryanodine receptors contribute to diaphragmatic weakness during mechanical ventilation. *Proceedings of the National Academy of Sciences of the United States of America, 113*, 9069–9074.

Mehra, D., Imtiaz, M. S., van Helden, D. F., Knollmann, B. C., & Laver, D. R. (2014). Multiple modes of ryanodine receptor 2 inhibition by flecainide. *Molecular Pharmacology, 86*, 696–706.

Mei, Y., Xu, L., Kramer, H. F., Tomberlin, G. H., Townsend, C., & Meissner, G. (2013). Stabilization of the skeletal muscle ryanodine receptor ion channel-FKBP12 complex by the 1,4-benzothiazepine derivative S107. *PloS One, 8*, e54208.

Meissner, G. (1994). Ryanodine receptor/Ca^{2+} release channels and their regulation by endogenous effectors. *Annual Review of Physiology, 56*, 485–508.

Meissner, G., & Lu, X. (1995). Dihydropyridine receptor-ryanodine receptor interactions in skeletal muscle excitation-contraction coupling. *Bioscience Reports, 15*, 399–408.

Meng, X., Wang, G., Viero, C., Wang, Q., Mi, W., Su, X. D., et al. (2009). CLIC2-RyR1 interaction and structural characterization by cryo-electron microscopy. *Journal of Molecular Biology, 387*, 320–334.

Molina-Navarro, M. M., Rosello-Lleti, E., Ortega, A., Tarazon, E., Otero, M., Martinez-Dolz, L., et al. (2013). Differential gene expression of cardiac ion channels in human dilated cardiomyopathy. *PloS One, 8*, e79792.

Morris, M. J., Craig, S. J., Sutherland, T. M., Board, P. G., & Casarotto, M. G. (2009). Transport of glutathione transferase-fold structured proteins into living cells. *Biochimica et Biophysica Acta, 1788*, 676–685.

Morris, M. J., Liu, D., Weaver, L. M., Board, P. G., & Casarotto, M. G. (2011). A structural basis for cellular uptake of GST-fold proteins. *PloS One, 6*, e17864.

Mosbah, A., Kharrat, R., Fajloun, Z., Renisio, J. G., Blanc, E., Sabatier, J. M., et al. (2000). A new fold in the scorpion toxin family, associated with an activity on a ryanodine-sensitive calcium channel. *Proteins, 40*, 436–442.

Most, P., Remppis, A., Weber, C., Bernotat, J., Ehlermann, P., Pleger, S. T., et al. (2003). The C terminus (amino acids 75-94) and the linker region (amino acids 42-54) of the Ca^{2+}-binding protein S100A1 differentially enhance sarcoplasmic Ca^{2+} release in murine skinned skeletal muscle fibers. *The Journal of Biological Chemistry, 278*, 26356–26364.

Murphy, R. M., Dutka, T. L., Horvath, D., Bell, J. R., Delbridge, L. M., & Lamb, G. D. (2013). Ca^{2+}-dependent proteolysis of junctophilin-1 and junctophilin-2 in skeletal and cardiac muscle. *The Journal of Physiology*, *591*, 719–729.

Nakai, J., Ogura, T., Protasi, F., Franzini-Armstrong, C., Allen, P. D., & Beam, K. G. (1997). Functional nonequality of the cardiac and skeletal ryanodine receptors. *Proceedings of the National Academy of Sciences of the United States of America*, *94*, 1019–1022.

Nakai, J., Tanabe, T., Konno, T., Adams, B., & Beam, K. G. (1998). Localization in the II-III loop of the dihydropyridine receptor of a sequence critical for excitation-contraction coupling. *The Journal of Biological Chemistry*, *273*, 24983–24986.

Oo, Y. W., Gomez-Hurtado, N., Walweel, K., van Helden, D. F., Imtiaz, M. S., Knollmann, B. C., et al. (2015). Essential role of calmodulin in RyR inhibition by dantrolene. *Molecular Pharmacology*, *88*, 57–63.

Orlova, E. V., Serysheva, I. I., van Heel, M., Hamilton, S. L., & Chiu, W. (1996). Two structural configurations of the skeletal muscle calcium release channel. *Nature Structural Biology*, *3*, 547–552.

Paolini, C., Quarta, M., D'Onofrio, L., Reggiani, C., & Protasi, F. (2011). Differential effect of calsequestrin ablation on structure and function of fast and slow skeletal muscle fibers. *Journal of Biomedicine & Biotechnology*, *2011*, 634075.

Park, H. Y., Kim, S. A., Korlach, J., Rhoades, E., Kwok, L. W., Zipfel, W. R., et al. (2008). Conformational changes of calmodulin upon Ca^{2+} binding studied with a microfluidic mixer. *Proceedings of the National Academy of Sciences of the United States of America*, *105*, 542–547.

Peralvarez-Marin, A., Tae, H., Board, P. G., Casarotto, M. G., Dulhunty, A. F., & Samso, M. (2011). 3D Mapping of the SPRY2 domain of ryanodine receptor 1 by single-particle cryo-EM. *PloS One*, *6*, e25813.

Pessah, I. N., & Feng, W. (2000). Functional role of hyperreactive sulfhydryl moieties within the ryanodine receptor complex. *Antioxidants & Redox Signaling*, *2*, 17–25.

Porta, M., Diaz-Sylvester, P. L., Neumann, J. T., Escobar, A. L., Fleischer, S., & Copello, J. A. (2012). Coupled gating of skeletal muscle ryanodine receptors is modulated by Ca^{2+}, Mg^{2+}, and ATP. *American Journal of Physiology. Cell Physiology*, *303*, C682–C697.

Proenza, C., Wilkens, C. M., & Beam, K. G. (2000). Excitation-contraction coupling is not affected by scrambled sequence in residues 681-690 of the dihydropyridine receptor II-III loop. *The Journal of Biological Chemistry*, *275*, 29935–29937.

Prosser, B. L., Hernandez-Ochoa, E. O., & Schneider, M. F. (2011). S100A1 and calmodulin regulation of ryanodine receptor in striated muscle. *Cell Calcium*, *50*, 323–331.

Prosser, B. L., Khairallah, R. J., Ziman, A. P., Ward, C. W., & Lederer, W. J. (2013). X-ROS signaling in the heart and skeletal muscle: Stretch-dependent local ROS regulates [Ca(2)(+)]i. *Journal of Molecular and Cellular Cardiology*, *58*, 172–181.

Protasi, F., Paolini, C., & Dainese, M. (2009). Calsequestrin-1: A new candidate gene for malignant hyperthermia and exertional/environmental heat stroke. *The Journal of Physiology*, *587*, 3095–3100.

Radermacher, M., Rao, V., Grassucci, R., Frank, J., Timerman, A. P., Fleischer, S., et al. (1994). Cryo-electron microscopy and three-dimensional reconstruction of the calcium release channel/ryanodine receptor from skeletal muscle. *The Journal of Cell Biology*, *127*, 411–423.

Raghunathan, S., Chandross, R. J., Kretsinger, R. H., Allison, T. J., Penington, C. J., & Rule, G. S. (1994). Crystal structure of human class mu glutathione transferase GSTM2-2 effects of lattice packing on conformational heterogeneity. *Journal of Molecular Biology*, *238*, 815–832.

Rebbeck, R. T., Karunasekara, Y., Board, P. G., Beard, N. A., Casarotto, M. G., & Dulhunty, A. F. (2014). Skeletal muscle excitation-contraction coupling: Who

are the dancing partners? *The International Journal of Biochemistry & Cell Biology, 48*, 28–38.
Rebbeck, R. T., Karunasekara, Y., Gallant, E. M., Board, P. G., Beard, N. A., Casarotto, M. G., et al. (2011). The beta(1a) subunit of the skeletal DHPR binds to skeletal RyR1 and activates the channel via its 35-residue C-terminal tail. *Biophysical Journal, 100*, 922–930.
Rebbeck, R. T., Nitu, F. R., Rohde, D., Most, P., Bers, D. M., Thomas, D. D., et al. (2016). S100A1 protein does not compete with calmodulin for ryanodine receptor binding but structurally alters the ryanodine receptor calmodulin complex. *The Journal of Biological Chemistry, 291*, 15896–15907.
Rebbeck, R. T., Willemse, H., Groom, L., Casarotto, M. G., Board, P. G., Beard, N. A., et al. (2015). Regions of ryanodine receptors that influence activation by the dihydropyridine receptor beta1a subunit. *Skeletal Muscle, 5*, 23.
Ritterhoff, J., Volkers, M., Seitz, A., Spaich, K., Gao, E., Peppel, K., et al. (2015). S100A1 DNA-based inotropic therapy protects against proarrhythmogenic ryanodine receptor 2 dysfunction. *Molecular Therapy, 23*, 1320–1330.
Ronjat, M., Feng, W., Dardevet, L., Dong, Y., Al Khoury, S., Chatelain, F. C., et al. (2016). In cellulo phosphorylation induces pharmacological reprogramming of maurocalcin, a cell-penetrating venom peptide. *Proceedings of the National Academy of Sciences of the United States of America, 113*, E2460–E2468.
Rullman, E., Andersson, D. C., Melin, M., Reiken, S., Mancini, D. M., Marks, A. R., et al. (2013). Modifications of skeletal muscle ryanodine receptor type 1 and exercise intolerance in heart failure. *The Journal of Heart and Lung Transplantation, 32*, 925–929.
Samarasinghe, K., Liu, D., Tummala, P., Cappello, J., Pace, S. M., Arnolda, L., et al. (2015). Glutathione transferase M2 variants inhibit ryanodine receptor function in adult mouse cardiomyocytes. *Biochemical Pharmacology, 97*, 269–280.
Schneider, M. F., & Chandler, W. K. (1973). Voltage dependent charge movement of skeletal muscle: A possible step in excitation-contraction coupling. *Nature, 242*, 244–246.
Schredelseker, J., Dayal, A., Schwerte, T., Franzini-Armstrong, C., & Grabner, M. (2009). Proper restoration of excitation-contraction coupling in the dihydropyridine receptor beta1-null zebrafish relaxed is an exclusive function of the beta1a subunit. *The Journal of Biological Chemistry, 284*, 1242–1251.
Schredelseker, J., Di Biase, V., Obermair, G. J., Felder, E. T., Flucher, B. E., Franzini-Armstrong, C., et al. (2005). The beta 1a subunit is essential for the assembly of dihydropyridine-receptor arrays in skeletal muscle. *Proceedings of the National Academy of Sciences of the United States of America, 102*, 17219–17224.
Shannon, T. R., Wang, F., & Bers, D. M. (2005). Regulation of cardiac sarcoplasmic reticulum Ca release by luminal [Ca] and altered gating assessed with a mathematical model. *Biophysical Journal, 89*, 4096–4110.
Sikkel, M. B., Collins, T. P., Rowlands, C., Shah, M., O'Gara, P., Williams, A. J., et al. (2013). Flecainide reduces Ca(2+) spark and wave frequency via inhibition of the sarcolemmal sodium current. *Cardiovascular Research, 98*, 286–296.
Smith, J. J., Vetter, I., Lewis, R. J., Peigneur, S., Tytgat, J., Lam, A., et al. (2013). Multiple actions of phi-LITX-Lw1a on ryanodine receptors reveal a functional link between scorpion DDH and ICK toxins. *Proceedings of the National Academy of Sciences of the United States of America, 110*, 8906–8911.
Smith, C. D., Wang, A., Vembaiyan, K., Zhang, J., Xie, C., Zhou, Q., et al. (2013). Novel carvedilol analogues that suppress store-overload-induced Ca^{2+} release. *Journal of Medicinal Chemistry, 56*, 8626–8655.
Sondergaard, M. T., Tian, X., Liu, Y., Wang, R., Chazin, W. J., Chen, S. R., et al. (2015). Arrhythmogenic calmodulin mutations affect the activation and termination of cardiac

ryanodine receptor-mediated Ca^{2+} release. *The Journal of Biological Chemistry, 290,* 26151–26162.

Sun, J., Xu, L., Eu, J. P., Stamler, J. S., & Meissner, G. (2001). Classes of thiols that influence the activity of the skeletal muscle calcium release channel. *The Journal of Biological Chemistry, 276,* 15625–15630.

Szentesi, P., Collet, C., Sarkozi, S., Szegedi, C., Jona, I., Jacquemond, V., et al. (2001). Effects of dantrolene on steps of excitation-contraction coupling in mammalian skeletal muscle fibers. *The Journal of General Physiology, 118,* 355–375.

Tae, H., Casarotto, M. G., & Dulhunty, A. F. (2009). Ubiquitous SPRY domains and their role in the skeletal type ryanodine receptor. *European Biophysics Journal, 39,* 51–59.

Tae, H. S., Cui, Y., Karunasekara, Y., Board, P. G., Dulhunty, A. F., & Casarotto, M. G. (2011). Cyclization of the intrinsically disordered alpha1S dihydropyridine receptor II-III loop enhances secondary structure and in vitro function. *The Journal of Biological Chemistry, 286,* 22589–22599.

Takano, K., Liu, D., Tarpey, P., Gallant, E., Lam, A., Witham, S., et al. (2012). An X-linked channelopathy with cardiomegaly due to a CLIC2 mutation enhancing ryanodine receptor channel activity. *Human Molecular Genetics, 21,* 4497–4507.

Tanabe, T., Beam, K. G., Adams, B. A., Niidome, T., & Numa, S. (1990). Regions of the skeletal muscle dihydropyridine receptor critical for excitation-contraction coupling. *Nature, 346,* 567–569.

Terentyev, D., Kubalova, Z., Valle, G., Nori, A., Vedamoorthyrao, S., Terentyeva, R., et al. (2008). Modulation of SR Ca release by luminal Ca and calsequestrin in cardiac myocytes: Effects of CASQ2 mutations linked to sudden cardiac death. *Biophysical Journal, 95,* 2037–2048.

Treves, S., Scutari, E., Robert, M., Groh, S., Ottolia, M., Prestipino, G., et al. (1997). Interaction of S100A1 with the Ca^{2+} release channel (ryanodine receptor) of skeletal muscle. *Biochemistry, 36,* 11496–11503.

Tripathy, A., Resch, W., Xu, L., Valdivia, H. H., & Meissner, G. (1998). Imperatoxin A induces subconductance states in Ca^{2+} release channels (ryanodine receptors) of cardiac and skeletal muscle. *The Journal of General Physiology, 111,* 679–690.

Tripathy, A., Xu, L., Mann, G., & Meissner, G. (1995). Calmodulin activation and inhibition of skeletal muscle Ca^{2+} release channel (ryanodine receptor). *Biophysical Journal, 69,* 106–119.

Van Petegem, F. (2015). Ryanodine receptors: Allosteric ion channel giants. *Journal of Molecular Biology, 427,* 31–53.

Vassilakopoulou, V., Calver, B. L., Thanassoulas, A., Beck, K., Hu, H., Buntwal, L., et al. (2015). Distinctive malfunctions of calmodulin mutations associated with heart RyR2-mediated arrhythmic disease. *Biochimica et Biophysica Acta, 1850,* 2168–2176.

Venturi, E., Galfre, E., O'Brien, F., Pitt, S. J., Bellamy, S., Sessions, R. B., et al. (2014). FKBP12.6 activates RyR1: Investigating the amino acid residues critical for channel modulation. *Biophysical Journal, 106,* 824–833.

Verburg, E., Dutka, T. L., & Lamb, G. D. (2006). Long-lasting muscle fatigue: Partial disruption of excitation-contraction coupling by elevated cytosolic Ca^{2+} concentration during contractions. *American Journal of Physiology. Cell Physiology, 290,* C1199–C1208.

Voss, A. A., Lango, J., Ernst-Russell, M., Morin, D., & Pessah, I. N. (2004). Identification of hyperreactive cysteines within ryanodine receptor type 1 by mass spectrometry. *The Journal of Biological Chemistry, 279,* 34514–34520.

Walweel, K., Li, J., Molenaar, P., Imtiaz, M. S., Quail, A., dos Remedios, C. G., et al. (2014). Differences in the regulation of RyR2 from human, sheep, and rat by Ca(2)(+) and Mg(2)(+) in the cytoplasm and in the lumen of the sarcoplasmic reticulum. *The Journal of General Physiology, 144,* 263–271.

Walweel, K., Oo, Y. W., & Laver, D. R. (2017). The emerging role of calmodulin regulation of RyR2 in controlling heart rhythm, the progression of heart failure and the antiarrhythmic action of dantrolene. *Clinical and Experimental Pharmacology & Physiology*, *44*(1), 135–142.

Waning, D. L., Mohammad, K. S., Reiken, S., Xie, W., Andersson, D. C., John, S., et al. (2015). Excess TGF-beta mediates muscle weakness associated with bone metastases in mice. *Nature Medicine*, *21*, 1262–1271.

Watanabe, H., Chopra, N., Laver, D., Hwang, H. S., Davies, S. S., Roach, D. E., et al. (2009). Flecainide prevents catecholaminergic polymorphic ventricular tachycardia in mice and humans. *Nature Medicine*, *15*, 380–383.

Wehrens, X. H., Lehnart, S. E., Huang, F., Vest, J. A., Reiken, S. R., Mohler, P. J., et al. (2003). FKBP12.6 deficiency and defective calcium release channel (ryanodine receptor) function linked to exercise-induced sudden cardiac death. *Cell*, *113*, 829–840.

Wehrens, X. H., Lehnart, S. E., Reiken, S. R., Deng, S. X., Vest, J. A., Cervantes, D., et al. (2004). Protection from cardiac arrhythmia through ryanodine receptor-stabilizing protein calstabin2. *Science*, *304*, 292–296.

Wei, L., Gallant, E. M., Dulhunty, A. F., & Beard, N. A. (2009). Junctin and triadin each activate skeletal ryanodine receptors but junctin alone mediates functional interactions with calsequestrin. *The International Journal of Biochemistry & Cell Biology*, *41*, 2214–2224.

Wei, L., Hanna, A. D., Beard, N. A., & Dulhunty, A. F. (2009). Unique isoform-specific properties of calsequestrin in the heart and skeletal muscle. *Cell Calcium*, *45*, 474–484.

Wei, L., Varsanyi, M., Dulhunty, A. F., & Beard, N. A. (2006). The conformation of calsequestrin determines its ability to regulate skeletal ryanodine receptors. *Biophysical Journal*, *91*, 1288–1301.

Weisleder, N., Brotto, M., Komazaki, S., Pan, Z., Zhao, X., Nosek, T., et al. (2006). Muscle aging is associated with compromised Ca^{2+} spark signaling and segregated intracellular Ca^{2+} release. *The Journal of Cell Biology*, *174*, 639–645.

Wium, E., Dulhunty, A. F., & Beard, N. A. (2016). Three residues in the luminal domain of triadin impact on Trisk 95 activation of skeletal muscle ryanodine receptors. *Pflügers Archiv*, *468*, 1985–1994.

Wu, J., Yan, Z., Li, Z., Qian, X., Lu, S., Dong, M., et al. (2016). Structure of the voltage-gated calcium channel Cav1.1 at 3.6 Å resolution. *Nature*, *537*, 191–196.

Wu, J., Yan, Z., Li, Z., Yan, C., Lu, S., Dong, M., et al. (2015). Structure of the voltage-gated calcium channel Cav1.1 complex. *Science*, *350*, aad2395.

Xu, L., Mann, G., & Meissner, G. (1996). Regulation of cardiac Ca^{2+} release channel (ryanodine receptor) by Ca^{2+}, H^{+}, Mg^{2+}, and adenine nucleotides under normal and simulated ischemic conditions. *Circulation Research*, *79*, 1100–1109.

Yamamoto, T., & Ikemoto, N. (2002). Spectroscopic monitoring of local conformational changes during the intramolecular domain-domain interaction of the ryanodine receptor. *Biochemistry*, *41*, 1492–1501.

Yan, Z., Bai, X. C., Yan, C., Wu, J., Li, Z., Xie, T., et al. (2015). Structure of the rabbit ryanodine receptor RyR1 at near-atomic resolution. *Nature*, *517*, 50–55.

Yin, C. C., Han, H., Wei, R., & Lai, F. A. (2005). Two-dimensional crystallization of the ryanodine receptor Ca^{2+} release channel on lipid membranes. *Journal of Structural Biology*, *149*, 219–224.

Zalk, R., Clarke, O. B., des Georges, A., Grassucci, R. A., Reiken, S., Mancia, F., et al. (2015). Structure of a mammalian ryanodine receptor. *Nature*, *517*, 44–49.

Zhong, X., Liu, Y., Zhu, L., Meng, X., Wang, R., Van Petegem, F., et al. (2013). Conformational dynamics inside amino-terminal disease hotspot of ryanodine receptor. *Structure*, *21*, 2051–2060.

Zhou, Q., Xiao, J., Jiang, D., Wang, R., Vembaiyan, K., Wang, A., et al. (2011). Carvedilol and its new analogs suppress arrhythmogenic store overload-induced Ca^{2+} release. *Nature Medicine*, *17*, 1003–1009.
Ziman, A. P., Ward, C. W., Rodney, G. G., Lederer, W. J., & Bloch, R. J. (2010). Quantitative measurement of Ca^{2+} in the sarcoplasmic reticulum lumen of mammalian skeletal muscle. *Biophysical Journal*, *99*, 2705–2714.
Zissimopoulos, S., Seifan, S., Maxwell, C., Williams, A. J., & Lai, F. A. (2012). Disparities in the association of the ryanodine receptor and the FK506-binding proteins in mammalian heart. *Journal of Cell Science*, *125*, 1759–1769.

FSC
www.fsc.org
MIX
Papier | Fördert
gute Waldnutzung
FSC® C083411

Kolibri 360 GmbH
Ferdinand-Jühlke-Straße 7
99095 Erfurt, Deutschland
produktsicherheit@kolibri360.de